Histopathological Image Analysis in Medical Decision Making

Nilanjan Dey
Techno India College of Technology, India

Amira S. Ashour
Tanta University, Egypt

Harihar Kalia
Seemantha Engineering College, India

R.T. Goswami
Techno India College of Technology, India

Himansu Das
KIIT University, India

A volume in the Advances in Medical Technologies and Clinical Practice (AMTCP) Book Series

IGI Global
DISSEMINATOR OF KNOWLEDGE

Published in the United States of America by
IGI Global
Medical Information Science Reference (an imprint of IGI Global)
701 E. Chocolate Avenue
Hershey PA, USA 17033
Tel: 717-533-8845
Fax: 717-533-8661
E-mail: cust@igi-global.com
Web site: http://www.igi-global.com

Library of Congress Cataloging-in-Publication Data

Names: Dey, Nilanjan, 1984- editor. | Ashour, Amira, 1975- editor. | Kalia, Harihar, editor. | Goswami, R. T., editor. | Das, Himansu, editor.
Title: Histopathological image analysis in medical decision making / Nilanjan Dey, Amira S. Ashour, Harihar Kalia, R.T. Goswami, and Himansu Das, editors.
Description: Hershey, PA : Medical Information Science Reference, [2019] | Includes bibliographical references.
Identifiers: LCCN 2018008106| ISBN 9781522563167 (hbk.) | ISBN 9781522563174 (ebook)
Subjects: | MESH: Histological Techniques | Image Processing, Computer-Assisted | Clinical Decision-Making | Pattern Recognition, Automated
Classification: LCC RC78.7.D53 | NLM QS 26.5 | DDC 616.07/54--dc23 LC record available at https://lccn.loc.gov/2018008106

This book is published in the IGI Global book series Advances in Medical Technologies and Clinical Practice (AMTCP) (ISSN: 2327-9354; eISSN: 2327-9370)

British Cataloguing in Publication Data
A Cataloguing in Publication record for this book is available from the British Library.

All work contributed to this book is new, previously-unpublished material.
The views expressed in this book are those of the authors, but not necessarily of the publisher.

For electronic access to this publication, please contact: eresources@igi-global.com.

Advances in Medical Technologies and Clinical Practice (AMTCP) Book Series

ISSN:2327-9354
EISSN:2327-9370

MISSION

Medical technological innovation continues to provide avenues of research for faster and safer diagnosis and treatments for patients. Practitioners must stay up to date with these latest advancements to provide the best care for nursing and clinical practices.

The **Advances in Medical Technologies and Clinical Practice (AMTCP) Book Series** brings together the most recent research on the latest technology used in areas of nursing informatics, clinical technology, biomedicine, diagnostic technologies, and more. Researchers, students, and practitioners in this field will benefit from this fundamental coverage on the use of technology in clinical practices.

COVERAGE

- Nutrition
- Patient-Centered Care
- Clinical Studies
- Biometrics
- Medical informatics
- Medical Imaging
- Nursing Informatics
- Telemedicine
- Neural Engineering
- Clinical Data Mining

IGI Global is currently accepting manuscripts for publication within this series. To submit a proposal for a volume in this series, please contact our Acquisition Editors at Acquisitions@igi-global.com or visit: http://www.igi-global.com/publish/.

Titles in this Series

For a list of additional titles in this series, please visit:
https://www.igi-global.com/book-series/advances-medical-technologies-clinical-practice/73682

Research Advancements in Pharmaceutical, Nutritional, and Industrial nzymology
Shashi Lata Bharati (North Eastern Regional Institute of Science and Technology, India) and Pankaj Kumar Chaurasia (Babasaheb Bhimrao Ambedkar Bihar University, India)
Medical Information Science Reference • ©2018 • 549pp • H/C (ISBN: 9781522552376) • US $255.00

Microbial Cultures and Enzymes in Dairy Technology
Şebnem Öztürkoğlu Budak (Ankara University, Turkey) and H. Ceren Akal (Ankara University, Turkey)
Medical Information Science Reference • ©2018 • 413pp • H/C (ISBN: 9781522553632) • US $265.00

Multifunctional Nanocarriers for Contemporary Healthcare Applications
Md. Abul Barkat (K.R. Mangalam University, India) Harshita A.B. (K.R. Mangalam University, India) Sarwar Beg (Jubilant Generics, India) and Farhan J. Ahmad (Jamia Hamdard, India)
Medical Information Science Reference • ©2018 • 602pp • H/C (ISBN: 9781522547815) • US $265.00

Biomedical Signal and Image Processing in Patient Care
Maheshkumar H. Kolekar (Indian Institute of Technology Patna, India) and Vinod Kumar (Indian Institute of Technology Roorkee, India)
Medical Information Science Reference • ©2018 • 312pp • H/C (ISBN: 9781522528296) • US $265.00

Next-Generation Mobile and Pervasive Healthcare Solutions
Jose Machado (University of Minho, Portugal) António Abelha (University of Minho, Portugal) Manuel Filipe Santos (University of Minho, Portugal) and Filipe Portela (University of Minho, Portugal)
Medical Information Science Reference • ©2018 • 286pp • H/C (ISBN: 9781522528517) • US $245.00

For an entire list of titles in this series, please visit:
https://www.igi-global.com/book-series/advances-medical-technologies-clinical-practice/73682

IGI Global
DISSEMINATOR OF KNOWLEDGE

701 East Chocolate Avenue, Hershey, PA 17033, USA
Tel: 717-533-8845 x100 • Fax: 717-533-8661
E-Mail: cust@igi-global.com • www.igi-global.com

Table of Contents

Detailed Table of Contents

In this chapter, the authors tried to develop a tool to automatize and facilitate the detection of Nosema disease. This work develops new technologies in order to solve one of the bottlenecks found on the analysis bee population. The images contain various objects; moreover, this work will be structured on three main steps. The first step is focused on the detection and study of the objects of interest, which are Nosema cells. The second step is to study others' objects in the images: extract characteristics. The last step is to compare the other objects with Nosema. The authors can recognize their object of interest, determining where the edges of an object are, counting similar objects. Finally, the authors have images that contain only their objects of interest. The selection of an appropriate set of features is a fundamental challenge in pattern recognition problems, so the method makes use of segmentation techniques and computer vision. The authors believe that the attainment of this work will facilitate the diary work in many laboratories and provide measures that are more precise for biologists.

Medical images have a larger size when compared to normal images. There arises a problem in the storage as well as in the transmission of a large number of medical images. Hence, there exists a need for compressing these images to reduce the size as much as possible and also to maintain a better quality. The authors propose a method for lossy image compression of a set of medical images which is based on Recurrent Neural Network (RNN). So, the proposed method produces images of variable compression rates to maintain the quality aspect and to preserve some of the important contents present in these images.

Digital pathology is one of the significant methods in the medicine field to diagnose and treat cancer. The cell morphology and architecture distribution of biopsies are analyzed to diagnose the spread and severity of the disease. Manual analyses are time-consuming and subjected to intra- and inter-observer variability. Digital pathology and computer-aided analysis aids in enormous applications including nuclei detection, segmentation, and classification. The major challenges in nuclei segmentation are high variability in images due to differences in preparation of slides, heterogeneous structure, overlapping clusters, artifacts, and noise. The structure of the proposed chapter is as follows. First, an introduction about digital pathology and significance of digital pathology techniques in cancer diagnosis based on literature survey is given. Then, the method of classification of histopathological images using deep learning for different datasets is proposed with experimental results.

In recent years, denoising has played an important role in medical image analysis. Image denoising is still accepted as a challenge for researchers and image application developers in medical image applications. The idea is to denoise a microscopic image through over-complete dictionary learning using a k-means algorithm and singular value decomposition (K-SVD) based on pursuit methods. This approach is good in performance on the quality improvement of the medical images, but it has low computational speed with high computational complexity. In view of the above limitations, this chapter proposes a novel strategy for denoising insight phenomena of the K-SVD algorithm. In addition, the authors utilize the technology of improved dictionary learning of the image patches using heap sort mechanism followed by dictionary updating process. The experimental results validate that the proposed approach successfully reduced noise levels on various test image datasets. This has been found to be more accurate than the best in class denoising approaches.

Fractal dimension is an emerging research area in order to characterize the complex or irritated objects found in nature. These complex objects are failed to analyze by classical Euclidian geometry. The concept of FD has extensively applied in many areas of application in image processing. The thought of the FD will work based upon the theory of self-similarity because it holds structures that are nested with one another. Over the last years, fractal geometry was applied extensively in medical image analysis in order to detect cancer cells in human body because our vascular system, nervous system, bones, and breast tissue are so complex and irregular in pattern, and also successfully applied in ECG signal, brain imaging for tumor detection, trabeculation analysis, etc. In order to analyze these complex structures, most of the researchers are adopting the concept of fractal geometry by means of box counting technique. This chapter presents an overview of box counting and its improved algorithms and how they work and their application in the field of medical image processing.

Image encryption is a main concern in digital transmission of data over communication network. As encryption and decryption of image has got considerable attention in the past decades, its effectiveness and compatibility need to be taken care of. The work reported in this chapter is mainly concerned with enhancement of dimension in image encryption technique. The work mainly deals with pixels shuffling of an image using Bogdanov chaotic map for both gray and color image, where encryption and decryption process are associated with the key. In color image, the image is divided into all three planes (RGB) individually. Scrambling is done with all three planes individually. All the three planes are summed up into a single plane which gives us the final result. In Bogdanov map, old pixel position is replaced with new pixel position. Further, the authors analyzed security of image encryption techniques with two parameters called NPCR and UACI. The efficacy of the encryption process can be seen in experimental results.

Down syndrome is a genetic disorder and the chromosome abnormality observed in humans that can cause physical and mental abnormalities. It can never be cured or rectified. Instead it has to be identified in the fetus and prevented from being born. Many ultrasonographic markers like nuchal fold, nasal bone hypoplasia, femur length, and EIF are considered to be the symptoms of Down syndrome in the fetus. This chapter deals with the creation of automatic and computerized diagnostic tool for Down syndrome detection based on EIF. The proposed system consists of two phases: 1) training phase and 2) testing phase. In training phase, the fetal images with EIF and Down syndrome is analyzed and characteristics of EIF are collected. In testing phase, detection of Down syndrome is performed on the fetal image with EIF based on the knowledge cluster obtained using ESOM. The performance of the proposed system is analyzed in terms of sensitivity, accuracy, and specificity.

Due to rapid development of multimedia communication and advancement of image acquisition process, there is a crucial requirement of high storage and compression techniques to mitigate high data rate with limited bandwidth scenario for telemedicine application. Lossless compression is one of the challenging tasks in applications like medical, space, and aerial imaging field. Apart from achieving high compression ratio, in these mentioned applications there is a need to maintain the original imaging quality along with fast and adequate processing. Predictive coding was introduced to remove spatial redundancy. The accuracy of predictive coding is based on the choice of effective and adaptive predictor which is responsible for removing spatial redundancy. Medical images like computed tomography (CT) and magnetic resonance imaging (MRI) consume huge storage and utilize maximum available bandwidth. To overcome these inherent challenges, the authors have reviewed various adaptive predictors and it has been compared with existing JPEG and JPEG LS-based linear prediction technique for medical images.

HE stain images are widely used in medical diagnosis and often considered a gold standard for histology and pathology laboratories. A proper analysis is needed to have a critical decision about the status of the diagnosis of the concerned patient. Segmentation is always considered as an advanced stage of image analysis where

Preface

INTRODUCTION

In image analysis, the computational improvement increases dramatically through the few last decades. New algorithms have endorsed the powerful computer-assisted analytical approaches development to radiological data. Digital scanners facilities the digitization and the storage of the tissue histopathology slide in the form of digital images. Therefore, digitized tissue histopathology become amenable to the computerized image analysis application as well as machine learning systems. Medical imaging leads to the development of the computer-assisted diagnosis (CAD) algorithms to counterpart the radiologist's opinion. The developed CAD algorithms assist the diagnosis, prognosis and the detection of disease, where the manual analysis of the microscopic digital images (MIRA) by the physicians is a very tedious process. Several factors directly to the importance of the CAD based microscopic image processing. Such limitations and challenges include the impractical examination of all regions of the tissue slide under the microscope at high magnifications (e.g., 40×). In addition, the resulting diagnosis varies considerably between different readers (oncologists) i.e. subjectivity issue. Moreover, uneven staining, occlusion, in homogeneity, multiple area of interest makes prognosis process a major impediment.

Consequently, the present proposed book includes the recent state of the art related to the CAD technology for digitized histopathology. A brief description of the improvement and application of innovative image analysis techniques for specific histopathology related problems are addressed. It provides interesting chapters related to the area of disease, preventive and corrective opinion to classify the particular grades of the lymphoma foe example. Furthermore, a complete prototype for extracting and for processing the information from images is provided. This book addresses the major techniques of segmentation, features extraction and classification and pattern recognition for the Histopathological images as well as their use to support the CAD.

OBJECTIVE OF THE BOOK

Medical image technologies have attracted much attention with the advancement of the medical equipment that devoted to use medical imaging. Microscopic imaging is one of the most significant visualization and interpretation methods in biology and medicine for cells and tissues. It solves real-world problems in decision making, pattern classification, diagnosis and learning will be achieved. In order to achieve all these necessities, feature extraction procedures are developed, which can be considered as a problem-oriented processing techniques in which an algorithm is used to be designed for a specific application. Progressions of this field will assist to intensify interdisciplinary discovery in microscopic image processing and CAD systems to aid physicians in diagnosis and early detection of diseases. The Computer aided system (CAD) can provide superior representation in the form of 3D and quantitative values to assist physicians to correctly diagnose the diseased tissue for further treatment planning. According to the pathology classification, cancer patients are classified into favourable and unfavourable histology based on the tissue morphology and to identify unfavourable histology at initial phase leads to increase the chance to recover the cancer quickly. In this book, an image analysis system that operates on digital Histopathological images is involved. Classification of the Histopathological images in terms of their extracted features such as the brightness, contrast, entropy, hue, saturation and value, size, texture, shape is also studied. Analysis of the histopathological images using artificial neural network and other machine learning techniques are also introduced.

ORGANIZATION OF THE BOOK

To achieve the objectives, this book contains 12 chapters contributed by promising authors that are organized as shown below.

Chapter 1

This chapter focuses on segmentation of Leukocyte Image with Shannon's Entropy. In this chapter a semi-automated approach is proposed by integrating the Shannon's Entropy and DRLS based segmentation procedure. It is used to extract the stained blood cell from digital PBC pictures. This chapter provides Cuckoo Search, SE based pre-processing and DRLS based post-processing procedure to examine the PBC pictures.

Chapter 2

This chapter focuses on microscopic image analysis for Nosema disease. This work develops new technologies in order to solve the bottleneck found on the analysis bee population. This chapter focuses on the detection and study of Nosema cells, extraction of characteristics, and compare the other objects with Nosema.

Chapter 3

This chapter introduces the lossy compression technique with LSTM networks for medical images. Generally medical images have larger in size which leads to a problem in the storage as well as in the transmission of such images. Hence, it is essential to compress these images to reduce the size and also to maintain a better quality. This chapter provides a method for lossy image compression of medical images based on recurrent neural network (RNN).

Chapter 4

This chapter focuses on identification of early cancer by using digital image analysis. To extract characteristic features from the digital images different techniques are used. In this chapter authors discusses some characteristics features of image processing techniques along with the different advanced analytical methods used in oncology.

Chapter 5

This chapter presents multi criteria decision making techniques for histopathological image classification. In this chapter different machine learning algorithms such as K-Nearest Neighbor, Random Forest, Support Vector Machine, Ensemble Learning, Multilayer Perceptron, Convolutional Neural Network are used for analysis. Further, Multi Criteria Decision Making (MCDM) methods such as SAW, WPM and TOPSIS are used to improve the efficiency of the decision making process.

Chapter 6

This chapter introduces the concept of histopathological image analysis for classification using deep learning method. It also introduces the digital pathology and significance of digital pathology techniques in cancer diagnosis. This chapter also provides the method of classification of histopathological images using deep learning for different datasets.

Chapter 7

This chapter describes the concept of K-SVD based algorithm for image denoising. This method is good in performance on the quality improvement of medical image. In addition, authors utilize the technology of improved dictionary learning of the image patches using heap sort mechanism followed by dictionary updation process.

Chapter 8

This chapter focuses on the analysis of medical images using fractal geometry concepts. It is generally applied extensively in medical image analysis in order to detect cancer cell, in human body because our vascular system, nervous system, and bones. It is also successfully applied in ECG signal, brain imaging for tumour detection, and trabeculation analysis.

Chapter 9

The chapter provides detailed analysis of color image encryption using multidimensional Bogdanov map. This chapter concerned with enhancement of dimension of image encryption which deals with pixels shuffling of an image using Bogdanov chaotic map for both gray and color image, where encryption and decryption process are associated with the key. This chapter also analyses the security of image encryption techniques with two parameters called NPCR and UACI.

Chapter 10

This chapter focuses on automatic diagnostic tool for down syndrome detection in Fetus. Down syndrome is a genetic disorder and the chromosome abnormality observed in humans that can cause physical and mental abnormalities. This chapter deals with the creation of automatic and computerised diagnostic tool for Down syndrome detection based on EIF.

Chapter 11

This chapter focuses on adaptive prediction methods for medical image or video compression in telemedicine. Due to rapid development of multimedia communication and advancement of Image acquisition process, there is a crucial requirement of high storage and compression techniques to mitigate high data rate with limited bandwidth scenario for Telemedicine application. Apart from achieving high compression ratio, there is a need to maintain the original imaging quality along with fast and adequate processing. To overcome these inherent challenges, this chapter reviewed various adaptive prediction techniques for medical images.

Chapter 12

This chapter discusses the concept of HE stain image segmentation concept using type-2 fuzzy set. Generally, most of the cells are colourless and transparent. So, it is difficult to analyse it. So, HE stain methodology is essential in histological section to make the cells distinct and visible which involves the usage of hematoxylin and eosin. Through segmentation, HE Stain image is divided into different segments and from those segments, it will be easy to analyse the particular ROI for which diagnosis will be conducted.

Topics presented in each chapter of this book are unique to this book and are based on unpublished work of contributed authors. In editing this book, we attempted to bring into the discussion all the new trends, experiments, and products that have made image processing in medical decision making as such a dynamic area. We believe the book is ready to serve as a reference for larger audience such as system architects, practitioners, developers, and researchers.

Nilanjan Dey
Techno India College of Technology, India

Amira S. Ashour
Tanta University, Egypt

Harihar Kalia
Seemanta Engineering College, India

R. T. Goswami
Techno India College of Technology, India

Himansu Das
KIIT University, India

Acknowledgment

We would like to thank everyone who participated in this project and made this book into a reality. In particular, we would like to acknowledge the hard work of authors and their cooperation during the revisions of their chapters.

We would also like to acknowledge the valuable comments of the reviewers which have enabled us to select these chapters out of the so many chapters we received and also improve the quality of the chapters.

Lastly, we appreciate the IGI Global team for their continuous support throughout the entire process of publication. Our gratitude is extended to the readers, who gave us their trust, and we hope this work guides and inspires them.

Nilanjan Dey
Techno India College of Technology, India

Amira S. Ashour
Tanta University, Egypt

Harihar Kalia
Seemanta Engineering College, India

R. T. Goswami
Techno India College of Technology, India

Himansu Das
KIIT University, India

Chapter 1
A Study on Segmentation of Leukocyte Image With Shannon's Entropy

N. Sri Madhava Raja
St. Joseph's College of Engineering, India

Hong Lin
University of Houston – Downtown, USA

S. Arunmozhi
Manakula Vinayagar Institute of Technology, India

Nilanjan Dey
Techno India College of Technology, India

V. Rajinikanth
St. Joseph's College of Engineering, India

ABSTRACT

In recent years, a considerable number of approaches have been proposed by the researchers to evaluate infectious diseases by examining the digital images of peripheral blood cell (PBC) recorded using microscopes. In this chapter, a semi-automated approach is proposed by integrating the Shannon's entropy (SE) thresholding and DRLS-based segmentation procedure to extract the stained blood cell from digital PBC pictures. This work implements a two-step practice with cuckoo search (CS) and SE-based pre-processing and DRLS-based post-processing procedure to examine the PBC pictures. During the experimentation, the PBC pictures are adopted from the database leukocyte images for segmentation and classification (LISC). The proposed approach is implemented by considering the RGB scale and gray scale version of the PBC pictures, and the performance of the proposed approach is confirmed by computing the picture similarity and statistical measures computed with the extracted stained blood cell with the ground truth image.

DOI: 10.4018/978-1-5225-6316-7.ch001

INTRODUCTION

Most of the infection/disease in human body is commonly assessed using bio-signals and images recorded with dedicated practices executed in a controlled environment. Compared to the medical imaging procedures, bio-signal based approaches are limitedly considered to evaluate the disease in human body; further it is normally adopted to examine the abnormality arising in vital human organs, such as brain, heart, muscles, digestive system, etc (Lin and Li, 2017; Paramasivam et al., 2017; Ranjan et al. 2018).

Recently, imaging methods are extensively adapted in medical domain to register internal and external organs of human body using approved imaging procedures. After recording these images, a clinical level evaluation is executed by means of a semi-automated and automated tool by an experienced imaging technician or the physician to get the pre-opinion regarding the infection/abnormality of the organ under assessment. Due to its importance and clinical significance, a variety of image processing methods are designed and considered to examine RGB and gray scale images recorded using a chosen imaging scheme. The imaging procedures, such as X-ray (Tuan et al., 2018), Magnetic Resonance Image (Palani et al., 2016; Rajinikanth et al., 2017; Rajinikanth and Satapathy, 2018), Magnetic Resonance Angiogram (Rajinikanth et al., 2018), Computed Tomography (Ashour et al., 2015; Fernandes et al., 2017; Naqi et al., 2018), Fundus imaging (Sudhan et al., 2017; Shree et al., 2018), Dermoscopy (Dey et al., 2018) etc., are widely discussed in the literature to examine infection in various organs of human body.

Along with the above said imaging procedures, clinical blood cell images recorded using Digital Microscope (DM) also play a vital role in medical field to identify the infection in a tissue/cell (Chakraborty et al., 2017). The DM images can be considered to inspect abnormal cell growth, blood infection due to cancer, AIDS, leukemia, malaria and other communicable diseases (Kamalanand and Jawahar, 2012; 2015; Hore et al., 2015; Lakshmi et al., 2015). The DM images of thick as well as thin blood smear are widely considered in the medical imaging literature to investigate a variety of diseases. Usually, the thin blood smear image is prepared in clinical level by means of collected blood samples from infected person and a staining agent, such as Leishman's stain, Giemsa stain, Jenner's stain, and Wright's stain. The staining medium is usually considered to differentiate a particular cell from the common group (Manickavasagam et al., 2014). After completing the preliminary recording task, the blood smear image is then registered with the DM in order to evaluate the infection by using a computer supported semi-automated/automated inspection practice.

The work of Rezatofighi and Zadeh (2011) confirm that, examination of Peripheral Blood Cell (PBC) by means of automated approach offers enhanced accuracy compared to other traditional techniques. Their work suggests that, an efficient assessment tool is necessary to examine the image to provide essential qualitative assessment and superior decision making during the segmentation and classification of white blood cell. Segmentation and classification of PBC is most important in hematological events. Their work also contributed a benchmark image dataset called Leukocyte Images for Segmentation and Classification (LISC); to test and validate the developed computer assisted blood cell examination and classification tools developed by the researchers.

In the literature, considerable schemes are proposed to examine the Region Of Interest (ROI) of Peripheral Blood Cell (PBC) pictures based on traditional and heuristic algorithm based methods (Manickavasagam et al., 2014). Previous research confirms that, heuristic approaches tender improved results contrast to the traditional schemes (Raja et al., 2014; Abhinaya and Raja, 2015; Balan et al., 2016; Anitha et al., 2017; Vishnupriya et al., 2017).

This chapter proposes a heuristic algorithm based methodology to segment the stained region of PBC image dataset of LISC using a two step procedure. The initial step implements Cuckoo Search (CS) and Shannon's multi-thresholding practice to improve the visibility in stained region by grouping the similar pixel values. Later, ROI from the thresholded picture is extracted using the segmentation procedure, called DRLS, discussed by Li et al. (2010). This tool is implemented on the gray scale as well as the RGB version of the PBC images of LISC. Finally, validation of the implemented procedure is done based on a relative examination among ROI and the Ground Truth (GT) image of LISC. The investigational outcome proves that, average result of image similarity measures (Jaccard and Dice) and statistical measures (sensitivity, specificity, accuracy and precision) obtained with the gray scale picture is superior compared to RGB scale picture. Further, this study also verifies that the average CPU time taken by the RGB scale picture is larger than gray scale image. Hence, in future, the PBC images can be examined in gray scale form to get better accuracy and evaluation time.

BACKGROUND

Because of its significance, variety of image analysing schemes are proposed and realized in literature to examine therapeutic images. The traditional picture examination procedures require operator's assistance during the inspection and sometimes it may offer sluggish result due to its computational complexity. Hence, heuristic methodology assisted image processing and classification procedures are widely implemented to attain enhanced results during medical image evaluation (Rajinikanth et al., 2016; 2017; 2018; Rani et al., 2017). Most of these schemes also assist to build the computer based semi/automated tool to evaluate medical pictures recorded using a class of imaging modalities.

Peripheral Blood Cell (PBC) images are widely used in medical field to evaluate the infection as well as disease active in the blood level. Physical assessment of PBC is a time consuming procedure and the final accuracy of the examination practice relies mainly on the experience of the doctor. In order to have improved accuracy during the PBC examination, most of the medical clinics employs computer assisted disease examination tool. These procedures work on a predefined programming methodology, which can efficiently support the enhancement, segmentation and classification of PBC registered using a Digital Microscope (DM). Moreover, these tools are efficient in analysing both the thin and thick blood smear images of DM.

Recently, a substantial amount of tools are developed to inspect blood infection, red blood cell and white blood cell. During the PBC analysis, detection and classification of Leukocytes plays significant task, since it is highly related with the immune system of human body. The leukocytes normally contain the lymphocytes, monocytes, eosinophils, basophils, and neutrophils (Rezatofighi and Zadeh, 2011; Chan et al., 2010). At some stage in infection as well as a sensitive trauma may boost or diminish the count of leukocytes. Improved proportions of neutrophils represent the cause of severe infection and the augmented proportion of lymphocytes represents chronic bacterial infectivity. These five leukocytes can be categorized based on its granule of cytoplasm, granule's stain property, cell dimension, relation between nuclease to the cytoplasmic substance, and the type of nucleolar lobe. The detection and classification of Leukocyte is essential to plan a proper treatment process to cure the infection.

Putzu and Ruberto (2013) proposed an approach to examine White Blood Cell (WBC) using DM images. Chan et al. (2010) implemented an automated approach to segment and evaluate Leukocyte nucleus and nucleus lobe and executed a dimensional analysis to identify the type of Leukocyte. Akramifard et al. (2012) proposed neural network assisted tool to extract, distinguish, and count the WBC from DM images. Wu et al. (2016) proposed an approach to assess the Leukocyte recorded with harmonic generation microscopy. Prinyakupt and Pluempitiwiriyawej (2015) proposed a segmentation and morphology based classification of WBC based on linear and naïve Bayes classifiers. Mathur et al. (2013) implemented a system for categorization of WBC from Leishman stained DM images. Costa (2015) developed a tool to evaluate PBC images of thin and thick blood smear. Ramesh et al. (2012) discussed a two-stage methodology to classify WBC from PBC images. The work of Rezatofighi and Zadeh (2011) implements the examination of PBC by means of an automated approach to for the qualitative assessment and superior decision making during the segmentation and classification of WBC. Recently, Shahin et al. (2018) proposed adaptive neutrosophic similarity score based WBC segmentation approach.

CONTRIBUTION

The main focus of this chapter is to develop an efficient semi-automated scheme to mine ROI of LISC dataset with improved accuracy. The recent works by Palani et al. (2016) and Rajinikanth et al. (2017) reported that, combination of thresholding and segmentation will help to achieve better result compared with solitary technique. Hence, in this chapter, well-organized procedure by integrating the Shannon's entropy based multi-thresholding and the DRLS assisted extraction is implemented to examine PBC images. The details of procedures considered in this chapter are presented below.

Cuckoo Search Algorithm

Among the existing meta-heuristic procedures, Cuckoo Search (CS) discussed by Yang and Deb (2009) is emerged as a successful soft computing technique. The mathematical expression is as follows;

The CS implemented with the subsequent assumptions (Brajevic et al., 2012; Chatterjee et al., 2017; Chakraborty et al., 2017; Li et al., 2017):

- Every bird leaves one egg in arbitrarily selected nest of host birds
- Nest of prominent living egg is passed to subsequent level. This egg hatches faster than host's eggs.
- In CS, for a chosen optimization task, the probability of identifying the egg by host bird is $p_a \in [0,1]$.

In CS, success in finding of resolution for a task mostly depends on its steering formula. Mostly it is driven by Lévy Flight (LF) and Brownian Walk (BW) strategy (Lakshmi et al., 2016).

In optimization exploration, fresh location ($X_i^{(t+1)}$) mostly rely on old position ($X_i^{(t)}$). In this chapter, the following expressions are considered to find updated location of cuckoo;

$$X_i^{(t+1)} = X_i^{(t)} + \alpha \oplus BW \tag{1}$$

where, $X_i^{(t+1)}$ is updated position, $X_i^{(t)}$ represents initial position, $\oplus$ denotes the entry wise multiplier, BW depicts the Brownian walk strategy. Normally, the $\alpha > 0$ and in this work, it is assigned as unity. Other details regarding CS can be found in (Yang, 2008).

In this chapter, the following parameters are assigned for the CS algorithm: agent's size is selected as 30, search dimension is assigned as 3 (tri-level thresholding), the entire iteration rate is fixed as 2000 and terminating criteria is assigned as maximized Shannon's entropy.

Multi-Thresholding With Shannon's Entropy

SE was developed by Kannappan (1972) and its related details entropy are available with Paul and Bandyopadhyay's work (2014).

The SE is described as:

Let M*N is image dimension, (x, y) gray pixel coordinates. It can be articulated as f (x, y), for

$x \in \{1,2,...,M\}$ and $y \in \{1,2,...,N\}$. If L denotes amount gray ranks in picture I_0 and {0,1,2,…, L-1} depict set of all gray ranks with symbolized term G, in such a way that:

$$f(x,y) \in G \ \forall (x,y) \in image \tag{2}$$

The standardized histogram of picture can be characterized as $H = \{h_0, h_1, \ldots, h_{L-1}\}$.

In the proposed work, a tri-level threshold is considered. Hence, this relation will be;

$$H(T) = h_0(t_1) + h_1(t_2) + h_2(t_3) \tag{3}$$

$$T^* = \max_T \ \{\mathrm{H(T)}\} \tag{4}$$

in which T^* is the optimal threshold (Rajinikanth et al. 2017).

Shannon's entropy should satisfy Eqn. 4.

Distance Regularized Level Set

From the year 1990's (Caselles et al., 1993; Malladi et al, 1995) Level Set (LS) technique has been largely used in traditional and medical image segmentation applications.

The chief merit of the LS technique compared with other approach is, it can create contours with multifaceted procedure to carry dividing and merging maneuver during the picture outline exploration.

This chapter employs modern edition of LS called or Distance Regularized LS (DRLS) proposed by Li et al. (2010) in order to extract the stained section from PBC pictures of LISC database. The DRLS technique has the following formula;

The arc development is =

$$\frac{\partial C^{'}(s,t)}{\partial t} = FW \tag{5}$$

where, $C^{'}$ - arc vector with spatial (s) and temporal (t) parameter, F - swiftness variable and W - deepest usual vector of arc C.

The arc progress of Eqn. (5) can be formed as DRLS by inserting $C^{'}(s,t)$ as zero LS of a time exciting LS utility $\phi\ (x,y,t)$. The variable ϕ presents negative standards inside the zero stage curve and positive value exterior.

The vector N is expressed as;

$$N = \frac{-\nabla\varphi}{\nabla\varphi} \tag{6}$$

where ∇ is the slope variable.

The LS development is;

$$\frac{\partial\varphi}{\partial t} = F\left|\nabla\varphi\right| \tag{7}$$

Related details on DRLS available in (Vaishnavi et al., 2014).

Evaluation of ROI with GT

The aim of the work is to extract the stained region from PBC picture and to calculate the texture features of leukocyte for additional examination. This work considers a benchmark PBC image dataset known as LISC, in which test pictures are allied with GT. After extracting the ROI (stained region) from the blood smear picture, a relative examination among the ROI and GT is performed and the values, like Jaccard, Dice, False Positive Rate (FPR), and False Negative Rate (FNR) are computed (Chaddad and Tanougast, 2016; Rajinikanth et al., 2017).

The mathematical expressions are presented in Eqn. 8-11;

$$JSC(I_{gt}, I_t) = I_{gt} \cap I_t / I_{gt} \cup I_t \tag{8}$$

$$DSC(I_{gt}, I_t) = 2\left(I_{gt} \cap I_t\right) / \left|I_{gt}\right| \cup \left|I_t\right| \tag{9}$$

$$FPR(I_{gt}, I_t) = \left(I_{gt} / I_t\right) / (I_{gt} \cup I_t) \tag{10}$$

$$FNR(I_{gt}, I_t) = \left(I_t / I_{gt}\right) / (I_{gt} \cup I_t) \tag{11}$$

where, I_{gt} represents the GT and I_t symbolize mined region.

Additionally, the image statistical values, such as sensitivity, specificity, accuracy, and precision are also computed (Lu et al., 2004; Moghaddam, & Cheriet, 2010).

Expression for these parameters are given in Eqn. 12 - 15:

$$Sensitvity = T_P / (T_P + F_N) \tag{12}$$

$$Specificity = T_N / (T_N + F_P) \tag{13}$$

$$Accuracy = (T_P + T_N) / (T_P + T_N + F_P + F_N) \tag{14}$$

$$\text{Precision} = T_P / (T_P + F_P) \tag{15}$$

where, I_{GT} is GT, I_S is ROI, T_N, T_P, F_N and F_P signifies related measures.

SOLUTIONS AND RECOMMENDATIONS

The proposed work considers a variety of leukocyte images available in LISC dataset. Preliminary examination is executed using the gray scale version of the stained basophil (Baso) images of the size 720 x 576 pixels. Later, similar procedure is executed on the RGB scale version of test image existing in LISC. Proposed experimentation is executed using the computer; AMD C70 Dual Core 1 GHz CPU with 4 GB of RAM and the software considered is MATLAB 7.

Figure 1 represents the different phases implemented in the proposed tool to mine stained sector of test picture. Firstly, Gray/RGB scale test picture is enhanced based on the tri-level thresholding procedure implemented using the CS and SE. After the pre-processing task on the considered test image, the ROI (stained cell) is then extracted using the DRLS segmentation procedure. Finally, the texture feature for the ROI is extracted using Haralick function. In future, these features can be considered to train and test the classifiers, which can group the considered PBC dataset in to various leukocyte categories.

Figure 2 shows the examination test pictures of basophil used in the initial evaluation. Here, Figure 2 (a) represents the pseudo name of the picture in LISC dataset, (b) depicts the test picture, (c) and (d) depicts the original and binary form of the GT.

Implemented two-step procedure is then executed on the test images with the Gray/RGB scale pictures. Initially, the CS+SE based thresholding is implemented using an assigned threshold value of three and then the DRLS based segmentation procedure is implemented using the operator assigned bounding box around the stained region of PBC image. After extracting the ROI, a comparative analysis is performed between the segmented section and the GT. Later, image likeness

Figure 1. Block diagram of implemented image examination scheme

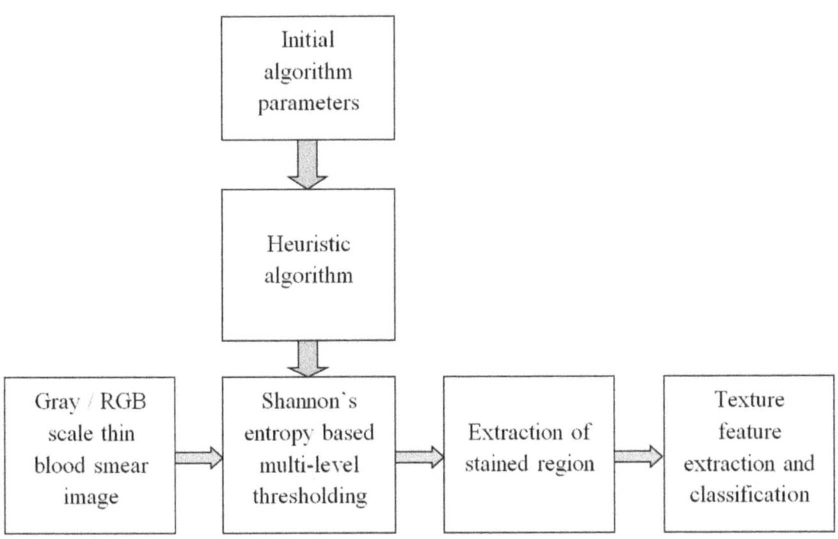

Figure 2. Example trial imagery adopted for initial examination. (a) Pseudo name, (b) RGB scaled test picture, (c) and (d) Presents the GT

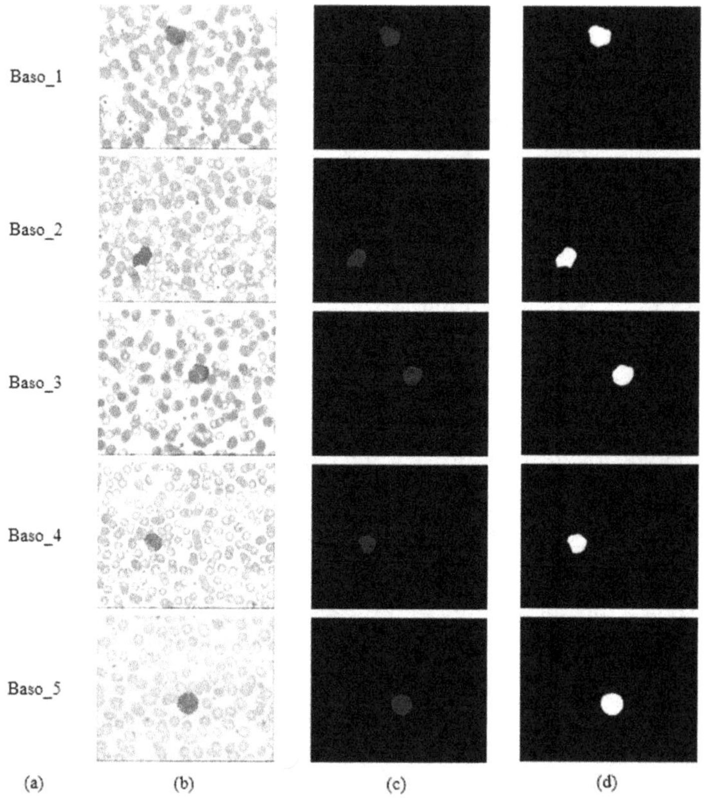

values and the statistical measures are computed and recorded for the considered images. During this procedure, the CPU time (sec) also recorded for both the gray and RGB scale pictures in order to validate the performance of proposed two-stage methodology on the considered test pictures.

Figure 3 depicts the outcome of implemented approach, in which (a) presented the operator assigned bounding box, (b) and (c) presents the initial and final version of DRLS on the gray scaled image. (d) Shows the 3D version of the extracted ROI and (e) and (f) depicts the extracted binary ROI and its complement image. Similar procedure is also executed for RGB scale images and the related outcome is clearly presented in Figure 3 (g) – (i).

Figure 4 presents GT of the chosen sample test pictures and the extracted ROI with gray and RGB scaled test pictures. Later, a comparative study among the GT and the ROI is executed and its corresponding outcomes, such as image likeness

Figure 3. Experimental outcome on a chosen WBC image (a) Operator assigned bounding box, (b) and (c) Initial and final LS function, (d) 3D version of WBC, (e) and (f) Segmented and complement images. (g) Processed RGB scale picture, (h) Initial LS function, (i) Final LS function

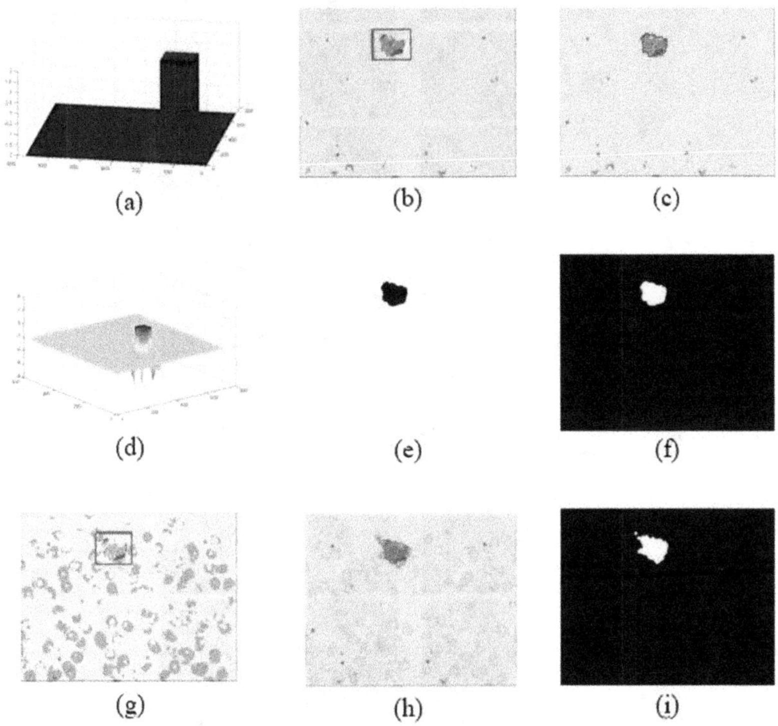

and statistical actions are recorded as presented in Table 1-4. The superiority of the proposed approach can be confirmed with these table values.

Table 1 presents the picture similarity measure values, such as TP, TN, True Positive rate (TPrate), True Negative rate (TNrate), False Positive rate (FPrate) and False Negative rate (FNrate) obtained from a comparative study between the GT and the ROI of gray scale basophil images. This table also presents the run time of the proposed tool in sec. In this table, average1 represents the mean value of obtained parameters for 10 test images and average2 represents the mean value of 53 basophil images of NISC database. Similar values are also recorded as in Table 2-4.

Table 2 presents the statistical measures obtained with the gray scale basophil images. Also Table 3 and Table 4 shows the picture likeness measures and statistical values attained with RGB scale version of the basophil test images. Same approach is executed with eosinophils (Eosi = 39 images), lymphocytes (Lymp = 52 images), monocytes (Mono=48 images) and neutrophils (Neut=50 images) and mixed cases

Figure 4. Outcome obtained for the chosen sample test images. (a) Pseudo name, (b) GT, (c) ROI of gray scale picture and (d) ROI obtained from RGB image

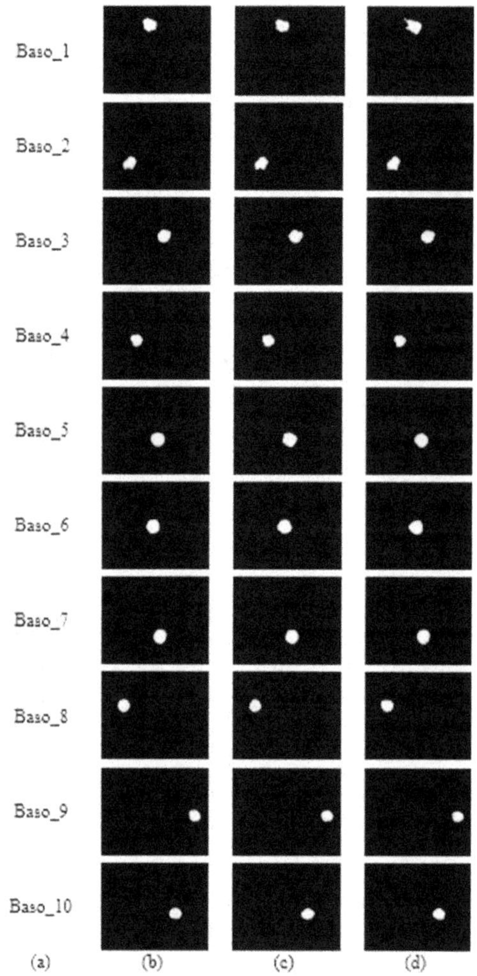

(Mixt =8 images) of NISC dataset is also executed and approximately similar result like basophil test case is attained for other PBC pictures. All the results are approximately identical, hence in this chapter, only the segmentation result of basophil alone is discussed.

From Table 2 and 4, one can observe that, implemented scheme is proficient in providing improved average values (>90%) for the Jaccard, Dice, sensitivity, specificity, accuracy and precision for both gray scale and the RGB test image cases. This result confirms the benefit of the proposed two step procedure with CS+SE and DRLS for the analysis of the PBC images. The above values are graphically

Table 1. Image similarity measures obtained with gray scale basophil image

Test Image	TP	TN	TPrate	TNrate	FPrate	FNrate	CPU Time (sec)
1	4316	398630	0.9507	0.9987	0.0023	0.0493	38.1464
2	4628	399438	0.9556	0.9997	0.0003	0.0444	31.0643
3	5141	398798	0.9438	0.9996	0.0004	0.0562	26.8421
4	4220	399793	0.9405	0.9997	0.0003	0.0595	42.0638
5	5928	397922	0.9503	0.9994	0.0006	0.0497	37.1974
6	5867	398010	0.9474	0.9995	0.0005	0.0526	46.7715
7	5586	398181	0.9683	0.9988	0.0012	0.0317	50.0532
8	4447	399474	0.9802	0.9990	0.0010	0.0198	29.6764
9	3971	399999	0.9489	0.9994	0.0006	0.0511	38.5527
10	4158	399828	0.9502	0.9995	0.0005	0.0498	33.9476
Average1	4826	399007	0.9536	0.9993	0.0007	0.0464	37.4315
Average2	4665	399203	0.9406	0.9991	0.0009	0.0594	36.0725

Table 2. Image statistical measures obtained for gray scale basophil image

Test Image	Jaccard	Dice	Sensitivity	Specificity	Accuracy	Precision
1	0.9152	0.9047	0.9789	0.9987	0.9987	0.9618
2	0.9297	0.9636	0.9556	0.9997	0.9991	0.9717
3	0.9151	0.9557	0.9438	0.9996	0.9988	0.9678
4	0.9128	0.9544	0.9405	0.9997	0.9990	0.9688
5	0.9128	0.9544	0.9503	0.9994	0.9986	0.9586
6	0.9159	0.9561	0.9474	0.9995	0.9987	0.9650
7	0.8959	0.9451	0.9683	0.9988	0.9984	0.9230
8	0.8998	0.9473	0.9802	0.9990	0.9988	0.9165
9	0.8990	0.9468	0.9489	0.9994	0.9989	0.9448
10	0.9063	0.9508	0.9502	0.9995	0.9989	0.9515
Average1	0.9102	0.9479	0.9564	0.9993	0.9988	0.9529
Average2	0.9085	0.9317	0.9486	0.9986	0.9972	0.9472

compared as shown in Figure 5. This figure confirms that, the gray scale version of PBC images offers improved performance compared with the RGB scale PBC images. Further the CPU time of gray scale picture (average = 36.0725 sec) is considerable smaller than RGB scale pictures (average = 63.6747 sec). The threshold

Table 3. Image similarity measures obtained with RGB scale basophil image

Test Image	TP	TN	TPrate	TNrate	FPrate	FNrate	CPU Time (sec)
1	3895	399947	0.9155	0.9912	0.0098	0.0845	71.6379
2	4655	399260	0.9221	0.9997	0.0003	0.0779	55.1684
3	5099	398959	0.9723	0.9995	0.0005	0.0277	49.0426
4	3994	399969	0.9777	0.9991	0.0009	0.0223	63.1685
5	5726	398045	0.9684	0.9989	0.0011	0.0316	68.0432
6	5757	398002	0.9452	0.9992	0.0008	0.0548	57.2664
7	5744	398108	0.9573	0.9992	0.0008	0.0427	70.5843
8	4528	399212	0.9279	0.9992	0.0008	0.0721	68.3774
9	3922	400055	0.9613	0.9993	0.0007	0.0387	47.0864
10	4176	399809	0.9463	0.9995	0.0005	0.0537	52.1782
Average1	4749	399136	0.9494	0.9984	0.0016	0.0506	60.2553
Average2	4714	399184	0.9338	0.9973	0.0027	0.0662	63.6747

Table 4. Image statistical measures obtained for RGB scale basophil image

Test Image	Jaccard	Dice	Sensitivity	Specificity	Accuracy	Precision
1	0.8752	0.8946	0.9163	0.9696	0.9448	0.9385
2	0.9028	0.9489	0.9221	0.9997	0.9988	0.9773
3	0.9344	0.9661	0.9723	0.9995	0.9991	0.9599
4	0.8981	0.9463	0.9777	0.9991	0.9989	0.9169
5	0.8988	0.9467	0.9684	0.9989	0.9984	0.9259
6	0.8976	0.9460	0.9452	0.9992	0.9984	0.9469
7	0.9106	0.9532	0.9573	0.9992	0.9986	0.9491
8	0.8701	0.9305	0.9279	0.9992	0.9983	0.9332
9	0.8993	0.9470	0.9613	0.9993	0.9989	0.9331
10	0.9064	0.9509	0.9463	0.9995	0.9989	0.9556
Average1	0.8993	0.9430	0.9495	0.9963	0.9933	0.9436
Average2	0.9004	0.9215	0.9403	0.9917	0.9952	0.9385

levels of RGB scale pictures are very complex than the gray scale pictures, so the RGB scale picture requires more computation time compared with the gray images. The computation time also depends on the size of the test images. Hence, in future, if the gray scale picture is considered for the examination, then the throughput of the implemented scheme will be good than the alternative.

Figure 5. Graphical representation of the statistical measure of gray and RGB scale basophil pictures

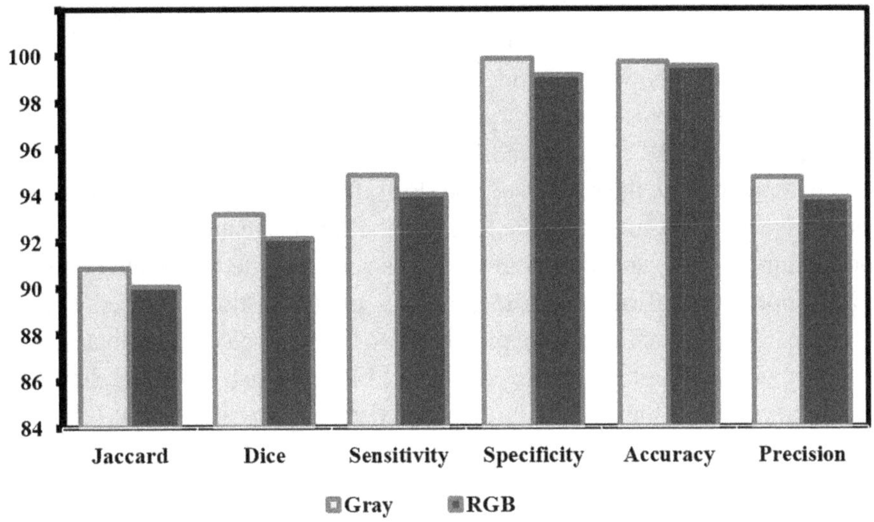

FUTURE RESEARCH DIRECTIONS

To identify the disease harshness and also to prepare for the additional treatment procedure, it is essential to analyze the PBC images with the help of medical experts. In recent years, most of the imaging centers have the capability to record DM images of PBC. In order to have a pre-opinion regarding the blood infection in clinical level, it is essential to use a suitable image processing tool to appraise the PBC images. The aim of the research work presented in this chapter is to develop a heuristic algorithm assisted two-step procedure to examine the PBC images of LISC dataset. The proposed work focuses on extracting the stained region from the considered PBC picture.

In future, the proposed work can be directed as follows: i) Implementation of recent heuristic algorithm to improve the pre-processing section, ii) Enhancing the results of the pre-processing by considering other thresholding procedures, such as Otsu's function, Kapur' entropy and Tsallis entropy, iii) Implementing the most famous ROI extraction procedures, like seed based region growing, watershed algorithm and active contour methods to enhance the picture likeness events and image statistical events, iv) Extracting the texture features of the PBC region to implement the classifier units for the automated detection and diagnose of the blood cell abnormalities.

CONCLUSION

The proposed method implements an evaluation tool by integrating Shannon's Entropy with Level Set segmentation to enhance the outcome during the PBC picture inspection. This work considers the well known datasets, known as LISC with five types of leukocytes. Firstly, proposed practice is experienced on gray scale version of the PBC picture and later it is implemented with the RGB scale picture. After extracting the stained region (ROI) from the leukocyte image dataset, a comparative assessment among the ROI and the GT image are performed and the famous picture likeness and statistical measures were recorded. The outcome of the proposed approach confirms that, the gray scale picture evaluation offers superior result compared with the RGB scale picture. Also the gray scale image examination provided superior throughput on the considered LISC dataset. In future, the texture features extracted from the ROI can be considered to develop an automated classified unit to classify the leukocytes of PBC images.

REFERENCES

Abhinaya, B., & Raja, N. S. M. (2015). Solving multi-level image thresholding problem—an analysis with cuckoo search algorithm. *Advances In Intelligent Systems And Computing*, *339*, 177–186. doi:10.1007/978-81-322-2250-7_18

Akramifard, H., Firouzmand, M., & Moghadam, R. A. (2012). Extracting, recognizing, and counting white blood cells from microscopic images by using complex-valued neural networks. *Journal of Medical Signals and Sensors*, *2*(3), 169–175. PMID:23717809

Anitha, P., Bindhiya, S., Abinaya, A., Satapathy, S. C., Dey, N., & Rajinikanth, V. (2017). RGB image multi-thresholding based on Kapur's entropy—A study with heuristic algorithms. *Second International Conference on Electrical, Computer and Communication Technologies (ICECCT)*. 10.1109/ICECCT.2017.8117823

Ashour, A. S., Samanta, S., Dey, N., Kausar, N., Abdessalemkaraa, W. B., & Hassanien, A. E. (2015). Computed tomography image enhancement using cuckoo search: A log transform based approach. *Journal of Signal and Information Processing*, *6*(3), 244–257. doi:10.4236/jsip.2015.63023

Balan, N. S., Kumar, A. S., Raja, N. S. M., & Rajinikanth, V. (2016). Optimal multilevel image thresholding to improve the visibility of plasmodium sp. in blood smear images. *Advances in Intelligent Systems and Computing*, *397*, 563–571. doi:10.1007/978-81-322-2671-0_54

Brajevic, I., Tuba, M., & Bacanin, N. (2012). Multilevel image thresholding selection based on the Cuckoo search algorithm. *Proceedings of the 5th International Conference on Visualization, Imaging and Simulation (VIS'12)*, 217–222.

Caselles, V., Catte, F., Coll, T., & Dibos, F. (1993). A geometric model for active contours in image processing. *Numerische Mathematik*, *66*(1), 1–31. doi:10.1007/BF01385685

Chaddad, A., & Tanougast, C. (2016). Quantitative evaluation of robust skull stripping and tumor detection applied to axial MR images. *Brain Informatics*, *3*(1), 53–61. doi:10.100740708-016-0033-7 PMID:27747598

Chakraborty, S., Chatterjee, S., Dey, N., Ashour, A. S., Ashour, A. S., Shi, F., & Mali, K. (2017). Modified cuckoo search algorithm in microscopic image segmentation of hippocampus. *Microscopy Research and Technique*, *80*(10), 1051–1072. doi:10.1002/jemt.22900 PMID:28557041

Chakraborty, S., Dey, N., Samanta, S., Ashour, A. S., Barna, C., & Balas, M. M. (2017). Optimization of non-rigid demons registration using cuckoo search algorithm. *Cognitive Computation*, *9*(6), 817–826. doi:10.100712559-017-9508-y

Chan, Y. K., Tsai, M. H., Zheng, Z. H., & Hung, K. D. (2010). Leukocyte nucleus segmentation and nucleus lobe counting. *BMC Bioinformatics*, *11*(1), 558. doi:10.1186/1471-2105-11-558 PMID:21073711

Chatterjee, S., Dey, N., Ashour, A. S., & Drugarin, C. V. A. (2017). Electrical energy output prediction using cuckoo search based artificial neural network. *Lecture Notes in Networks and Systems*, *18*, 277–285. doi:10.1007/978-981-10-6916-1_26

Da Costa, L. (2015). Digital image analysis of blood cells. *Clinics in Laboratory Medicine*, *35*(1), 105–122. doi:10.1016/j.cll.2014.10.005 PMID:25676375

Dey, N., Rajinikanth, V., Amira, S., Ashour, A. S., & Tavares, J. M. R. S. (2018). Social Group Optimization Supported Segmentation and Evaluation of Skin Melanoma Images. *Symmetry*, *10*(2), 51. doi:10.3390ym10020051

Fernandes, S. L., Gurupur, V. P., Lin, H., & Martis, R. J. (2017). A novel fusion approach for early lung cancer detection using computer aided diagnosis techniques. *Journal of Medical Imaging and Health Informatics*, *7*(8), 1841–1850. doi:10.1166/jmihi.2017.2280

Hore, S., Chakroborty, S., Ashour, A. S., Dey, N., Ashour, A. S., Sifaki-Pistolla, D., ... Chaudhuri, S. R. (2015). Finding contours of hippocampus brain cell using microscopic image analysis. *Journal of Advanced Microscopy Research, 10*(2), 93–103. doi:10.1166/jamr.2015.1245

Kamalanand, K., & Jawahar, P. M. (2012). Coupled jumping frogs/particle swarm optimization for estimating the parameters of three dimensional HIV model. *BMC Infectious Diseases, 12*(1), 82. doi:10.1186/1471-2334-12-S1-P82 PMID:22471518

Kamalanand, K., & Jawahar, P. M. (2015). Prediction of Human Immunodeficiency Virus-1 Viral Load from CD4 Cell Count Using Artificial Neural Networks. *Journal of Medical Imaging and Health Informatics, 5*(3), 641–646. doi:10.1166/jmihi.2015.1430

Kannappan, P. L. (1972). On Shannon's entropy, directed divergence and inaccuracy. *Probability Theory and Related Fields, 22*, 95–100.

Lakshmi, V.S., Tebby, S.G., Shriranjani, D., & Rajinikanth, V. (2016). Chaotic cuckoo search and Kapur/Tsallis approach in segmentation of T.cruzi from blood smear images. *Int. J. Comp. Sci. Infor. Sec., 14*, 51-56.

Li, C., Xu, C., Gui, C., & Fox, M. D. (2010). Distance regularized level set evolution and its application to image segmentation. *IEEE Transactions on Image Processing, 19*(12), 3243–3254. doi:10.1109/TIP.2010.2069690 PMID:20801742

Li, Z., Dey, N., Ashour, A. S., & Tang, Q. (2017). Discrete cuckoo search algorithms for two-sided robotic assembly line balancing problem. *Neural Computing & Applications*, 1–12. doi:10.100700521-017-2855-5

Lin, H., & Li, Y. (2017). Using EEG data analytics to measure meditation. *Lecture Notes in Computer Science, 10287*, 270–280. doi:10.1007/978-3-319-58466-9_25

LISC. (n.d.). Retrieved from http://users.cecs.anu.edu.au/~hrezatofighi/Data/Leukocyte%20Data.htm

Lu, H., Kot, A. C., & Shi, Y. Q. (2004). Distance-reciprocal distortion measure for binary document images. *IEEE Signal Processing Letters, 11*(2), 228–231. doi:10.1109/LSP.2003.821748

Malladi, R., Sethian, J. A., & Vemuri, B. C. (1995). Shape modeling with front propagation: A level set approach. *IEEE T. Pattern Anal. Mac. Int., 17*(2), 158–175. doi:10.1109/34.368173

Manickavasagam, K., Sutha, S., & Kamalanand, K. (2014). Development of systems for classification of different plasmodium species in thin blood smear microscopic images. *Journal of Advanced Microscopy Research*, *9*(2), 86–92. doi:10.1166/jamr.2014.1194

Mathur, A., Tripathi, A. S., & Kuse, M. (2013). Scalable system for classification of white blood cells from Leishman stained blood stain images. *Journal of Pathology Informatics*, *4*(2), S15. doi:10.4103/2153-3539.109883 PMID:23766937

Moghaddam, R. F., & Cheriet, M. (2010). A multi-scale framework for adaptive binarization of degraded document images. *Pattern Recognition*, *43*(6), 2186–2198. doi:10.1016/j.patcog.2009.12.024

Naqi, S. M., Sharif, M., Yasmin, M., & Fernandes, S. L. (2018). Lung nodule detection using polygon approximation and hybrid features from CT images. *Current Medical Imaging Reviews*, *14*(1), 108–117. doi:10.2174/1573405613666170306114320

Palani, T. K., Parvathavarthini, B., & Chitra, K. (2016). Segmentation of brain regions by integrating meta heuristic multilevel threshold with Markov random field. *Current Medical Imaging Reviews*, *12*(1), 4–12. doi:10.2174/1573394711666150827203434

Paramasivam, A., Kamalanand, K., Sundravadivelu, K., & Mannar, J. P. (2017). Effect of electrode contact area on the information content of the recorded electrogastrograms: An analysis based on Rényi entropy and Teager-Kaiser Energy. *Polish Journal of Medical Physics and Engineering*, *23*(2), 37–42.

Paul, S., & Bandyopadhyay, B. (2014). A novel approach for image compression based on multi-level image thresholding using Shannon entropy and differential evolution. *Students' Technology Symposium (TechSym), IEEE*, 56 – 61. 10.1109/TechSym.2014.6807914

Prinyakupt, J., & Pluempitiwiriyawej, C. (2015). Segmentation of white blood cells and comparison of cell morphology by linear and naïve Bayes classifiers. *Biomedical Engineering Online*, *14*(1), 63. doi:10.118612938-015-0037-1 PMID:26123131

Putzu, L., & Ruberto, C. D. (2013). White blood cells identification and counting from microscopic blood image. *International Journal of Medical and Health Sciences*, *7*(1), 20–27.

Raja, N. S. M., Rajinikanth, V., & Latha, K. (2014). Otsu based optimal multilevel image thresholding using firefly algorithm. Modelling and Simulation in Engineering, Article ID 794574.

Rajinikanth, V., Dey, N., Satapathy, S. C., & Ashour, A. S. (2018). An approach to examine magnetic resonance angiography based on Tsallis entropy and deformable snake model. *Future Generation Computer Systems*, *85*, 160–172. doi:10.1016/j.future.2018.03.025

Rajinikanth, V., Fernandes, S. L., Bhushan, B., & Sunder, N. R. (2018). Segmentation and analysis of brain tumor using Tsallis entropy and regularised level set. *Lecture Notes in Electrical Engineering*, *434*, 313–321. doi:10.1007/978-981-10-4280-5_33

Rajinikanth, V., Raja, N. S. M., & Satapathy, S. C. (2016). Robust color image multi-thresholding using between-class variance and cuckoo search algorithm. *Advances in Intelligent Systems and Computing*, *433*, 379–386. doi:10.1007/978-81-322-2755-7_40

Rajinikanth, V., Raja, N. S. M., Satapathy, S. C., & Fernandes, S. L. (2017). Otsu's multi-thresholding and active contour snake model to segment dermoscopy images. *Journal of Medical Imaging and Health Informatics*, *7*(8), 1837–1840. doi:10.1166/jmihi.2017.2265

Rajinikanth, V., & Satapathy, S. C. (2018). Segmentation of ischemic stroke lesion in brain MRI based on social group optimization and fuzzy-Tsallis entropy. *Arabian Journal for Science and Engineering*, 1–14. doi:10.100713369-017-3053-6

Rajinikanth, V., Satapathy, S. C., Dey, N., & Vijayarajan, R. (2018). DWT-PCA image fusion technique to improve segmentation accuracy in brain tumor analysis. *Lecture Notes in Electrical Engineering*, *471*, 453–462. doi:10.1007/978-981-10-7329-8_46

Rajinikanth, V., Satapathy, S. C., Fernandes, S. L., & Nachiappan, S. (2017). Entropy based segmentation of tumor from brain MR images–A study with teaching learning based optimization. *Pattern Recognition Letters*, *94*, 87–94. doi:10.1016/j.patrec.2017.05.028

Ramesh, N., Dangott, B., Salama, M. E., & Tasdizen, T. (2012). Isolation and two-step classification of normal white blood cells in peripheral blood smears. *Journal of Pathology Informatics*, *3*(1), 13. doi:10.4103/2153-3539.93895 PMID:22530181

Rani, J., Kumar, R., Talukdar, F. A., & Dey, N. (2017). The Brain tumor segmentation using Fuzzy C-Means technique: A study. In Recent Advances in Applied Thermal Imaging for Industrial Applications. IGI Global.

Ranjan, R., Arya, R., Fernandes, S. L., Sravya, E., & Jain, V. (2018). A fuzzy neural network approach for automatic k-complex detection in sleep EEG signal. *Pattern Recognition Letters*. doi:10.1016/j.patrec.2018.01.001

Rezatofighi, S. H., & Zadeh, H. S. (2011). Automatic recognition of five types of white blood cells in peripheral blood. *Computerized Medical Imaging and Graphics*, *35*(4), 333–343. doi:10.1016/j.compmedimag.2011.01.003 PMID:21300521

Shahin, A. I., Guo, Y., Amin, K. M., & Sharawi, A. A. (2018). A novel white blood cells segmentation algorithm based on adaptive neutrosophic similarity score. *Health Inf. Sci. Syst.*, *6*(1), 1. doi:10.100713755-017-0038-5 PMID:29279774

Shree, V. T. D., Revanth, K., Raja, N. S. M., & Rajinikanth, V. (2018). A hybrid image processing approach to examine abnormality in retinal optic disc. *Procedia Computer Science*, *125*, 157–164. doi:10.1016/j.procs.2017.12.022

Sudhan, G. H. H., Aravind, R. G., Gowri, K., & Rajinikanth, V. (2017). Optic disc segmentation based on Otsu's thresholding and level set. *International Conference on Computer Communication and Informatics (ICCCI)*. 10.1109/ICCCI.2017.8117688

Tuan, T. M. (2018). Dental diagnosis from X-Ray images: An expert system based on fuzzy computing. *Biomedical Signal Processing and Control*, *39*, 64–73. doi:10.1016/j.bspc.2017.07.005

Vaishnavi, G. K., Jeevananthan, K., Begum, S. R., & Kamalanand, K. (2014). Geometrical analysis of schistosome egg images using distance regularized level set method for automated species identification. *J. Bioinformatics Intell. Cont*, *3*(2), 147–152. doi:10.1166/jbic.2014.1080

Vishnupriya, R., Raja, N. S. M., & Rajinikanth, V. (2017). An efficient clustering technique and analysis of infrared thermograms. *Third International Conference on Biosignals, Images and Instrumentation (ICBSII)*, 1-5. 10.1109/ICBSII.2017.8082275

Wu, C.-H., Wang, T.-D., Hsieh, C.-H., Huang, S.-H., Lin, J.-W., Hsu, S.-C., ... Liu, T.-M. (2016). Imaging Cytometry of Human Leukocytes with Third Harmonic Generation Microscopy. *Scientific Reports*, *6*(1), 37210. doi:10.1038rep37210 PMID:27845443

Yang, X. S. (2008). *Nature-Inspired Metaheuristic Algorithms*. Frome, UK: Luniver Press.

Yang, X. S., & Deb, S. (2009). Cuckoo search via Lévy flights. In *Proceedings of World Congress on Nature and Biologically Inspired Computing (NaBIC 2009)*. IEEE Publications. 10.1109/NABIC.2009.5393690

ADDITIONAL READING

Ackerman, M. J., Filart, R., Burgess, L. P., Lee, I. & Poropatich, R. K. (2010). Developing next-generation telehealth tools and technologies: patients, systems, and data perspectives. Telemed. *e-Health*, 16(1):93–95.

Ahmed, S., Dey, N., Ashour, A. S., Sifaki-Pistolla, D., Bălas-Timar, D., Balas, V. E., & Tavares, J. M. R. S. (2017). Effect of fuzzy partitioning in Crohn's disease classification: A neuro-fuzzy-based approach. *Medical & Biological Engineering & Computing*, *55*(1), 101–115. doi:10.100711517-016-1508-7 PMID:27106754

Arslan, S., Ozyurek, E., & Gunduz-Demir, C. (2014). A color and shape based algorithm for segmentation of white blood cells in peripheral blood and bone marrow images. *Cytometry. Part A*, *85*(6), 480–490. doi:10.1002/cyto.a.22457 PMID:24623453

Beck, C. (2009). Generalised information and entropy measures in physics. *Contemporary Physics*, *50*(4), 495–510. doi:10.1080/00107510902823517

Binh, H. T. T., Hanh, N. T., Quan, L. V., & Dey, N. (2016). Improved Cuckoo search and chaotic flower pollination optimization algorithm for maximizing area coverage in wireless sensor networks. *Neural Computing & Applications*, 1–13. doi:10.100700521-016-2823-5

Bokhari, F., Syedia, T., Sharif, M., Yasmin, M., & Fernandes, S. L. (2018). Fundus Image Segmentation and Feature Extraction for the Detection of Glaucoma: A New Approach. *Current Medical Imaging Reviews*, *14*(1), 77–87. doi:10.2174/157340 5613666170405145913

Borra, S., Thanki, R., Dey, N., & Borisagar, K. (2018). *Secure transmission and integrity verification of color radiological images using fast discrete curvelet transform and compressive sensing*. Smart Health; doi:10.1016/j.smhl.2018.02.001

Chatterjee, S., Dey, N., Shi, F., Ashour, A. S., Fong, S. J., & Sen, S. (2018). Clinical application of modified bag-of-features coupled with hybrid neural-based classifier in dengue fever classification using gene expression data. *Medical & Biological Engineering & Computing*, *56*(4), 709–720. doi:10.100711517-017-1722-y PMID:28891000

Cheriguene, S., Azizi, N., Dey, N., Ashour, A. S., & Ziani, A. (2018). A new hybrid classifier selection model based on mRMR method and diversity measures. *International Journal of Machine Learning and Cybernetics*, 1–16. doi:10.100713042-018-0797-6

Dănilă, E., Moraru, L., Dey, N., Ashour, A. S., Shi, F., Fong, S. J., ... Biswas, A. (2018). Multifractal analysis of ceramic pottery SEM images in Cucuteni-Tripolye culture. *Optik (Stuttgart)*, *164*, 538–546. doi:10.1016/j.ijleo.2018.03.052

Dey, N., Ashour, A. S., Beagum, S., Pistola, D. S., Gospodinov, M., Gospodinova, E. P., & Tavares, J. M. R. S. (2015). Parameter optimization for local polynomial approximation based intersection confidence interval filter using genetic algorithm: An application for brain MRI image de-noising. *Journal of Imaging*, *1*(1), 60–84. doi:10.3390/jimaging1010060

Dey, N., Ashour, A. S., Shi, F., Fong, S. J., & Sherratt, R. S. (2017). Developing residential wireless sensor networks for ECG healthcare monitoring. *IEEE Transactions on Consumer Electronics*, *63*(4), 442–449. doi:10.1109/TCE.2017.015063

Dey, N., Ashour, A. S., Shi, F., Fong, S. J., & Sherratt, R. S. (2017). Developing residential wireless sensor networks for ECG healthcare monitoring. *IEEE Transactions on Consumer Electronics*, *63*(4), 442–449. doi:10.1109/TCE.2017.015063

Dey, N., Ashour, A. S., Shi, F., Fong, S. J., & Tavares, J. M. R. S. (2018). Medical cyber-physical systems: A survey. *Journal of Medical Systems*, *42*(4), 74. doi:10.100710916-018-0921-x PMID:29525900

Dey, N., Ashour, A. S., Shi, F., Fong, S. J., & Tavares, J. M. R. S. (2018). Medical cyber-physical systems: A survey. *Journal of Medical Systems*, *42*(4), 74. doi:10.100710916-018-0921-x PMID:29525900

Dey, N., Ashour, A. S., Shi, F., & Sherratt, R. S. (2017). Wireless capsule gastrointestinal endoscopy: Direction-of-arrival estimation based localization survey. *IEEE Reviews in Biomedical Engineering*, *10*, 2–11. doi:10.1109/RBME.2017.2697950 PMID:28459696

Dorini, L. B., Minetto, R., & Leite, N. J. (2013). Semiautomatic white blood cell segmentation based on multiscale analysis. *IEEE Journal of Biomedical and Health Informatics*, *17*(1), 250–256. doi:10.1109/TITB.2012.2207398 PMID:22855228

Fredo, A. R. J., Kavitha, G., & Ramakrishnan, S. (2015). Automated segmentation and analysis of corpus callosum in autistic MR brain images using fuzzy-c-means-based level set method. *Journal of Medical and Biological Engineering*, *35*(3), 331–337. doi:10.100740846-015-0047-2

Goswami, S., Roy, P., Dey, N., & Chakraborty, S. (2016). Wireless body area networks combined with mobile cloud computing in healthcare: A survey. Class. *Clust. Biomed. Sign. Proc.*, *7*, 388.

Kamal, S., Dey, N., Nimmy, S. F., Ripon, S. H., Ali, N. Y., Ashour, A. S., ... Shi, F. (2018). Evolutionary framework for coding area selection from cancer data. *Neural Computing & Applications*, *29*(4), 1015–1037. doi:10.100700521-016-2513-3

Li, Y., Zhu, R., Mi, L., Cao, Y. & Di Yao, D. (2016). Segmentation of white blood cell from acute lymphoblastic leukemia images using dual-threshold method. *Computational and Mathematical Methods in Medicine*, vol. 2016, Article ID 9514707, 12 pages. Doi:.10.1155/2016/9514707

Li, Z., Dey, N., Ashour, A. S., Cao, L., Wang, Y., Wang, D., ... Shi, F. (2017). Convolutional Neural Network Based Clustering and Manifold Learning Method for Diabetic Plantar Pressure Imaging Dataset. *J. Med. Imaging Health Inform*, *7*(3), 639–652. doi:10.1166/jmihi.2017.2082

Machado, J.A.T. (2012). Shannon entropy analysis of the genome code. *Mathematical Problems in Engineering*, vol. 2012, Article ID 132625, 12 pages. Doi:10.1155/2012/132625

Machado, J. T. (2010). Entropy analysis of integer and fractional dynamical systems. *Nonlinear Dynamics*, *62*(1-2), 371–378. doi:10.100711071-010-9724-4

Manic, K. S., Rajinikanth, V., Ananthasivam, S., & Suresh, U. (2015). Design of controller in double feedback control loop–an analysis with heuristic algorithms. *Chemical Product and Process Modeling*, *10*(4), 253–262. doi:10.1515/cppm-2015-0005

Martis, R. J., & Fernandes, S. L. (2017). A special section on early cancer detection and machine vision. *Journal of Medical Imaging and Health Informatics*, *7*(8), 1823–1824. doi:10.1166/jmihi.2017.2274

Metzler, R., & Klafter, J. (2000). The random walk's guide to anomalous diffusion: A fractional dynamics approach. *Physics Reports*, *339*(1), 1–77. doi:10.1016/S0370-1573(00)00070-3

Moraru, L., Moldovanu, S., Dimitrievici, L. T., Ashour, A. S., & Dey, N. (2016). (2016). Texture anisotropy technique in brain degenerative diseases. *Neural Computing & Applications*. doi:10.100700521-016-2777-7

Naik, A., Satapathy, S. C., Ashour, A. S., & Dey, N. (2016). Social group optimization for global optimization of multimodal functions and data clustering problems. *Neural Computing & Applications*. doi:10.100700521-016-2686-9

Nurzaman, S. G., Matsumoto, Y., Nakamura, Y., Shirai, K., Koizumi, S., & Ishiguro, H. (2011). From Lévy to Brownian: A computational model based on biological fluctuation. *PLoS One*, *6*(2), e16168. doi:10.1371/journal.pone.0016168 PMID:21304911

Pal, G., Acharjee, S., Rudrapaul, D., Ashour, A. S., & Dey, N. (2015). Video segmentation using minimum ratio similarity measurement. *Int J Image Min.*, *1*(1), 87–110. doi:10.1504/IJIM.2015.070027

Palani, T., & Parvathavarthini, B. (2017). Multichannel interictal spike activity detection using time–frequency entropy measure. *Australasian Physical & Engineering Sciences in Medicine*, *40*(2), 413–425. doi:10.100713246-017-0550-6 PMID:28409335

Preethi, B. J., & Rajinikanth, V. (2014). Improving segmentation accuracy in biopsy cancer cell images using Otsu and Firefly Algorithm. *Int J Appl Eng Res*, *9*(24), 8502–8506.

Raja, N. S. M., Kavitha, G., & Ramakrishnan, S. (2012). Analysis of vasculature in human retinal images using particle swarm optimization based Tsallis multi-level thresholding and similarity measures. *Lecture Notes in Computer Science*, *7677*, 380–387. doi:10.1007/978-3-642-35380-2_45

Raja, N. S. M., & Rajinikanth, V. (2014). Brownian distribution guided bacterial foraging algorithm for controller design problem, in ICT and Critical Infrastructure: Proceedings of the 48th Annual Convention of Computer Society of India-Vol I, *Advances in Intelligent Systems and Computing*, 248:141–148. Doi: 10.1007/978-3-319-03107-1_17

Rajaram, R., Castellani, B. & Wilson, A.N. (2017). Advancing Shannon Entropy for Measuring Diversity in Systems, *Complexity*, vol. 2017, Article ID 8715605, 10 pages. Doi:.10.1155/2017/8715605

Rajinikanth, V., & Couceiro, M. S. (2015). RGB histogram based color image segmentation using firefly algorithm. *Procedia Computer Science*, *46*, 1449–1457. doi:10.1016/j.procs.2015.02.064

Rajinikanth, V., Raja, N. S. M., & Kamalanand, K. (2017). Firefly algorithm assisted segmentation of tumor from brain MRI using Tsallis function and Markov random field. *Journal of Control Engineering and Applied Informatics*, *19*(2), 97–106.

Rajinikanth, V., Raja, N. S. M., & Latha, K. (2014). Optimal multilevel image thresholding: An analysis with PSO and BFO algorithms. *Australian Journal of Basic and Applied Sciences*, *8*, 443–454.

Roopini, I. T., Vasanthi, M., Rajinikanth, V., Rekha, M., & Sangeetha, M. (2018). Segmentation of tumor from brain mri using fuzzy entropy and distance regularised level set. *Lecture Notes in Electrical Engineering*, *490*, 297–304. doi:10.1007/978-981-10-8354-9_27

Samanta, S., Ahmed, S., Salem, M. A.-M. M., Nath, S. S., Dey, N., & Chowdhury, S. S. (2014). Haralick features based automated glaucoma classification using back propagation neural network. *Advances in Intelligent Systems and Computing*, *327*, 351–358. doi:10.1007/978-3-319-11933-5_38

Saraswat, M., & Arya, K. V. (2014). Automated microscopic image analysis for leukocytes identification: A survey. *Micron (Oxford, England)*, *65*, 20–33. doi:10.1016/j.micron.2014.04.001 PMID:25041828

Sarkar, S., & Das, S. (2013). Multilevel image thresholding based on 2D histogram and maximum Tsallis entropy—a differential evolution approach. *IEEE Transactions on Image Processing*, *22*(12), 4788–4797. doi:10.1109/TIP.2013.2277832 PMID:23955760

Satapathy, S. C., Raja, N. S. M., Rajinikanth, V., Ashour, A. S., & Dey, N. (2016). Multi-level image thresholding using Otsu and chaotic bat algorithm. *Neural Computing & Applications*, 1–23. doi:10.100700521-016-2645-5

Shriranjani, D., Tebby, S. G., Satapathy, S. C., Dey, N., & Rajinikanth, V. (2018). Kapur's entropy and active contour-based segmentation and analysis of retinal optic disc. *Lecture Notes in Electrical Engineering*, *490*, 287–295. doi:10.1007/978-981-10-8354-9_26

Suganthi, S., & Ramakrishnan, S. (2014). Semiautomatic segmentation of breast thermograms using variational level set method. *IFMBE Proceedings*, *43*, 231–234. doi:10.1007/978-3-319-02913-9_59

Thanaraj, P., Roshini, M., & Balasubramanian, P. (2016). Integration of multivariate empirical mode decomposition and independent component analysis for fetal ECG separation from abdominal signals. *Technology and Health Care*, *24*(6), 783–794. doi:10.3233/THC-161224 PMID:27315149

Tuba, M. (2014). Multilevel image thresholding by nature-inspired algorithms: A short review. *Computer Science Journal of Moldova*, *22*, 318–338.

Varlamis, I., Apostolakis, I., Sifaki-Pistolla, D., Dey, N., Georgoulias, V., & Lionis, C. (2017). Application of data mining techniques and data analysis methods to measure cancer morbidity and mortality data in a regional cancer registry: The case of the island of Crete, Greece. *Computer Methods and Programs in Biomedicine*, *145*, 73–83. doi:10.1016/j.cmpb.2017.04.011 PMID:28552128

Wang, D., He, T., Li, Z., Cao, L., Dey, N., Ashour, A. S., ... Shi, F. (2016). Image feature-based affective retrieval employing improved parameter and structure identification of adaptive neuro-fuzzy inference system. *Neural Computing & Applications*, 1–16. doi:10.100700521-016-2512-4

Wang, D., He, T., Li, Z., Cao, L., Dey, N., Ashour, A. S., ... Shi, F. (2018). Image feature-based affective retrieval employing improved parameter and structure identification of adaptive neuro-fuzzy inference system. *Neural Computing & Applications*, *29*(4), 1087–1102. doi:10.100700521-016-2512-4

Xing, Y. & Wu, J. (2013). Controlling the shannon entropy of quantum systems. *The Scientific World Journal*, vol. 2013, Article ID 381219, 13 pages. Doi:.10.1155/2013/381219

Chapter 2
Microscopic Image Processing for the Analysis of Nosema Disease

Soumaya Dghim
Universidad de Las Palmas de Gran Canaria, Spain

Carlos M. Travieso-Gonzalez
Universidad de Las Palmas de Gran Canaria, Spain

Mohamed Salah Gouider
Université de Tunis, Tunisia

Melvin Ramírez Bogantes
Costa Rica Institute of Technology, Costa Rica

Rafael A. Calderon
National University of Costa Rica, Costa Rica

Juan Pablo Prendas-Rojas
Costa Rica Institute of Technology, Costa Rica

Geovanni Figueroa-Mata
Costa Rica Institute of Technology, Costa Rica

ABSTRACT

In this chapter, the authors tried to develop a tool to automatize and facilitate the detection of Nosema disease. This work develops new technologies in order to solve one of the bottlenecks found on the analysis bee population. The images contain various objects; moreover, this work will be structured on three main steps. The first step is focused on the detection and study of the objects of interest, which are Nosema cells. The second step is to study others' objects in the images: extract characteristics. The last step is to compare the other objects with Nosema. The authors can recognize their object of interest, determining where the edges of an object are,

DOI: 10.4018/978-1-5225-6316-7.ch002

counting similar objects. Finally, the authors have images that contain only their objects of interest. The selection of an appropriate set of features is a fundamental challenge in pattern recognition problems, so the method makes use of segmentation techniques and computer vision. The authors believe that the attainment of this work will facilitate the diary work in many laboratories and provide measures that are more precise for biologists.

INTRODUCTION

Nowadays, microscopic image analysis has become increasingly important for the recognition and classification of diseases. Several tools are available to process and analyze images in the medical and biological fields, but their relevance cannot adapt with certain problems.

Diagnosis is one of the most commonly used methods in the verification of contagious diseases in food producing animals such as bees, and has always been the most important. This method makes it possible to test and analyze the key characteristics and then define the disease by providing the necessary information on its type and classification. In the late 1990s, Nosemosis, a parasitic disease, affected European and Asian bee populations. Nosema Apis (N. Apis) was the most likely cause of Nosema. Biologists have devoted many of their studies that treat the disease and describe its molecular and genetic characteristics.

Honeybees are very important for the honey they produce and for their vital role as agricultural pollinators. Biologists considered that the human diet can be directly related to bee pollination, also they estimated the economic value of pollination to several billion dollars (“Colony Collapse”, 2009; “Bee Mortality”, 2008), and furthermore, they considered the honeybee health a great impact on economy and biodiversity worldwide.

Honeybees (*Apismellifera*) are social insects, which form colonies composed of three classes of individuals: the queen, thousands of workers and, when there is greater nectar flow, several hundred drones. The colony population can vary between 30,000 to 60,000 individuals, depending on the time of year, with each individual performing a specific function (Espina et al, 1984). The queen is the only fertile female of the hive, her main function being egg laying. The workers are in charge of feeding the young, building honeycombs, protecting and defending the hive, and collecting food, among other functions. The drones participate mainly in the fertilization of the queen and in maintaining the internal temperature of the hive (Crane, 1990).

The breeding and management of honeybees is known as “Beekeeping”, an activity practiced almost anywhere in the world with a great ecological and socioeconomic importance. Different products are obtained from beekeeping: honey, pollen, propolis, royal jelly, wax, venom, among others. However, the main benefit of bees is the pollination of different plant species, including forest trees, which ensures their reproduction. They also participate in the pollination of agricultural crops (Sanchez et al, 2009). It is estimated that about 30% of the food consumed by the world population is derived from bee-pollinated crops (Slaa et al, 2006). Therefore, the conservation of these insects is vital for the productivity of agricultural systems and the dynamics of ecosystems (Melendez et al, 2008).

Mellifera bees are affected by different etiological agents such as viruses, bacteria, fungi and parasites. More than 35 diseases associated with this bee species have been described and most of them cause considerable damage to world beekeeping (Ritter, 2001). According to Calderón and Sánchez (2001), the diseases with the highest prevalence in honeybee hives in Costa Rica are European locha, Varroasis (parasitoids caused by the Varroa destructor mite) and Nosemosis (caused by the Microsporidium Nosema spp.).

Nosemosis,Nosemiasis or Nosematosisisconsidered one of the diseases of major economic impact worldwide. (Calderon et al, 2010) This disease can be caused by two species of microsporidia, *Nosemaapis* and *Nosemaceranae* (Microspora, Nosematidae), which form spores and infect the intestinal epithelial cells of adult bees (Traver et al, 2011; Bravo et al, 2014). Previously, Nosemosis in *A. mellifera* bees was considered strictly caused by *N. apis* (see Figure 1), while the Asian bee *A. cerana* was infected by *N. ceranae* (see Figure 2).

However, in European countries, the existence of *N. ceranae* has been determined in *A. mellifera* bees, where it has caused considerable damage due to its high pathogenicity (Higes et al, 2006).

N. ceranae and *N. apis* presented small differences in size as shown in Figure 3.

In Costa Rica, Nosemosiswas first described in 1985 (Calderon et al, 2011). However, it was not reported as a problem until 2009, when very high levels of infection were found in hives of different apicultural areas (Servicio, 2012). Since then, a large number of samples of adult bees have been analyzed, with the presence of Nosema spores with levels of infection ranging from mild to severe (Calderon et al, 2011).

Nosema spores are ingested by young workers when they perform cleaning activities on contaminated combs, whereas the queen is infected through royal jelly provided by sick mother bees and the drones are infected when they receive contaminated food from the workers, by way of trofalaxis (mouth to mouth). Once the spores are ingested by the bee, they quickly pass into the intestine, where they develop and form a large amount of spores (Calderon et al, 2011).

Figure 1. Apis cerana (N.ceranae)

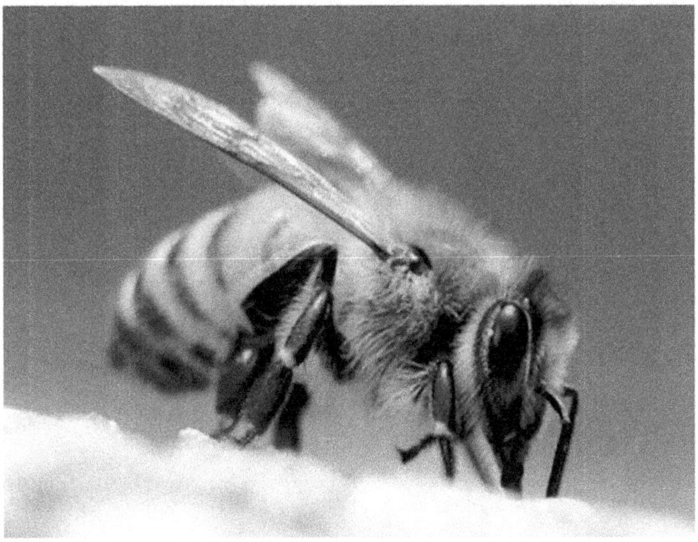

Figure 2. Apis mellifera (N.mellifera/ N.apis)

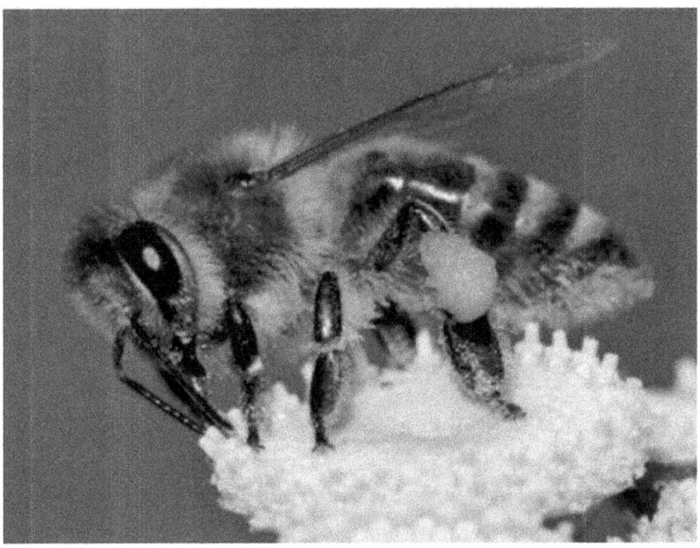

According to some studies, Nosemosis infection causes degeneration of the digestive tissue, causing severe malnutrition in the honey-producing bee and, as a consequence, premature death. In addition, it can affect flight behavior and thereby decrease the number of bees (Eiri et al, 2015).

Figure 3. (A) Nosema ceranae and (B)Nosema apis

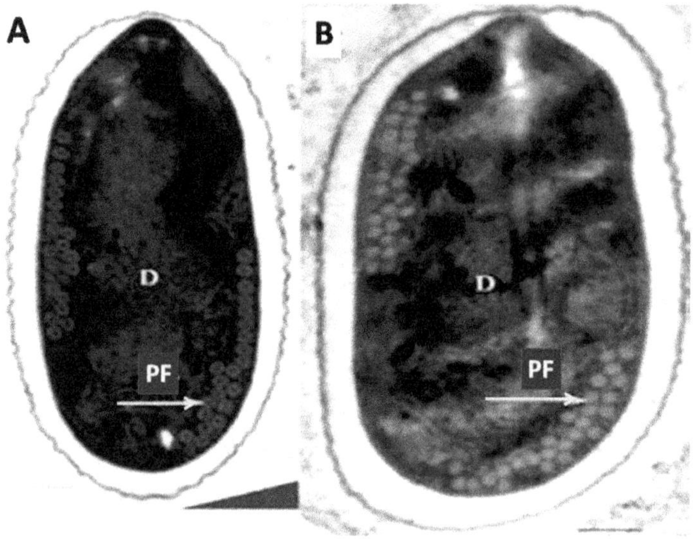

Due to the above, this disease has negative repercussions on the diversity of plant species and crop productivity, causing pollination deficiencies and causing significant economic losses in honey production (Gisder et al, 2017).

Image processing is a discipline of computer science and mathematics that studies on digital images, possible improvements, enhancements, transformations, etc., in order to have better quality or extract information.The image processor manipulates mainly digital images on a level of pixel. It also has intermediate data of various kinds: maps of regions, lists of related points, tables of measured values, etc.By analogy with mathematical operators, image-processing operators are referred to as more or less complex processes taking as input an image or a set of information relating to an image and producing an image or a set of information relating to the data Initials.Operators are generally classified into different families, depending on the information they accept as input and which they output, and according to the transformations they make to the data.

The use of the tools of image processing and computer vision becomes very important in order to facilitate on different fields. In particular, on biology, one of application is the detection of diseases on microscopic images; in addition, these tools became necessary for thediagnosis and classification of diseases. In this work, we will try to study the microscopic images of Nosema disease with infect honeybees. It is a dangerous particular and virulent agent, can affect an entire colonies health. Bees produce honey and are vital pollinators of agricultural and horticultural crops, they are estimated to provide one-third of human food and an economic value that can be billions of dollars. Therefore, any danger threatens bees, will constitute a global economic threat as well as a biodiversity threat. For this reason, many biological works have been ruled out of the study of this disease, but this is not enough, because it is necessary that the computer scientists also make importance on this subject and try to give help to the biologists and facilitate their work.

In summary, the most of actual works develop manual approaches to study the Nosema disease. This research work focuses on the use of image processing on image processing stage and extraction feature stage; and the use of artificial intelligent to do automatic decisions.

BIOLOGICAL WORK

Techniques for the Diagnosis of Nosemosis

Identification of the Agent

In some dangerous cases of the disease, bees unable to fly, bees with a distended abdomen, dead bees on the ground in front of the peckercan be seen, as well as brown fecal marks on the combs and on the front of the hive (Higes et al, 2006; Calderon et al, 2011). However, most colonies do not show clear signs of infection, even when the disease is enough to cause important losses in honey production and pollination efficiency ("OIE", 2013). Because of the above, an accurate diagnosis of Nosemosiscan only be made by microscopic examination of the adult bee's abdomen or ventricle, either by molecular means (polymerase chain reaction-PCR) or by transmission electron microscopy ("OIE", 2013).

Laboratory Tests for the Diagnosis of Nosemiasis

In order to determine the presence of Nosemosis, a sample of bees should be obtained from the peck of the hive, which guarantees older bees, where there is a greater probability of infection (Higes et al, 2010). Collecting a minimum of 60 workers in order to define 5% of diseased bees with 95% confidence is recommended (Medina et al, 2014).

Cantwell Method

To make the diagnosis of Nosema spp. in the lab, adult bees are analyzed using the Cantwell Method (Molina et al, 1990) 30 adult bees are taken and placed on absorbent paper. Subsequently, the abdomens are separated from the bees and placed in a mortar to be macerated, and 1.0 ml of distilled water is added for each abdomen (total: 30 ml). The macerate is homogenized by constant stirring for one minute, and then a drop of the suspension is put on a slide and examined under a microscope at a magnification of 40x to identify microsporidia spores, characterized by being oval, bright and refractive.

Hemocytometer Method

To measure the presence of spores of Nosema sp. in the sample, the level of infection is determined by the Hemocytometer method, which allows the quantification of the number of spores through the Neubauer chamber. The sample supernatant is mechanically agitated with a micropipette to homogenize it, a 10μl aliquot is taken, placed in the hemocytometer and allowed to stand for 2 minutes, in order for the spores to settle. The sample is then observed under a microscope at a 40x magnification and the spore count is performed. All spores framed by double lines are counted, including all counters touching the double lines on the left and top sides of each block, but not those touching the bottom double lines and those on the right side of the block. To obtain a good average, the spores of five blocks, the four corner blocks and the central block are counted by hemocytometer.

According to Molina et al. (2013), the following formula is used to calculate the number of spores per bee:

$$(\text{Total number of spores counted} \div 80) \times 4{,}000{,}000 = \text{Spores number per bee} \qquad (1)$$

Subsequently, the spores' number determined by the formula is compared to the Jaycox table (Table 1) to know the intensity of the infection.

It should be noted that this procedure is laborious and the experience of the person observing the sample is important, since the appearance of the spores can be mistaken for yeast, fungal spores, fatty bodies or cysts of *Malpighamoebamellificae*

Table 1. Jaycox table to determine the level of Nosemosis infection in bees (Molina et al, 1990)

Intensity of Infection	Number of Spores Per Bee
Very light	10 000 - 1 000 000
Light	1 000 000 - 5 000 000
Moderate	5 000 000 - 10 000 000
Strong	10 000 000 - 20 000 000
Very strong	Exceeding 20 000 000

(Amebiasis) or other structures. In addition, in samples with large amounts of spores, counting is time consuming.

Polymerase Chain Reaction

The Polymerase Chain Reaction (PCR) technique is used in molecular biology for the identification of viruses, bacteria and microsporidia, which makes it possible to obtain millions of copies of a DNA fragment (it multiplies or amplifies small amounts of DNA). Therefore, it provides a very sensitive test for the detection of Nosemosis, since it can detect the spores at very low levels of infection and allows simultaneous differentiation of the two nemat species that parasitize honeybees (Heathe et al, 2015; Nabian et al, 2011).

To make the difference between *N. apis* from *N. ceranae*, different methods have been developed. However, in any of the methodologies used, the key components in the process are the primers, which are small DNA fragments containing specific sequences that serve as a starting point for their replication, and the enzyme DNA polymerase that leads to Synthesis of a new DNA Wisp. To replicate the strands of genetic material, a thermocycler is required where cycles of high and low temperatures are developed. At the end of the cycles, this ensures that the DNA has replicated to twice the original amount and thus twice the detection of microsporidia in the samples.

THE PROPOSAL

In the biological side,the study of the Nosema diseaseis developed on many works. For the computer side, there area few works, which occupied a general view of honeybees. For example, in (Giuffre et al, 2017) implements tools of imaging processing that was usedtostudythe autogrooming behavior of honeybee. In (Tu et al, 2016),they use tools of video analysis to monitor the honeybeebehavior and detect the bee disturbance. In (Kvieisa et al, 2015) focuses on different automatic monitoring system architectures for real-time beehive temperature monitoring, to provide useful information for people associated with beekeeping and help them to manage their honey bee (*Apismellifera*) colonies. In (Alaverz-Ramos et al, 2013), it is only shown a work, which is focused on the study of Nosema disease;they use the tools of imaging processing and implement an automatic approach to classify the Nosema pathogenic Agent.

The current process on biological studies is developed on manual way; the automatic approach of this work is the study of Nosema microscopic images, the possible objects are detected on the images, and later, an automatic segmentation is implemented based on bioinspired characteristics of the Nosema cell to recognize our object of interest using the tools of imaging processing.

Extraction for Nosema Microscopic images

The problem of used images is that contain many kinds of objects, Nosema cells and other kinds of cells. The location of the Nosema cell inside the images is itself a problem. Thus, the cell image is cropped manually from the digital image (see Figure 4). The region of interest is selected (ROI), then, it is automatically preprocessed to detect the shape of the cell. Since our images are charged by many objects and we can say they are very blurry and noisy, we select the Nosema cell, by cropping a Nosema image wich is clearly isolated from other objects. Thus, every Nosema cell sub-image contains only one clear cell.

An example of others objects can be seen in Figure 5.

Processing and Segmentation

This proposal applied the Otsu method (Otsu, 1979), in order to have an automatic object block on the color image, using the binarization information from Otsu method.

Figure 4. Nosema cells shown in the yellow rectangles

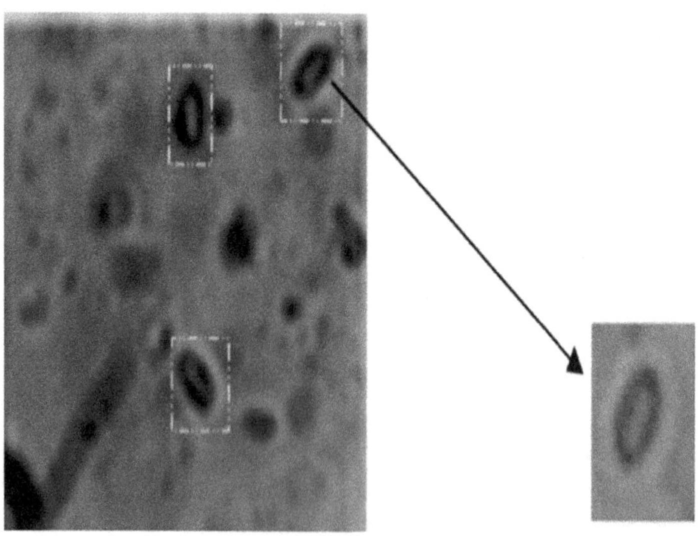

Figure 5. (a). Nosema cell and (b), (c), (d), (e): other kinds of cells in the microscopique images

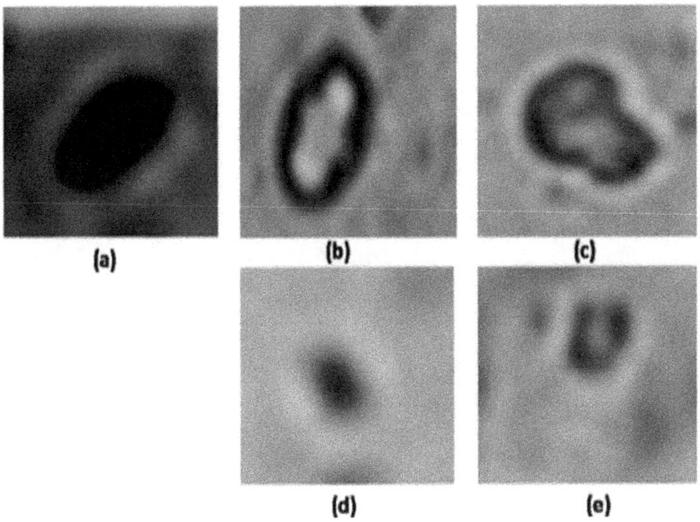

First, the gray scale image of the Nosema cell colored image was calculated. Then, a binarization block (Otsu Method) is applied for the microscopic images. After, we applied some dilatation operators on the image in order to enhace it and to reduce the noise. Finally, we filled the cell hole and the Nosema cell was very clear and prepared to be studied.

The technique used to separate the object or the region of interest from its background is the first part of the segmentation process, see figure 6.

1. **Selection:** As we montioned above, we select the Nosema cell manually by using a predefined Matlab function.
2. **Thresholding:** It consists of performing the level 255 at the pixels whose value is greater than a threshold s and 0 the level of the others.
3. **Binarization:** The binarization of an image consist of transform each pixel's value to '0' or'1' depending on whether it has a value lower or higher (respectively) than a set threshold. The resulting image is used for geometrical feature extraction.
4. **Masks:** Finally, we calculating the HSV masks of the Nosema cell. The resulting masks then are used for color feature extraction.

Figure 6. Automatic processing steps for Nosema cell extraction

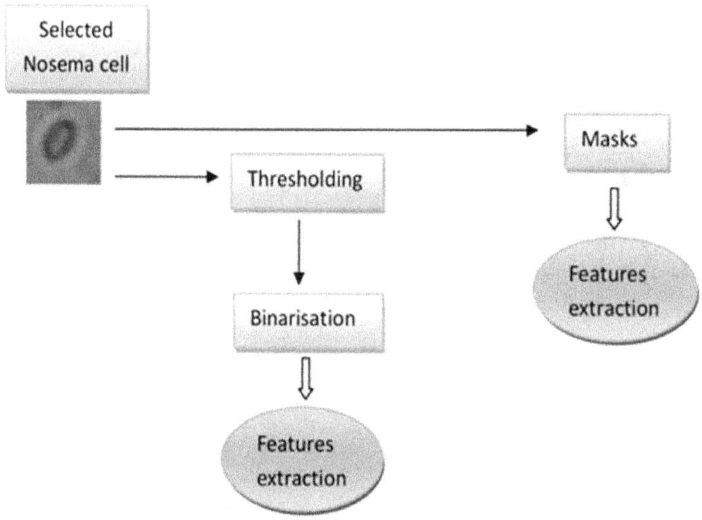

Features Extraction

The type of microscopic images did not provide clearinformation for the task of automatic recognition and detection of Nosema cells. However, they contain the needed information. That information is distributedon the image and hiddenunder other objects.

A number of n features from the Nosemacell imageswere extracted, the features we see more useful for our approach. These features were geometric and color parameters, with information about size, area, shape, and texture, with information about pixel intensities and their distribution on the image. Certainly, color may be a high source of information, in this particular case,because the yellow color is intrinsic to the definition of the cell. The featureextraction was divided in two steps wich are described in thenext sections:

Geometrical Features

Geometric features are very useful and in addition have been used extensively in almost every work related to the recognition and classification of objects. The perimeter of the cell, its area and its convex area have been calculated, these three parameters provide an important part of the basic information about Nosema cell. The convex area is very useful information, because the shape of the Nosema cell is like an ellipse. It consists of the number of pixels in the binary image that specifies the convex hull. The perimeter is the distance between each adjoining pair of pixels around the border of the cell; the area is the number of pixels inside the region. In addition, we calculated many other geometric parameters likesolidity, which is the portion of the area of the convex region contained in the cell; and eccentricity, which is relation between the distance of the focus of the ellipse and the length of the principal axis.

Colour Features

The Nosema cell original image is represented by a matrix with dimensions $(M \times N \times 3)$ where $M \times N$ represents the image dimensions of each colour channel and the number 3 represent the blue, red and green colors. We considered only the the Nosema cell region and we calculated the averages of R (Red), B (Blue), G (Green) channels. The Gray Level Co-occurrence (Sebastian et al, 2012) of HSV channels were used in order to obtain the contrast of every channel.

Then, we studied the other kinds of object, which are not Nosema cells, present in our microscopic images in the same way and we extracted their features. Finally, we had a database with Nosema cells object feautures and other kind of object features.

Experimental Methodologies and Recognition

The last step is to apply the automatic decision. We divided our database into two parts: the first one for learning the system and the second one to do the test. For it, Artificial Neural Network (ANN) are used to recognize the Nosema cell from its characterization with the feature extraction. Different works, especially in medicine and biology, use them because they are successful in solving intelligent tasks. The principles of ANN are closely related to such areas as pattern recognition, signal processing, and artificial intelligence. The neural networks are excellent when modeling incomplete or noisy data. Neural networks often treat these kinds of problems better than statistical methods. For microscopic images of Nosema cell has many noisy objects and the definition of cell is open, therefore, this classifier is a very good option for this application.

In this work, we used a Multi-Layer Perceptron NN trained by Back Propagation algorithm (MLP-BP) where we have put the same number of neurons in the input layer as the number of our features, so, the numbers of neurons in the output layer was "n", that is, the number of features . In our case, it was determined to use one hidden layer. Since weights of neurons in the input layer were initialized randomly, 30 NNs were trained by holding–out validation method. Then, determine if it is Nosema cell or not. Finally, we repeated each experiment 20 times in order to get a valid, stable and robust measure of the performance of our system and results are given in terms of mean percentage.

Figure 7. Architecture of used ANN (Multi-Layer Perceptron)

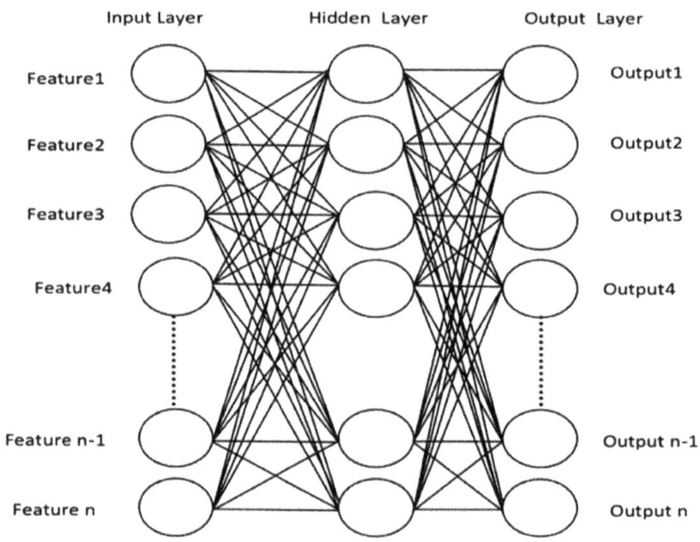

RESULTS

After learning our system and testing our object, the ANN model we implemented gave us a percentage of 96% of success in Nosema cells recognition. This result was very encouraging. In the other hand, we can optimize the number of hidden units of ANN by searching for the found point. As a result, 35 units of hidden neurons were chosen as the optimal point, reaching an accuracy of 96%.

CONCLUSION

Microscopic images are quite useful in the recognition and classification of diseases in natural and medical sciences. In this approach, we applied some technique of imaging processing (dilatation, thresholding, binarisation, Masks,ect…) to the microscopic images of Nosema, a dangerous disease, which affects bees. This work is focused on implementing an automatic process to extract the main features of the interested object (geometrical and color features). Finally, we implemented a Back propagation Perceptron to learn and test the system; then recognize our objects of interest. The result was very encouraging in the recognition and detection of the disease, reaching a 96% of success. As a future work, we can increase the number of extracted futures and the database can be increased with larger objects and this maybe can give us a better result.

ACKNOWLEDGMENT

This work has been supported by the Ministry of Economy and Competitiveness (TEC2016-77791-C4-1-R).

REFERENCES

Alvarez-Ramos, C. M., Niño, E., & Santos, M. (2013). Automatic Classification of Nosema Pathogenic Agents through Machine Vision techniques and Kernel-based Vector Machines. *IEEE, 8th Computing Colombian Conference.*

Anonymous. (2008). Bee mortality and bee surveillance in Europe. *EFSA Journal, 154*, 1–28.

Anonymous. (2009). *Colony Collapse Disorder Progress Report.* CCD Steering Committee.

Bravo, J., Carbonell, V., Valdebenedito, J. T., Figueroa, C., Valdovinos, C. E., Martín-Hérnandez, R., ... Delporte, C. (2014). Identification of Nosemaceranaein the Valparaíso District, Chile. *Archivos de Medicina Veterinaria, 46*(3), 487–491. doi:10.4067/S0301-732X2014000300021

Calderón, R. A., & Pichardo, J. (2011). *Nosemiasis en abejas melíferas: diagnóstico, control y prevalencia.* Heredia.

Calderón, R. A., & Ramírez, F. (2010). *Enfermedades de las abejas melíferas, con énfasis en abejas africanizadas* (Vol. 125). Heredia, Costa Rica: Ed. CINAT-UNA.

Calderón, R. A., & Sánchez, L. (2001). Diagnóstico de enfermedades en colmenas de abejas africanizadas en Costa Rica: Prevalencia y distribución de setiembre a noviembre del 2007. *Agronomia Costarricense, 35*, 49–60.

Crane, E. (1990). *Bees and beekeeping: science, practice and world resources.* London, UK: HeinemannNewnes.

Eiri, D., Suwannapong, G., Endler, M., & Nieh, J. (2015). Nosemaceranae can infect honeybee larvae and reduces subsequentadult longevity. *PLoS One, 10*(5), 1–17. doi:10.1371/journal.pone.0126330 PMID:26018139

Elizabeth, C., Heathe, H., Cresswell, J., & Tyler, C. (2015). Interactive effects of pesticideexposure and pathogen infection on bee health - a critical analysis: Pesticide-pathogen interactions on bee health. *Biological Reviews of the Cambridge Philosophical Society.*

Espina, D., & Ordetx, G. (1984). Apicultura tropical. *Tecnológica de Costa Rica*, 506.

Gisder, S., Schüler, V., Horchler, L. L., Groth, D., & Genersch, E. (2017). Long-Term28 Temporal Trends of Nosema spp. Infection Prevalence in Northeast Germany: Continuous Spread of Nosemaceranae, an Emerging Pathogen of Honeybees (Apismellifera), but No General Replacement of Nosemaapis. *Frontiers in Cellular and Infection Microbiology*.

Giuffre, C., Lubkin, S. R., & Tarpy, D. R. (2017). Automated Assay and Differential Model Of Western Honey Bee (Apis Mellifera) Autogrooming Using Digital Image Processing. *Computers and Electronics in Agriculture*, *135*, 338–344. doi:10.1016/j.compag.2017.02.003

Gonzalez, R. C., & Woods, R. E. (2008). *Digital Image Processing*. Pearson Prentice Hall.

Higes, M., Martin, R., & Meana, A. (2006). Nosemaceranae, a new microsporidian parasite in honeybees in Europe. *Journal of Invertebrate Pathology*, *92*(2), 93–95. doi:10.1016/j.jip.2006.02.005 PMID:16574143

Higes, M., Martin-Hernández, R., & Meana, A. (2010). Nosema ceranae in Europe: Anemergenttype C Nosemosis. *Apidologie*, *41*(3), 375–392. doi:10.1051/apido/2010019

Kviesisa, A., & Zacepinsa, A. (2015). System Architectures for Real-time Bee Colony Temperature Monitoring. *Procedia Computer Science*, *43*, 86–94. doi:10.1016/j.procs.2014.12.012

Marr, D., & Hildreth, E. (1980). Theory of Edge Detection. *Proceedings of the Royal Society of London*, *207*(1167), 187–217. doi:10.1098/rspb.1980.0020 PMID:6102765

Medina, C., Guzmán, E., Espinosa, L., Uribe, L., Gutiérrez, R., & Gutiérrez, F. (2014). Frecuencia de Varrosis y Nosemosis en colonias de abejas melíferas (*Apis mellifera*) en el estado de Zacatecas, México. *Revista Chapingo Serie Ciencias Forestales y del Ambiente*, 30–36.

Meléndez, V., Parra, V., Delfín, H., Ayala, R., Reyes, E., & Manrique, P. (2008). Abejas silvestres: Diversidad, el papel como polinizadores y la importancia de su conservación. *Bioagrociencias*, *1*, 38–45.

Molina, A., Guzmán, E., Message, D., Jong, D., Pesante, D., Mantilla, C., . . . Alvarado, F. (1990). Enfermedades y plagas de la abeja melífera occidental. OIRSA-BID, 147.

Nabian, S., Ahmadi, K., Nazem-Shirazi, M. H., & Gerami-Sadeghian, A. (2011). First detection of Nosemaceranae, a microsporidian protozoa of european honeybees (Apismellifera) in Iran. *Iranian Journal of Parasitology*, *6*, 89–95. PMID:22347302

Organización Mundial de Sanidad Animal (OIE). (2013). Manual de las Pruebas de Diagnóstico y de las Vacunas para los Animales Terrestres. *Capítulo 2.2.4 Nosemosis de las abejas melíferas.*

Otsu, N. (1979). A threshold selection method from gray-level histograms. *IEEE Transactions on Systems, Man, and Cybernetics*, *9*(1), 62–66. doi:10.1109/TSMC.1979.4310076

Pirk, C., Miranda, J. C., Kramer, W., Murray, T. E., Nazzi, F., Shutler, D., ... Dooremalen, C. (2013). Statistical guidelines for Apismellifera research. *Journal of Apicultural Research*, *52*(4), 1–24. doi:10.3896/IBRA.1.52.4.13

Ritter, W. (2001). Enfermedades de las abejas. Acribia, Zaragoza, 146.

Sánchez, L., & Herrera, E. (2009). Importancia de la biodiversidad apícola para la seguridad alimentaria de Costa Rica. *Memorias del X Congreso Nacional de Apicultura: Apicultura y su impacto en la seguridad alimentaria*, 66.

Sebastian, B., Unnikrishnan, A., & Balakrishnan, K. (2012). Grey Leve Co-Occurrence Matrices: Generalization and Some New Features. *International Journal of Computer Science, Engineering and Information Technology*, *2*(2), 151–157.

Servicio Nacional de Salud Animal (SENASA). (2012). *Protocolo Vigilancia Epidemiológica de Nosemosis*. Programa Nacional de Sanidad Apícola.

Slaa, J., Sánchez, L., Malagodi-Braga, K., & Hofstede, F. (2006). Stingless bees in applied pollination: Practice and perspectives. *Apidologie*, *37*(2), 293–315. doi:10.1051/apido:2006022

Traver, B., & Fell, R. D. (2011). Prevalence and infection intensity of Nosema in honeybee (ApismelliferaL) colonies in Virginia. *Journal of Invertebrate Pathology*, *107*(1), 43–49. doi:10.1016/j.jip.2011.02.003 PMID:21345338

Tu, G. J., Hansen, M. K., Kryger, P., & Ahrendt, P. (2016). Automatic behaviour analysis system for honeybees using computer vision. *Computers and Electronics in Agriculture*, *122*, 10–18. doi:10.1016/j.compag.2016.01.011

ADDITIONAL READING

Borra, S., Thanki, R., Dey, N., & Borisagar, K. (2018). *Secure transmission and integrity verification of color radiological images using fast discrete curvelet transform and compressive sensing*. Smart Health.

Dan, W., He, T., Li, Z., Cao, L., Dey, N., Ashour, A. S., & Balas, V. E. (2018). Image feature-based affective retrieval employing improved parameter and structure identification of adaptive neuro-fuzzy inference system. *Neural Computing & Applications*, *29*(4), 1087–1102. doi:10.100700521-016-2512-4

Das, H., Jena, A. K., Badajena, J. C., Pradhan, C., & Barik, R. K. (2018). Resource Allocation in Cooperative Cloud Environments. In Progress in Computing, Analytics and Networking (pp. 825-841). Springer, Singapore. doi:10.1007/978-981-10-7871-2_79

Das, H., Jena, A. K., Nayak, J., Naik, B., & Behera, H. S. (2015). A novel PSO based back propagation learning-MLP (PSO-BP-MLP) for classification. In *Computational Intelligence in Data Mining-Volume 2* (pp. 461–471). New Delhi: Springer. doi:10.1007/978-81-322-2208-8_42

Das, H., Naik, B., & Behera, H. S. (2018). Classification of Diabetes Mellitus Disease (DMD): A Data Mining (DM) Approach. In Progress in Computing, Analytics and Networking (pp. 539-549). Springer, Singapore.

Dey, N., Ashour, A. S., Shi, F., Fong, S. J., & Tavares, R. S. (2018). Medical cyber-physical systems: A survey. *Journal of Medical Systems*, *42*(4), 74. doi:10.100710916-018-0921-x PMID:29525900

Dey, N., Rajinikanth, V., Ashour, A. S., & Tavares, J. M. (2018). Social Group Optimization Supported Segmentation and Evaluation of Skin Melanoma Images. *Symmetry*, *10*(2), 51. doi:10.3390ym10020051

Luminiţa, M., Moldovanu, S., Culea-Florescu, A. L., Bibicu, D., Dey, N., Ashour, A. S., & Sherratt, S. (2018). Texture spectrum coupled with entropy and homogeneity image features for myocardium muscle characterization. *Current Bioinformatics*.

Mishra, B. B., Dehuri, S., Panigrahi, B. K., Nayak, A. K., Mishra, B. S. P., & Das, H. (2018). Computational Intelligence in Sensor Networks, vol. 776, Studies in Computational Intelligence, Springer

Mishra, B. S. P., Das, H., Dehuri, S., & Jagadev, A. K. (2018). *Cloud Computing for Optimization: Foundations, Applications, and Challenges* (Vol. 39). Springer. doi:10.1007/978-3-319-73676-1

Nayak, J., Naik, B., Jena, A. K., Barik, R. K., & Das, H. (2018). Nature Inspired Optimizations in Cloud Computing: Applications and Challenges. In *Cloud Computing for Optimization: Foundations, Applications, and Challenges* (pp. 1–26). Cham: Springer. doi:10.1007/978-3-319-73676-1_1

P. K. Pattnaik, S. S. Rautaray, H. Das, & J. Nayak (Eds.). (2018). Progress in Computing, Analytics and Networking: *Proceedings of ICCAN 2017* (Vol. 710). Springer.

Pradhan, C., Das, H., Naik, B., & Dey, N. (2018). *Handbook of Research on Information Security in Biomedical Signal Processing* (pp. 1–414). Hershey, PA: IGI Global. doi:10.4018/978-1-5225-5152-2

Rajinikanth, V., Dey, N., Satapathy, S. C., & Ashour, A. S. (2018). An approach to examine magnetic resonance angiography based on Tsallis entropy and deformable snake model. *Future Generation Computer Systems*, *85*, 160–172. doi:10.1016/j.future.2018.03.025

Reddy, K. H. K., Das, H., & Roy, D. S. (2017). *A Data Aware Scheme for Scheduling Big-Data Applications with SAVANNA Hadoop. Futures of Network.* CRC Press.

Sahani, R., Rout, C., Badajena, J. C., Jena, A. K., & Das, H. (2018). Classification of Intrusion Detection Using Data Mining Techniques. In Progress in Computing, Analytics and Networking (pp. 753-764). Springer, Singapore. doi:10.1007/978-981-10-7871-2_72

Sarkhel, P., Das, H., & Vashishtha, L. K. (2017). Task-Scheduling Algorithms in Cloud Environment. In *Computational Intelligence in Data Mining* (pp. 553–562). Singapore: Springer. doi:10.1007/978-981-10-3874-7_52

Sarwar, K., Dey, N., Nimmy, S. F., Ripon, S. H., Ali, N. Y., Ashour, A. S., ... Shi, F. (2018). Evolutionary framework for coding area selection from cancer data. *Neural Computing & Applications*, *29*(4), 1015–1037. doi:10.100700521-016-2513-3

Shriranjani, D., Tebby, S. G., Satapathy, S. C., Dey, N., & Rajinikanth, V. (2018). Kapur's Entropy and Active Contour-Based Segmentation and Analysis of Retinal Optic Disc. In *Computational Signal Processing and Analysis* (pp. 287–295). Singapore: Springer. doi:10.1007/978-981-10-8354-9_26

Simon, F., Li, J., Song, W., Tian, Y., Wong, R. K., & Dey, N. (2018). Predicting unusual energy consumption events from smart home sensor network by data stream mining with misclassified recall. *Journal of Ambient Intelligence and Humanized Computing*, 1–25.

Chapter 3
Medical Image Lossy Compression With LSTM Networks

Nithin Prabhu G.
JSS Science and Technology University, India

Trisiladevi C. Nagavi
JSS Science and Technology University, India

Mahesha P.
JSS Science and Technology University, India

ABSTRACT

Medical images have a larger size when compared to normal images. There arises a problem in the storage as well as in the transmission of a large number of medical images. Hence, there exists a need for compressing these images to reduce the size as much as possible and also to maintain a better quality. The authors propose a method for lossy image compression of a set of medical images which is based on Recurrent Neural Network (RNN). So, the proposed method produces images of variable compression rates to maintain the quality aspect and to preserve some of the important contents present in these images.

DOI: 10.4018/978-1-5225-6316-7.ch003

INTRODUCTION

The process of reducing the size of any data file is referred as data compression. It is essential as most of the real world data is rich and redundant in nature. Major types of data compression are either lossless or lossy. The compression that condenses the binary data by recognizing and removing statistical redundancy is referred as lossless data compression. Generally no information will be missing in case of lossless data compression. On the contrary, the process that reduces binary data by removing less important or noisy information is said to be lossy data compression. Further, compression is applied on various types of digital media such as text, image, audio and video for reducing storage and transmission cost.

Here the authors are interested in medical images and its associated compression operations. Medical image compression is a process in which the compression of data is executed where in few bits are encoded into the actual image. Decreasing the irrelevance redundancy of data present in images is the main purpose of it. The medical image transmission speed is slower when the actual image is transmitted, but the compression techniques help to increase the speed of transmission. Medical image compression mainly concentrates on reducing the image data size and attempts to retain most of the necessary details.

The core objective of compressing the medical images is to show these images in terms of small quantity of bits without losing the needed content of information within the actual image. This is because each and every medical image has important information that should not be lost while decreasing the volume of the image. By the expeditious growth of the technology, there is a need for managing a large quantity of medical image data and also to store those images in the right way by the use of fruitful techniques. This normally results in compressing the images. So again there arises an issue regarding the different approaches to optimally compress the medical images. Again there are two major techniques to compress images as seen in data compression. Hence image compression can also be either lossy or lossless. There are many algorithms and methodologies for image compressions which deal with the elimination of different data redundancies like inter pixel, coding and psycho visual, etc. Even though the lossless technique is about not losing the major data present in images, it fails to compress the images in an optimal way.

Therefore the authors are trying to use lossy compression technique to compress a set of medical images and also to show that it is a better technique to compress medical images when compared to other approaches.

However, following a normal method for lossy image compression will not yield the desired results. To accomplish the aforementioned results, advanced neural network architecture called as Recurrent Neural Network (RNN) is adopted for lossy compression. The traditional neural networks cannot use its power of reasoning about the previously occurred events to decide the events that may occur in future, at every point of time of that event. RNN stands different as it overcomes this drawback by allowing the information to stay for a long time by making use of its loop. In other words, the network forms loops within itself. The RNN's can be imagined where in multiple copies of the existing network loops within itself there by passing the information and evaluating as many times as required. Most important feature of RNN is the ability to connect the information that has occurred in the previous event to the ongoing event.

In case of lossy compression of medical images RNN's are used to provide the knowledge of the previously processed image block to understand the present block of image. This also helps in different phases of lossy compression to preserve the quality of image. The size of the image is reduced significantly but the quality of the image is preserved even after n iterations of compression. Hence, only a very small difference in the quality can be observed when compared to the original medical image. Therefore loss in the data present in medical images is highly reduced. Another advantage of RNN is that it can reduce the number of parameters by the method of weight sharing as the depth of the network increases after different time steps. Also when there is some kind of sequential data in images, RNN's are very useful in compression.

BACKGROUND

A neural network is an information processing system, whose algorithm and hardware design was inspired by biological neurons. It has the capacity to assimilate by examples that makes it highly flexible and also powerful. Artificial neural networks are simplified models of the neural networks. There are different types of neural networks based on functionalities. Some of them are feed forward, convolutional, recurrent, radial basis function, modular, and so on.

Here the authors are making use of RNN to compress medical images. A RNN is one of the artificial neural network type in which connections between processing units or neurons form a directed cycle. RNNs utilize their internal memory to execute arbitrary sequences of inputs. These are the most prominent and effective sense of neural network, they are even applicable to images which may be decomposed into a range of patches and viewed as a sequence. RNNs have three different varieties of layer. These include input layer, hidden layer and output layer. The input layer accepts the input, activation functions are processed at hidden layer and finally the output is received. There are multiple hidden layers present and each of them is characterized through their very own weights together with biases.

Several neural networks methodologies have been utilized for the purpose of medical image compression. The below section involves the literature survey of various techniques available for medical image compression using neural networks and their views on the topic.

Medical image compression technique using adaptive neural network is proposed by the authors Moorthi & Amutha (2012). Back propagation neural network was proposed in this article for data compression. Further, it advocates parallel processing of data. The training procedure enables the network suitable for different kinds of data. The authors have attempted to produce better quality images than normal image compression techniques. This approach doesn't produce high quality image results as compared to that of the current architecture proposed by the same authors.

Using feed forward neural network, grayscale medical image compression was achieved by authors Yeo et al. (2011). The approach makes use of feed forward neural network trained with back propagation algorithm. It is projected for compressing grey scale medical images only. In order to compress MRI image authors have employed a three hidden layer Feed Forward Network (FFN) as the focal compression algorithm. However it produces good results only for grey scale medical images. It has a simple neural network architecture which cannot be applied to compress different sorts of medical images efficiently.

System for medical radiographs compression using neural networks and Haar wavelet is presented in the paper authored by Khashman and Dimililer (2009). It uses wavelet transform based compression using simple neural networks. However this architecture is not able to choose an optimum compression ratio to different sets of medical images. It is trained to compress only radiograph medical image contents and hence not suitable for other medical images. Also the neural network architecture is very simple and can't handle large datasets.

Base et al. (2005), outlines medical image compression by implementing vector quantization and topology-preserving neural networks with probability distribution methods. A transformation-based procedure is implemented as an element of the encoder on the block-decomposed image. Also makes use of Kohonen's feature map or the Linde Buzo Gray (LBG) algorithm. It is not able to produce better results when compared to other neural network methodologies as it uses only vector quantization approach. Also, it is observed that the method proposed falls short in producing optimal results to different types of medical images.

A new approach based on back propagation neural network for image compression is shown in the paper Dimililer (2013). It also uses Haar wavelet and discrete cosine transforms. Here, initially neural network is trained with the X-ray image for relating with ideal compression method and their optimum compression ratio. It is able to produce average results on few of the medical images. Similar compression ratio was not obtained after applying the proposed compression method. Hence the overall results are not so significant when compared to proposed Long Short Term Memory (LSTM) architecture.

Most of these research works focus mainly on various lossless techniques of image compressions using basic sets of neural networks. But the architecture explained by the authors concentrates on lossy method of image compressions using deep neural networks. This makes it very special and unique from the rest of the works. Even the result of this method is better and efficient when compared to rest of the medical image compression techniques. Also using recurrent neural network architecture it is possible to achieve slightly better performance than JPEG.

MAIN FOCUS OF THE CHAPTER

Objectives of the Chapter

- Further minimize the size of various medical images, as a result ensures no additional large storage and brings down the expected transmission time.
- Generate a neural network that is competitive across a variety of compression rates on medical images arbitrary dimensions.
- Provide a high compression ratio with minimal distortion.
- Achieve desirable compression rate for 64 X 64 images, which is confined to 32 X 32 images in the existing research.
- Focus on low resolution images. Since, existing compression techniques focuses on large images.
- Proposed RNN will result in improved compression outcomes across number of iterations as it involves progressive method of compression.
- To show the difference between the original image, compressed image, and decompressed image.

Issues and Problems

- There is no proper methodology proposed for the efficient compression of various medical images up to date.
- The size of each medical image is very large and the storage capacity required to store such large sets of medical images is also very large.
- Lossy image compression technique compresses the images to very large extent but this method of compression is not yet applied to medical images as it leads to the loss of major components of the image. But using suitable techniques of neural networks it is still possible to adopt lossy image compression techniques for medical images.

- Most of the image compression techniques that use neural networks adopt compression rate which is fixed and it is established depending upon the bottleneck layer's size Simoncelli et al. (2016). The proposed method enhances the previous approaches by facilitating variable compression rates as required depending upon the type of images to be compressed.
- Application of modern types of neural network architecture to compress various medical images are not yet into implementation as medical people are not aware of the power of such modern neural network architectures.

SOLUTIONS AND RECOMMENDATIONS

For the above discussed problems there are few solutions that can be applied in order to obtain well compressed low size medical images. Here the authors use RNN as the solution to address this issue. The recurrent units of RNN used here are LSTM units Hochreiter and Schmidhuber (1997).The arrangement of a general LSTM unit is made up of a cell state which is mainly composed of three different gates. The first gate is an input gate which is generally made up of a sigmoid layer. The second gate is an output gate which also has a sigmoid layer with $\tanh$ layer. The third gate is a forget gate which also has a sigmoid layer that decides which data has to be stored and the irrelevant data in that particular context is removed. The cell state has an important function of remembering different values from the given data over random time intervals. Because of this reason LSTM has the term memory in it. The terminology long short term inlet signifies that it is a representation of the short term memory that will remain for a very long interval of time without any changes. An LSTM is a most suitable model in classification and approximation of time series problem for a given time interval between main actions.

The LSTM units are absolutely capable of handling long term dependencies through which the encoding and decoding phases of medical images are handled in an easy manner. Various different medical images are accessed from various sources on which this method of compression is tried in. The image datasets were extracted from sources like NIH, TCIA, OASIS, Kaggle, Medical Imagenet, MIMIC, SMIR, ADNI, MIDAS, FITBIR, etc.

The authors also took into account the different types of medical images such as Computed Tomography, Positron Emission Tomography, Magnetic Resonance Imaging, PET-CT, X-Ray, Molecular Imaging, Histopathological images, etc.

As it is a field of medical image compression that uses lossy compression technique more validation criteria is provided by authors to justify the method that is chosen. So the reasons are as follows:

- **Highly Size is Reduced:** Size of each medical image is large. Using lossy compression techniques the size can be highly reduced and since RNN is made use of it is possible to decide how much to reduce in order to maintain the quality of image and minimizing the loss of data from image.
- **Still Better Quality is Ensured:** Generally there is a myth that lossy compression will lead to decrease in the quality of the image but since we use RNN, the parameters are set in such a way that important data is not lost but only the unwanted noise is removed ensuring high quality of image even after compression.
- **Storage and Transmission is Easy:** As the image size highly reduces it becomes easy to store millions of images in the hospital database. Transmission of images mainly depends upon the size of the images. Larger size takes more time for transmission but low size images can be transmitted very quickly. Since the size is highly reduced transmission becomes faster.
- **Results of Compression Indicate it:** No other image compression techniques whether its lossy or lossless methods yield better results as our work suggests. Table 1 in Appendix part clearly shows that the lossy compression techniques using LSTM is able to yield high ratio of PSNR-HVS and MS-SSIM which indicates that image quality after compression is still better.
- Without the usage of neural networks, lossy image compression is surely not suitable for medical image compression. But as the authors have made use of advance neural network architecture, i.e, LSTM it's possible to generate low size, high quality compressed image. Understanding the LSTM architecture in depth will help anyone understand why lossy compression technique yields better results.

METHODOLOGY

Here the authors describe the overall architecture used to compress medical images. The architecture is depicted using Figure 1. This lossy compression networks consists of Recurrent Neural Network components of LSTM Toderici et al. (2016) which includes an encoding network (E) consisting of encoder, a decoding network (D) consisting of decoder and a binarizer (B) So by having these components, the authors begin first by encoding the input images which is then followed by generating binary codes through the process of transformation of these medical images that can be transmitted to the next phase i.e., decoder or it can be stored.

The decoder network on receiving the binary code generates an approximation of the original medical image input and also by remembering the earlier values through LSTM cells. Authors repeat this process by using residual error which is nothing but

Figure 1. Overall architecture of compression network

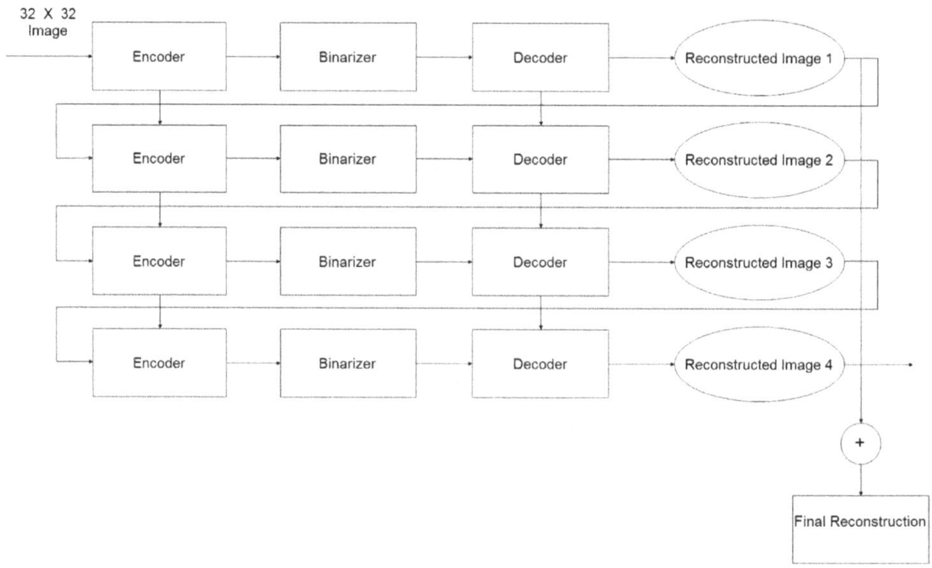

the difference between the original medical image and the reconstructed image from the decoder by a process called as auto gain additive reconstruction, until required form of the image is obtained that is well compressed and also having a better quality. Here the single iteration of the neural network architecture which the authors have described in Figure 1 and the same is represented using the following equations:

$$b_t = B(E_t(r_{t-1})) \tag{1}$$

$$\hat{x}_t = d_t(b_t) + \mu\hat{x}_{t-1} \tag{2}$$

$$r_{t-1} = x - \hat{x}_t, r_0 = x, \hat{x}_0 = 0 \tag{3}$$

where d_t and E_t indicates the states of decoder in the decoding network and encoder in the encoding network at time iteration of 't' respectively which represents the process that happens inside the two vital phases of the network, that is decoder and encoder, b_t indicates the progressive binary depiction of image phase that happens in decoder with the help of auto gain additive reconstruction; This b_t makes use of residual r_t from the encoder and binarizer B phase, $\hat{x}_t$ indicates the original image x that is reconstructed progressively with $\mu = 1$for additive gain reconstruction and r_t indicates the residual between the original image x and the reconstructed $\hat{x}_t$. In each of the iteration, a binarized stream of bits will be produced by B i.e, $b_t \in \{-1, 1\}^m$ where m stands for the number of bits generated after each iteration which follows the perspective that is outlined in Todericiet et al. (2015). These equations are used in the entire process of compression and the importance of each of them is covered even in the next phases of methodology described.

Initially the number of input and output neurons is decided depending upon the number of two dimensional arrays of pixels of a medical image. The image that will be used to compress will have the pixel values that range from 0 to 255. Blocks of size 8×8 pixels are extracted from each of the medical image, i.e. 64 pixels of values are presented to input layer. Then the activation function for the network is selected. Here the authors select sigmoidal function as the activation function which requires each neuron to be in the range of 0 to 1. Soon after this normalization process is carried out through division of pixel values with its highest possible value i.e., 255. Then by the process of linearization, the two dimensional blocks of medical image is converted into one dimensional vector which helps to represent the inputs into neural network.

In order to simplify the learning process, the segmentation process can be used where in the rows or columns of the matrix are divided into blocks that are of equal size which are non-overlapping in nature. This helps in simplifying the representation of image making it more meaningful and easy for analysis. This process is optional.

After this two weight matrices are selected for training of network where the first matrix indicates the weight connections that are present between the input layer and the hidden layer. The second matrix indicates the weight connections that are present between the hidden layer and the output layer. The values inside both the weight matrices range from 0.1 to 0.9. Optimal values that are neither too small nor too large must be present inside these matrices as the larger values may lead to instability of the network while the smaller values can cause excessive slow learning.

The first stage of LSTM architecture is compression process wherein encoder has a major role to play in. The encoder is intended to discard the various redundancies and to create the main process of lossy compression of the medical image. After the network training, new inputs and expected outputs are transferred into the network input layer. The first stage of encoding is called mapping. Here a mapper is used to reduce some data redundancies like spatial redundancies, statistical redundancies, temporal redundancies, etc. This process is reversible in nature. The amount of data that is required to illustrate the image by the mapper may or may not be directly reduced.

The main advantage for which LSTM units are made use of for lossy image compression technique is explained here. It is mainly due to the quality aspect that has to be well preserved during the entire lossy compression process & also minimize the loss in the data. The LSTM units loop within themselves thereby remembering different values and patterns until a long time. This property is very important and is made use of in many phases. So during the mapping of the image, the LSTM cells remember various noises, colour codes and patterns which help in quick and smart encoding of image thereby saving a lot of time, making the process reversible and increasing the quality of compressed image by just maintaining a low size image. With the stored weights, hidden layer output is calculated and then attained values are binarized with 8 bits and remembered. This process of remembering is utilized in coming phases which saves a lot of time. Next stage for compressing the image is called the binarizer. Binarizer reduces psycho visual redundancies. It is irreversible unlike the mapper and the symbol encoder. Keeping the irrelevant information is its goal out of the compressed representation. As the LSTM units can remember the events for a long time, binarizers work is also eased out. It is not considered when the desired error-free compression has been attained.

The third and the final step involves generating a fixed length code to represent the binarizer output and map the output in accordance with the code. The required stored information in LSTM cells will be used up in this process. The LSTM equations Zaremba et al. (2014) are outlined as following:

Let C_t, x_t and h_t indicates the cell, the input, and the hidden states respectively in every t iteration. These are taken into consideration as each LSTM unit is connected to each other using the cell state C_t which has 3 main layers, the input layer, the hidden layer and the output layer. Initially the input and the hidden layer are considered. Then the new cell state C_t and the new hidden state h_t are computed by making use of the given current input x_t, the previous cell state C_{t-1}, and the previous hidden state h_{t-1}, as

$$[f, i, 0, j]^T = [\sigma, \sigma, \sigma, \tanh]^T((Wx_t + Uh_{t-1}) + b) \tag{4}$$

$$C_t = f \odot C_{t-1} + i \odot j \tag{5}$$

$$h_t = 0 \odot \tanh(C_{t-1}) \tag{6}$$

where $\odot$ denotes multiplication that is done element wise, and b forms the bias of the network. Element wise multiplication is necessary to calculate hidden states at the initial stage. The complexity will not increase as it is done only once and also when certain set of values repeat while multiplication the LSTM cells are able to remember the product value obtained at the previous iterations thereby multiplication is ignored by directly taking the known value. For example, initially for the first image, element wise multiplication is done for values ranging between 0.1 to 0.9, this element wise multiplication need to be carried out for values in a different block of image. LSTM can remember the previously multiplied values which is stored in forget gate as well as provided to its input gate. Thereby directly the values are taken/accessed without this process of element wise multiplication.

The activation function σ chosen here is the sigmoid function which is given by the equation,

$$\sigma(x) = 1 \,/\, (1 + \exp(-x)) \tag{7}$$

The output at each iteration t of LSTM network is denoted by h_t . W and U denotes the convolutional linear transformations applied to x_t and h_{t-1} respectively at the given iteration t to calculate the function that is utilized further in calculating new cell state. These equations are important as they decide the feature of remembrance of LSTM units which is its power.

The second stage of LSTM architecture is decompression process wherein decoder is used to decompress the medical image. Decompression is the reverse path of compression which involves reconstruction of the compressed image. This reconstruction involves reading the stored data (compressed image) which is to be set as hidden layer outputs. After this the network is calculated by using the previously stored weight matrices, with the input to the output layer and also the weights between hidden and output layer. This technique of reconstructing the medical image is called as post processing.

The decoder has two main stages which are as follows. A symbol decoder and an inverse mapper form the integral parts here which will be handled by LSTM units. The saved information required for decoding process will be made use of with the help of LSTM cells. The recurrent units of LSTM are able to connect previous information to the present task of decompression. The decoder does not have binarizer because the binarizer is irreversible, so this block is no longer included in the general decoder model. In addition to different recurrent units of LSTM, an auto-gain additive reconstruction is used as shown in Figure 2 to create the final image reconstruction from the decoder outputs. This automatic gain control would scale the residual from encode phase and also undo the scaling when trying to decode image.

Here the authors consider the reconstruction process of the previously obtained residual image, r_{t-1}, and for each blotch of the residual image gain multiplier is derived. After this the authors multiply the gain which is obtained from the previous step's processed output with the residual target that is fed into the on-going iteration. Finally the Equation 1 converts to:

$$g_t = G(\hat{x}_t),\, b_t = B(E_t(r_{t-1} \odot ZOH(g_{t-1}))) \tag{8}$$

$$r_{(t-1)} = d_t(b_t)\varphi ZOH(g_{t-1}) \tag{9}$$

$$\hat{x}_t = \hat{x}_{t-1} + r_{t-1}, r_t = x - \hat{x}_t \tag{10}$$

$$g_0 = 1, r_0 = x \tag{11}$$

where φ denotes division that is done element wise and ZOH indicates the spatial up-sampling done using the mathematical model called as zero-order hold. Estimation of the gain factor g_t is indicated by $G(\cdot)$, using a convolutional network consisting of five layers that is of feed forward type, where each layer is made up of two astrides. So finally the authors have obtained the required additive gain factor to decide the accuracy and quality of the results, also the final progressive binary depiction of the required image b_t is obtained there by the phase of decoder comes to an end.

The authors use automated gate control which makes use of gain block in Figure 2. It is actually a neural network which will take as input the currently decoded image and it will predict what gain factor to use. As it only depends upon the decoding image as opposed to the input for the residual which is unknown, it is able to have zero impact in terms of data. So by using this, the authors try to minimize the problems induced by its varying statistics of residuals changing.

There are enough validation or performance criteria to evaluate the proposed model. Also authors have compared the performance of the proposed work with the existing works.

There is a dearth of work on lossy compression techniques using Recurrent Neural Networks applied on medical images. But using RNN it is possible to compress the medical images to a smaller size with quality of image still remaining the same. The results clearly indicate it. First part of the result consists of two graphs. Figure

Figure 2. Auto-gain additive reconstruction

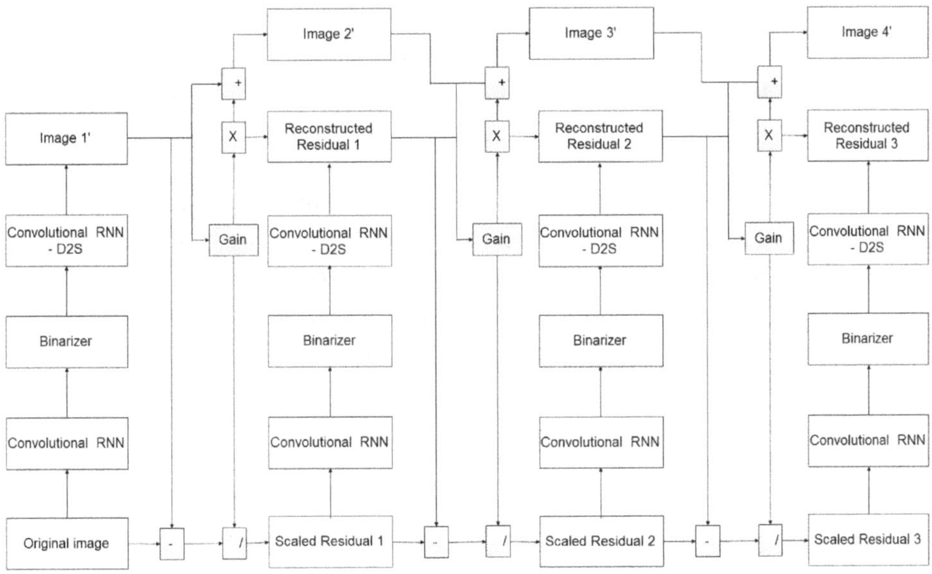

3 and Figure 4 depicts the *Comparison of compression ratios in terms of MS-SSIM* and *PSNR-HVS* respectively for different types of medical images. It can be observed that the lines coincide with each other clearly states that the quality after compression remains same for different varieties of medical images after certain number of epochs. Further, these two figures illustrate that the initial quality and the quality of the image after compression is same. In both these cases, higher values imply a closer match between the test and reference images. Both the evaluation metrics are computed for different sets of medical images over the reconstructed images after each iteration.

RESULTS AND DISCUSSIONS

In order to assess the recurrent units of LSTM architecture, the authors have used training data which are of 2 different sets. The first type of dataset consists of medical images of "32×32" dimension dataset. The other dataset utilizes a random sample of many images of 1280×720 type that are fed from certain sources. Here these medical images are fragmented into non overlapping 32×32 slabs and represents 64 slabs that have very poor quality of compression ratio that are measured using different lossless compression algorithms and techniques like PNG method. Here the authors plan to create data that is very compact to compress using the current medical image dataset. This is done by selecting the blotches which are known to compress the least under lossless compression algorithms. The overall intention of this work is to obtain a superior compression model that involves the training on such blotches that are very compact or difficult to compress. This dataset is referred to as the High Entropy dataset as it helps to evaluate the performance of training in a better way.

The LSTM network architecture used here was trained by making use of the deep learning frameworks of Tensorflow API Abadi et al. (2015) and SciPy library. Different learning rates were used to train each of the networks in order to achieve higher accuracy. The authors also make use of evaluation metrics in order to evaluate the performance of the LSTM model in different scenarios. Here the authors make use of an intuitive image metric that contrasts the uncompressed original images with that of the compressed, devalued ones. It is essential to consider the fact that there is no consent in the field for which the metric is able to depict the human perception in a better way. So the best alternative that can be accomplished is to group from the existing options while admitting the existence that each evaluation metric is bound to have different advantages as well as disadvantages.

The authors make use of an appropriate metric that compares algorithms which are used for lossy image compression called as Multi-Scale Structural Similarity (MS-SSIM) Bovik et al. (2003) and the Peak Signal to Noise Ratio - Human Visual System (PSNR-HVS) Gupta et al. (2011). The authors apply MS-SSIM independently to different sets of medical images and then find the average of the results. The PSNR-HVS is utilized for the purpose of determining the information related to colours in the image which is measured in terms of decibels. MS-SSIM provides a statistical score that ranges in-between 0 and 1. The comparison of compression ratios for three different types of images in terms of MS-SSIM and PSNR-HVS is shown in Figure 3 and Figure 4 respectively. The higher values obtained in those two cases clearly suggest that there exist a replica which is very close enough to the test image as well as to the reference images. For all the models after each iteration, both these ratio metrics are determined over the auto gain additive reconstructed images. Area under the rate distortion curve (AUC) is used in order to rank the models by addressing the difficulty of determining the minimal number of binary digits per symbol which has to be transmitted over a medium, so that at the receiver end it is possible to approximately reconstruct the source image without crossing a given deformity.

The lines in both the comparison plots are almost overlap with each other and this is the indication that the lossy compression techniques for various datasets of medical images is able to produce almost the same ratio of evaluation metrics and it also indicates that the quality of images are also preserved with minimal loss in data as the higher values obtained clearly shows that the tested images that are compressed is very same as reference image.

The dataset that were used for the compression were never compressed with a lossy algorithm ever before but few attempts were made using lossless image compression techniques and desirable output was not obtained. So the authors here have used neural network architectures consisting of Residual GRU, Recurrent LSTM units and Auto gain additive reconstruction to outline the results for the model that performs the best after many steps of training of the medical images dataset. More analysis is reported in Appendix 1 where the performance on the medical image dataset is clearly explained.

FUTURE RESEARCH DIRECTIONS

The future for medical image compressions is by using various deep learning methodologies to efficiently compress the images to maximum extent possible with higher degree of quality. Various forms of LSTM like Associative LSTM or Gated Recurrent units can be used to further increase the efficiency of results obtained. Different image reconstruction methods like one shot reconstruction methods, residual rescaling methods can be tried in decoder units to obtain different results as required for applications associated with it.

Figure 3. Comparison of compression ratios in terms of MS-SSIM

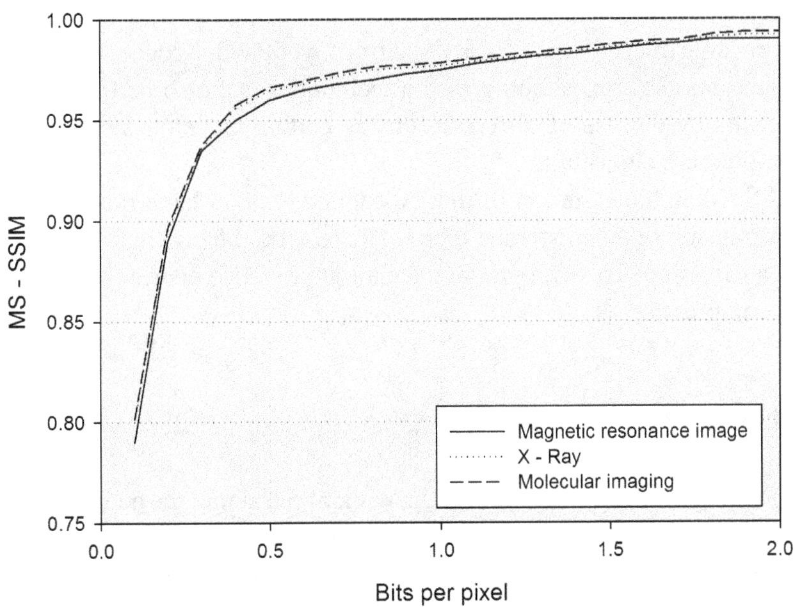

Figure 4. Comparison of compression ratios in terms of PSNR-HVS

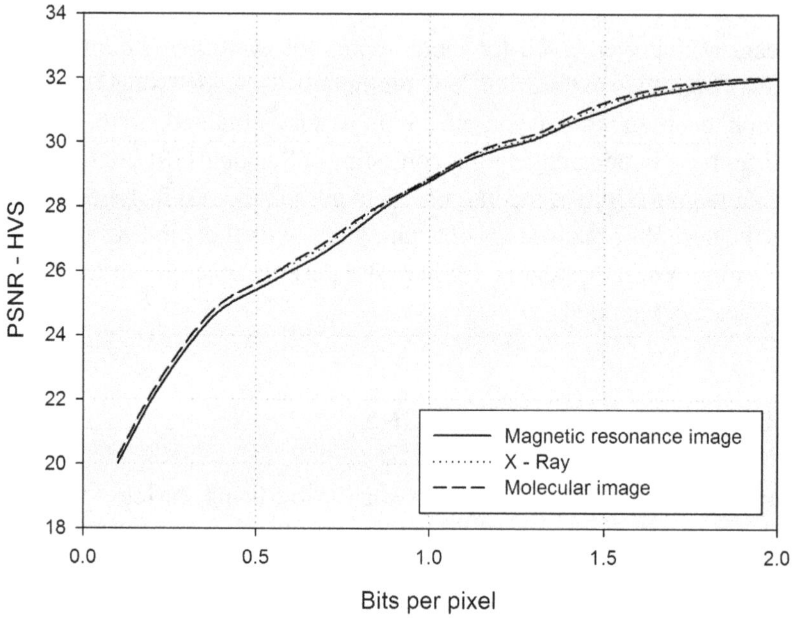

There are many research opportunities in medical image compressions using lossy compression techniques with the use of various machine learning models. White box machine learning methods like support vector machines can also be used to compress these images.

The next challenge in this research field will be to choose the best compression methods on large images which are derived from WebP video codec. A combination of lossy and lossless image compression techniques can also be tried to achieve higher results by the use of different entropy coding techniques combined with lossy compression algorithms.

This LSTM architecture can further be applied to other large images which are prone for transmission and storage thereby increasing the efficiency of storage as well as transmission. This compression technique can also be tried over videos for efficient compression.

CONCLUSION

The proposed system tries to eliminate the work of retraining the network again and again. The loops that each RNN unit is bound to, eliminates this step of retraining by remembering all the required values that are obtained in the first step itself. So, each network needs to be trained only once which helps in saving time to a very large extent. This RNN architecture consists of an encoder, a binarizer, a decoder and auto-gain additive reconstruction architecture. The authors make use of an important RNN type that is LSTM network in order to efficiently compress the medical images. Here the neural network architecture tries to surpass JPEG across most bitrates at image compression on the rate distortion curve, without the intervention of entropy coding. Generally there is a myth that lossy compression will lead to decrease in the quality of the image but since we use RNN, the parameters are set in such a way that important data is not lost but only the unwanted noise is removed ensuring high quality of image even after the compression. No other image compression techniques whether its lossy or lossless methods yield better results as our work suggests. Table 1 in Appendix 1 clearly shows that the lossy compression technique using LSTM is able to yield high ratio of PSNR-HVS and MS-SSIM. It also indicates that image quality after compression is still better.

REFERENCES

Abadi, M., Agarwal, A., Barham, P., Brevdo, E., Chen, Z., Citro, C., … Zheng, X. (2015). *TensorFlow: Large-scale machine learning on heterogeneous systems.* Available from tensorflow.org

Balle, J., Laparra, V., & Simoncelli, E. P. (2016). End-to-end optimization of nonlinear transform codes for perceptual quality. In *Proceedings of Picture Coding Symposium (PCS)*, (*vol. 16*, pp. 1-5). Academic Press. 10.1109/PCS.2016.7906310

Base, A. M., Jancke, K., Wismuller, A., Foo, S., & Martinetz, T. (2005). Medical image compression using topology-preserving neural networks. *International Journal of Engineering Applications of Artificial Intelligence*, *18*(4), 383–392. doi:10.1016/j.engappai.2004.10.004

Bovik, A. C., Wang, Z., & Simoncelli, E. P. (2003). Multiscale structural similarity for image quality assessment. In *Proceedings of the Thirty-Seventh Asilomar Conference on Signals, Systems and Computers* (vol. 2, pp. 1398–1402). IEEE.

Dimililer, K. (2013). Back propagation neural network implementation for medical image compression. *International Journal of Applied Mathematics.*

Gupta, P., Srivastava, P., Bhardwaj, S., & Bhateja, V. (2011). A modified PSNR metric based on HVS for quality assessment of color images. In *Proceedings of International Conference on Communication and Industrial Application* (pp. 1-4). IEEE Xplore. 10.1109/ICCIndA.2011.6146669

Hochreiter, S., & Schmidhuber, J. (1997). Long short-term memory. *International Journal of Neural Computation*, *9*(8), 1735–1780. doi:10.1162/neco.1997.9.8.1735 PMID:9377276

Khashman, A., & Dimililer, K. (2009). Medical radiographs compression using neural networks and Haar wavelet. In *Proceedings of International Conference on IEEE EUROCON* (pp. 1448-1453). IEEE.

Moorthi, M., & Amutha, R. (2012). Medical image compression using adaptive neural network. In *Proceedings of International Conference on Emerging Trends in Science, Engineering and Technology (INCOSET)* (pp. 222-227). Academic Press. 10.1109/INCOSET.2012.6513909

Toderici, G., O'Malley, S. M., Hwang, S. J., Vincent, D., Minnen, D., Baluja, S., ... Sukthankar, R. (2015). Variable rate image compression with recurrent neural networks. *Proceedings of International Conference on Learning Representations.*

Toderici, G., Vincent, D., Johnston, N., Hwang, S. J., Minnen, D., Shor, J., & Covell, M. (2016). *Full Resolution Image Compression with Recurrent Neural Networks.* CVF.

Yeo, W. K., & David, F. W., & Oh, T.H. (2011).Grayscale medical image compression using feed forward neural networks. *Proceedings of IEEE International Conference on Computer Applications and Industrial Electronics (ICCAIE)*, 633-638. 10.1109/ICCAIE.2011.6162211

Zaremba, W., Sutskever, I., & Vinyals, O. (2014). *Recurrent Neural Network Regularization.* Computing Research Repository (CoRR) which is part of arXiv e-print service.

ADDITIONAL READING

Bovik, A. C. (2005). *Handbook of Image and video processing*. Burlington: Academic Press.

Bruylants, T., Munteanu, A., & Schelkens, P. (2015). Wavelet based volumetric medical image compression. *Signal Processing Image Communication*, *31*, 112–133. doi:10.1016/j.image.2014.12.007

Dougherty, G. (Ed.). (2011). *Medical Image Processing Techniques and Applications.* Springer-Verlag New York. doi:10.1007/978-1-4419-9779-1

Geetha, P. (2017). Survey of Medical Image Compression Techniques and Comparative Analysis. In I. Management Association (Ed.), Medical Imaging: Concepts, Methodologies, Tools, and Applications (pp. 1165-1198). Hershey, PA: IGI Global. doi:10.4018/978-1-5225-0571-6.ch048

Hans, W. B., & Gregory, A. B. (2016). *Audio, Image, Video Coding, and Transmission*. Wiley Telecom.

Hantao, L., & Zhou, W. (2017). Perceptual Quality Assessment of Medical Images. In *Reference Module in Biomedical Sciences*. Elsevier.

Hochreiter, S., & Schmidhuber, J. (1997). Long Short Term Memory. *Neural Computation*, *9*(8), 1735–1780. doi:10.1162/neco.1997.9.8.1735 PMID:9377276

Hussain, A. J., Al-Fayadh, A., & Radi, N. (2018). Image compression techniques: A survey in lossless and lossy algorithms. *Neurocomputing*, 1–26.

Isaac, B. (Ed.). (2009). *Handbook of Medical Image Processing and Analysis*. Burlington: Academic Press.

Jain, A. K., Mao, J., & Mohiuddin, K. M. (1996). Artificial neural networks: A tutorial. *Computer*, *29*(3), 31–44. doi:10.1109/2.485891

Jaiswal, R. R., & Gaikwad, A. N. (2015). Neural Network Assisted Effective Lossy Compression of Medical Images. *IETE Technical Review*, *23*(2), 119–126. doi:10.1080/02564602.2006.11657937

Kai, X., Jie, Y., Min, Z. Y., & Liang, L. X. (2005). HVS-based medical image compression. *European Journal of Radiology*, *55*(1), 139–145. doi:10.1016/j.ejrad.2004.09.007 PMID:15950111

Lucas, L. F. R., Rodrigues, N. M. M., da Silva Cruz, L. A., & de Faria, S. M. M. (2017). Lossless Compression of Medical Images Using 3-D Predictors. *IEEE Transactions on Medical Imaging*, *36*(11), 2250–2260. doi:10.1109/TMI.2017.2714640 PMID:28613165

Morgan, P., & Frankish, C. (2009). Image quality, compression and segmentation in medicine. *The Journal of Audiovisual Media in Medicine*, *25*(4), 149–154. doi:10.1080/0140511021000051135 PMID:12554293

Parikh, S. S., Ruiz, D., Kalva, H., Escribano, G. F., & Adzic, V. (2018). High Bit-Depth Medical Image Compression With HEVC. *IEEE Journal of Biomedical and Health Informatics*, *22*(2), 552–560. doi:10.1109/JBHI.2017.2660482 PMID:28141538

Ramaswamy, A., & Mikhael, W. B. (1996). A mixed transform approach for efficient compression of medical images. *IEEE Transactions on Medical Imaging*, *15*(3), 343–352. doi:10.1109/42.500143 PMID:18215915

Sarma, K. K. (2016). Learning Aided Digital Image Compression Technique for Medical Application. In N. Kamila (Ed.), *Handbook of Research on Emerging Perspectives in Intelligent Pattern Recognition, Analysis, and Image Processing* (pp. 400–422). Hershey, PA: IGI Global. doi:10.4018/978-1-4666-8654-0.ch019

Singh, M., Kumar, S., Chouhan, S.S., & Shrivastava, M. (2016). Various Image Compression Techniques: Lossy and Lossless. *International Journal of Computer Applications*, 142(6), 0975 – 8887.

Singh, S., Kumar, V., & Verma, H. K. (2007). DWT–DCT hybrid scheme for medical image compression. *Journal of Medical Engineering & Technology*, *31*(2), 109–122. doi:10.1080/03091900500412650 PMID:17365435

Tick, H. O. (2010). JPEG2000 and JPEG: Image Quality Comparison of Compressed Medical Modalities. *International Journal of Computers and Applications*, *32*(4), 393–398.

Venugopal, D., Mohan, S., & Raja, S. (2016). An efficient block based lossless compression of medical images, *Optik - International Journal for Light and Electron Optics*, 127(2), 754-758.

KEY TERMS AND DEFINITIONS

Binarizer: The process of quantizing the data according to a threshold value is called binarizer.

Compression: The process of reducing the volume of data is called as compression.

Data Compression: The process of reducing the number of bits that is required to represent the data is called as data compression.

Decoder: Decoder is a compression unit or an algorithm that decodes the information from one given format to a different format. It is opposite to that of encoder.

Encoder: Encoder is a compression unit or an algorithm that converts information from one given format to a different format. Here some large data is converted into small data.

Entropy Coding: The method of lossless data compression which is independent of the features of the medium in which it is present is called as entropy coding.

Feed Forward Network: A feed forward neural network is an artificial neural network that has connections between the units which do not form a closed cycle.

Image Compression: The process of encoding or minimizing the size of the image without degrading its quality is called as image compression.

Long Short-Term Memory (LSTM): The variant of recurrent neural networks that is capable of learning long term dependencies in sequence.

Rate Distortion: The information theory that solves the problem of deciding the minimal number of bits per symbol that must be sent over the given channel so that the input can be roughly reconstructed at the destination without exceeding the distortion specified.

Recurrent Neural Network: A recurrent neural network is an artificial neural network that has connections between the units which do form a closed directed cycle.

Residual: A residual is the difference between the observed value and the predicted value by the model.

APPENDIX

Performance on the Medical Image Dataset

The authors mentioned that they have used evaluation metrics to evaluate the results obtained as AUC. MS-SSIM and PSNR-HVS are two such evaluation metrics used. We see that values of MS-SSIM for different datasets of medical images remains almost 1.8 for all of them with very small differences in the values. This indicates that the structural similarity after compression is same for all the different types of images. So the RNN is able to maintain a balance between different kinds of medical images. PSNR-HVS gives the color code information and quality ratio information. The constant values of PSNR-HVS among the different sets of medical images indicate that even after compression the quality is still better without any loss in the medical data that is really important. Also the higher values that are obtained in both the evaluation metrics i.e, MS-SSIM and PSNR-HVS clearly suggest that there exist a replica which is very close enough to the test image as well as to the reference images. This helps us to know that the quality of image is well preserved even after lossy compression because of the usage of LSTM units.

Table 1. Implementation on the medical image dataset (32X32 images) evaluated for the designated metric as Area Under the Curve (AUC). All models are trained up for a large number of training steps. Without the intervention of entropy coding the images were compressed

Types of Medical Images	MS-SSIM AUC	PSNR-HVS AUC
Computed Tomography	1.8080	52.34
Magnetic Resonance Imaging	1.8064	52.30
Positron Emission Tomography	1.8067	52.31
PET-CT	1.8054	52.28
X-Ray	1.8074	52.32
Molecular Imaging	1.8066	52.31
Histopathological images	1.8072	52.32

Chapter 4
Digital Image Analysis for Early Diagnosis of Cancer:
Identification of Pre-Cancerous State

Durjoy Majumder
West Bengal State University, India

Madhumita Das
West Bengal State University, India

ABSTRACT

Cancer diagnoses so far are based on pathologists' criteria. Hence, they are based on qualitative assessment. Histopathological images of cancer biopsy samples are now available in digital format. Such digital images are now gaining importance. To avoid individual pathologists' qualitative assessment, digital images are processed further through use of computational algorithm. To extract characteristic features from the digital images in quantitative terms, different techniques of mathematical morphology are in use. Recently several other statistical and machine learning techniques have developed to classify histopathological images with the pathologists' criteria. Here, the authors discuss some characteristic features of image processing techniques along with the different advanced analytical methods used in oncology. Relevant background information of these techniques are also elaborated and the recent applications of different image processing techniques for the early detection of cancer are also discussed.

DOI: 10.4018/978-1-5225-6316-7.ch004

INTRODUCTION

Today digital images plays an immense importance in entire medical process and health care - from disease diagnosis to intervention and treatment (Tolxdorff et al, 2004). Different advanced image processing and analysis techniques are now have a wide spread use in different branches of life sciences as well as in medicine. In both the areas, captured data of images are widely used for scientific and clinical investigations to identify pathological changes and thereby help in an understanding of pathophysiological changes. Thus, medical images provide information that are becoming an indispensable part of today's patients care for disease diagnosis and thereby treatment procedure. Hence, different medical institutions across the globe capture large amount of image data. As the number of image data are increasing, so its management and thereby getting of meaningful interpretation out of them are becoming a challenge for scientists and engineers.

Today, cancer constitutes a major health problem. Global data suggest that approximately 1 out of every 2 men and 1 out of every 3 women are affected with cancer at some point during their lifetime. Such malefic scenario are correlated with increase in tobacco use and changes to urban and sedentary life-style. Fortunately, due to availability of several advanced medicines have significantly increase the life-span of the cancer patients. Moreover, early diagnosis and selection of proper treatment protocol become another two crucial factors for increased survival rate of cancer patients. Therefore, detection of pre-cancerous state becomes crucial for clinical management of cancer. Moreover, identification of malignancy level is also important in the selection of therapy. Traditionally, malignancy level is readily identified by pathologists using of histopathological images of biopsy samples, however, through empirical judgments through an assessment of the deviations in the cellular and/or tissue morphology. Overall, such assessment is subjective, and hence have a considerable variation of interpretation (Ismail et al, 1989; Andrion et al, 1995).

Empirical assessment is unreliable and hence, needs second pathologist opinion. This would make an unnecessary delay in the initiation of treatment procedure which in turn could be detrimental for the patient. So, it is very much pertinent to develop computational tools and for cancer diagnosis an automated method would be preferred. Moreover this procedure provides inferences in a quantitative manners. During the last two decades, due to availability of digital image capturing procedures, a tremendous amount of research works have initiated to conduct for automated cancer diagnosis. Though this approach holds great promise for reliable cancer diagnosis and treatment follow-up; however, it is not a straight-forward procedure and numerous challenges need to overcome.

Digital image is represented in a two-dimensional function, $f(x,y)$ where x and y are spatial coordinates of all finite, discrete quantities, and the amplitude f represent a pair of coordinates (x,y) in finite, discrete quantities. Finite set of digital value of image is called pictual elements, image elements, and pixels. A convenient tool for image processing is MatLab® (Gonzalez et al, 2009). There are many variety of disciplines and fields in science and technology such as photography, remote sensing, forensic science, industrial inspection and medical diagnosis where image processing is used. For bio-medical applications followings issues are the concern: (i) extraction of quantitative information from the acquired images, (ii) Translation of the information for developing decision support system and (iii) storage and exchange of image data without altering of meaningful information in a robust, efficient and accurate manner.

DIFFERENT LEVELS OF BIOMEDICAL IMAGE ACQUISITION

Biomedical image including cancer biopsy image data are generally occur at three levels – organ level, cell/tissue level and molecular level.

Organ Level Images

There are two different sources medical images - archival images and personal images. First one have the different image sources of the same organ while second one consisting of huge amount of image data of an individual. Now-a-days most the images are captured in digital format with increasing resolution; therefore, image processing technology are facing difficulties to provide newer medical interpretation. However, due to improvement in image acquisition technology in terms of pixel (for example, 200 nm in nano-tomogram) and reconstruction (for example, in computed tomogram 8000 × 8000 pixel per slice with 0.7 μm isotropic with 64 MB per slice), the size of image data of medical relevance increased from KB to TB. With this increment in the amount of data, information technology face difficulty regarding its storage and/or sharing through network (Tolxdorff et al, 2004).

As par Society of Nuclear Medicine and Molecular Imaging (SNMMI), the objective interest of biomedical imaging is targeted to visualize, characterize, and measure biological processes both at the molecular and cellular levels in all the living systems including human being (Mankoff, 2007). Molecular imaging captures image data at 3D and thereby makes quantitative analysis with respect to time. It is a noninvasive procedure and used to diagnose diseases of different organs and tissues like cancer, brain and cardiovascular disorders. Presently different imaging modalities like Positron Emission Tomography (PET), Magnetic Resonance Imaging (MRI),

Computed Tomography (CT), Single Photon Emission Computed Tomography (SPECT), Optical imaging, and Ultrasound (US) are included as molecular imaging modalities. Among these modalities, PET and SPECT access tissue's functional behavior while others are inclined towards structural elucidation. Sometimes hybrid imaging modalities like, hybrid PET/CT, PET/MRI, PET/SPECT/CT help to substantiate the structure and function correlation (Townsend et al, 2004; Pichler et al, 2010; Magota et al, 2011). Hence images captured with different imaging modalities require different data handling methods.

Molecular Level Images

With the extension of genomic science, scientists are getting involved in the understanding of the functional assay of whole genome. So high dimensional gene expression system (micro-array) is developed. This may have significance with respect to diagnosis and prognostic significance in terms of molecular function; hence, are able to make distinction between normal versus disease cells.

Cell/Tissue Level Image Data

Histopathological tissue are analyzed for two purposes – for confirmation of the disease and its grade. Grading of diseases is the empirical way of denoting disease progression. This procedure is routinely practiced in clinic for cancer diagnosis. In such cases, computational image analysis not only help in faster diagnosis but also may provide quantitative statement (Gurcan et al 2009). Majority of the above mentioned imaging data acquisition methods are costly. Cost can be reduced if meaningful information can be extracted from cellular and/or tissue level. However due to loss of data acquisition beyond microscopic focus area cell/tissue level image processing are not being readily done. However, recently whole slide imaging technique is available increases the chance to get a meaningful information from analyzing images at this level (Yu et al, 2016).

CLASSIFICATION OF DIGITAL IMAGES

The images are classified as binary, gray-scale, color, and multi spectral (Demirkaya et al, 2009). Binary images can only take two values like black and white, or OFF and ON. A binary image takes only 1-bit to represent each pixel. In the applications where minimum level of information are required this types of images are frequently used for example, optical character recognition (OCR). Sometimes threshold operation is applied to convert a gray-scale image into a binary image. In such operation every pixel above a certain limit is converted to white ('1'), and below of that are considered as black ('0'). Gray-scale images have monochrome or one-color because it has no color information. The number of bits in each pixel denotes the gray levels information. Each pixel in gray-scale image carries 8 bits, which allows maximum of 256 different gray levels. In medical images, generally 12 or 16 bits/pixel are used. Sometimes extra gray levels information is used in digital imaging for denoting and clarifying detail information with the use of a small portion of an image that is made much larger.

Color images have three-band monochrome data and hence each band data represents to different color; however, each spectral band store information at the gray-level. In digital technology, color images are denoted through red, green, and blue (RGB) system. For each color 8-bit monochrome is used as standard, therefore color image would have 24 bits/pixel (8-bits for each of the three color bands i.e., red, green, and blue). Multispectral images obtained by infrared, ultraviolet, and/or X-ray are not directly visible by the human eye but are readily used in medical imaging procedures. However, information obtained by these procedures are often transformed to different spectral bands to RGB components through mapping procedures.

HISTOLOGY IMAGE ANALYSIS

In pathological laboratory, images of tissue sections of biopsy samples on glass slides are captured digitally. Such images are known as histological images. These are further utilized for analysis by the pathologists. Disease grading is done by viewing these histological images. In cancer histological grading represents the level of morphological deformity of cells thus functionality of cancer at cellular and molecular level which in turn, may denote the aggressiveness and/or drug sensitivity of cancer. Therefore assigning of grade is very important as this information may be used for its treatment planning. This information is sometimes correlated with cancer prognosis. Henceforth quantitative assessment of histological images may aid in further decision making (Ali et al, 2016).

The histopathological image are generally captured at different magnifications (100×, 200×, and 1000×). Such images are utilized by different computational tools to get further information at the pixel level. Such data are further analyzed by different computational and analytical tools like multivariate statistical analysis for diagnostic classification (Demir and Yener, 2005). Prior to data analysis histopathology images are gone through different image preprocessing methods. Though for most of the images, processing methods follow the same steps of algorithm; however depending on the images from different diseases these steps may vary during morphological processing, selection of region and boundary within an image, thresholding for feature extraction followed by disease classification.

The processes of digital pathology has developed immensely that may assist to pathologist in interpreting the large number of samples within a short duration. Thus the area needs further development in terms of interpretation of result in a more quantitative manner and with little intervention of user. Recently an automated computerized image analysis algorithms successfully detect neuroblastoma (Gurcan et al, 2006). For diagnosis of renal cancer, recent time the application of different statistical methods like Bayesian classifier, k-means algorithm help to overcome the observer variability and thus help to reach to a confirmed pathological decision (Waheed at al 2007). Using histopathological images captured at 200X magnification 98% classification accuracy was achieved. Neuroblastoma histopathological images are classified with the likelihood function estimation and the detection sensitivity was 81.1% (Sertel et al, 2009). Breast cancer was diagnosed in a quantitative manner using color image with boundary based segmentation algorithm. This algorithm uses geodesic active contours and weighted mean shift normalization for detection of object boundary (Xu et al, 2010; Basavanhallya et al, 2011).

MATHEMATICAL MORPHOLOGY

Mathematical morphology (MM) is commonly used for processing and analysis of spatial and geometrical structures like graphs, surface meshes, solids. This method relies on set theory, lattice theory, topology, and random functions. It can also applied to digital images for morphological image processing which consists of a set of operations. Though it was originally applied in binary images but later grayscale images are analyzed with this technique. With this, binary images are considered as sets and thereby a large number of binary operations and techniques like erosion, dilation, opening, closing, granulometry, skeletonization and others are applied to it. Several other operations like morphological gradients, top-hat transform and the Watershed have also included as MM (Ledda et al 2000; Gonzalez et al, 2009; Renato et al, 2010).

Operations are performed with the combinations of a basic set of numerical manipulations between an image A and a much smaller object (compared to A) B, called structuring element and is represented through a matrix of 0s and 1s. The object B, act as probe to scan A to modify it with some specific rule that define the characteristics of the process to perform. In morphological image processing dilation and erosion are the fundamental operations. Both are defined in terms of the interaction of the original image A to be processed with the structuring element B.

Morphological erosion. For erosion operation, two sets of image data are processed where the data of image A is eroded by B, the small structuring element. Such operation is expressed as Minkowski substraction:

$$A \ominus B = \{r \mid (r + b) \in A \; \forall \; b \in B\}$$

The set intersection erosion can be expressed as:

$$A \ominus B = \cap_{b \in B} T_{-b}(A)$$

Morphological dilation. The dilation operation is performed with a structuring element for probing and then expands its shapes in the input image. It is the set union of the objects A obtained after the translation of the original image for each coordinate pixel b in the structuring element B.

$$A \oplus B = \cup_{b \in B} T_{b}(A)$$

Binary dilation can be interpreted as the combination of two sets by using the vector additions of set elements, called the *Minkowshi Addition.* This operation is expressed as:

$$A \oplus B = \{r \mid r = a+b \; \forall \; a \in A \text{ and } b \in B\}$$

Opening filter. The morphological opening of A by B ($A \circ B$) is simply erosion of A by B, followed by dilation by B:

$$A \circ B = (A \ominus B) \oplus B$$

In above expression, $\ominus$ and $\oplus$ denote erosion and dilation, respectively.

Though dilation tries to reverse erosion process, but during this process, detailing of closely related the element that matches with the shape and size of structuring element will vanish. The consequence of erosion is that if any object is disappeared by this operation cannot be recovered.

Closing Filter. Morphological closing operation is the dual of opening, performed by dilation and erosion process with the same structuring element:

$$A \bullet B = (A \oplus B) \ominus B$$

Opening and closing filters are used as discriminators for filtering, segmentation, edge detection, differential counting, and numerical analysis of shapes.

Edge detection. Edge detection is an algorithm for identifying points in a digital image, thus features in a digital image is detected and extracted. With this operation image brightness changes sharply. This helps in capturing important changes and events through discontinuities in image brightness. Thus depth, surface orientation, variation in illumination and material properties are likely to be disclosed. In the process a set of curves are being applied and thus object boundary and/or surface are defined. As a result of edge detection, only important structural elements are retained while less important structural features are being filter out. Therefore, there is reduction of data amount for further processing. However, applying of edge detection algorithm becomes difficult in real life images. Extracted edges from such images are often not connected or denote false edges, this is known as *fragmentation*. So it complicates the subsequent task. Sobel method is the popular edge detection method in image processing.

Top-hat transform. Top-hat transform operation exhibits details by extracting small elements from a specific images. Top-hat transform are of two types - white top-hat and black top-hat. Former operation is the result of the difference between the input image and its opening (○) by the structuring element, while the later is the difference between the closing (●) and the input image.

Let f: E $\rightarrow$R be a gray scale image, where the mapping points from an Euclidean space or discrete grid E (such as R^2 or Z^2) into the real line

Let $b(x)$ is the gray scale structuring element.

Then, the white top-hat transform of f is given by: $T_w(f) = f - f \circ b$

The black top-hat transform of f is given by: $T_w(f) = f \bullet b - f$

Top-hat transforms are helpful in feature extraction, background equalization, image enhancement, and others (Gillibert and Jeulin, 1994). The white top-hat transform becomes operative to an image that have brighter structuring element than their surroundings; while white top-hat transform becomes operative to an image that have brighter structuring element than their surroundings. In both the cases image should contain objects that have smaller than the structuring elements and return images that contain only non-negative pixel values. During top-hat transforms the structuring element b controls the size or width of the extracted elements thus controlling of b govern the size of the elements. With increase in size of b, the extracted elements will be larger in size.

Morphological operation was used for precise selection of red blood cells (*RBCs*) among mixture of cell types through process of segmentation using grey scale granulometries, boundary calculation and texture. The segmented image is used for detection of malarial parasite among the selected cells (Di Ruberto et al, 2000; Di Ruberto et al, 2002). Further it is shown that morphological segmentation is more precise than water shed algorithm (Chatap and Shibu, 2014).

IMAGE PROCESSING: OVERVIEW OF METHODS

Digital Image Processing methods are versatile, and have repeatability while preserves the original data. The different image processing techniques are elaborated as below:

Image Preprocessing

Image preprocessing is done to change pixel brightness values of an image to improve its visual impact. Available algorithms for this are generally interactive and application dependent.

Pre-processing operations are applied prior to extraction of information and data analysis of an image. Such functions are grouped into two - radiometric or geometric corrections. Radiometric corrections are applied to reduce sensor irregularities and noise; as a result, transformation can distinctly be noted between two images. There are many types of noise in images like salt and pepper noise, film grains etc. Removing noise to improve image quality is done with enhancement techniques which are as below:

Contrast Stretching. The contrast stretching methods are applied to stretch the narrow range to the whole of the available range.

Noise Filtering. Noise is the unnecessary information that is introduced in image either during its acquisition or transmission. There are several types of noise in an image: Impulse noise (Salt and pepper noise), Amplifier noise (Gaussian noise), Shot noise, Quantization noise (uniform noise), Film grain, isotropic noise, Multiplicative noise (Speckle noise) and Periodic noise. Different filtering algorithms are used to remove such noise, of which median filter is popularly used.

Histogram modification. Contrast of an image is enhanced with histogram equalization. This method redistributes pixels with each value within a range so that contrast is enhanced at the peaks and decreased at the tails.

Image Segmentation

Segmentation process makes several subdivisions of an image into several parts or objects. Depending upon the problem to solve, subdivision is applied.

Feature Extraction

Features are the characteristic items of an image. The characteristic features such as size, shape, composition, location etc. are extracted first and these are subjected to perform classification of the target image with the help of high-level analysis.

The above mentioned processes may be helpful in the automation process of cancer diagnosis. In the preprocessing step, noise is eliminated to improve the image quality thus, selection of the focal areas of an image can easily be determined. Along with this nucleus/cell segmentation would be helpful to extract cell level information. It is the most vital step for different features extraction as this would ultimately help in diagnosis.

After preprocessing step, different features either at the cell or tissue-level are extracted depending on the image and choice of interest. In the effort to extract cellular-level features, the properties of the elements in individual cells are quantitated, thus morphology, texture, fractal, granularity or intensity of the elements are generally be extracted. For tissue-level, feature extraction quantifies cellular distribution across the tissue i.e., it focuses on the spatial dependency of the cells. This is denoted through gray-level dependency of the pixels. Like cell level, textural, fractal, and/or topological features can also be extracted at tissue level.

Image Classification

Generally image is classified based on extracted features. As features were extracted in terms of a pixel therefore, image classification depends on pixel or a group of pixels in grey value. Sometimes image is classified based on multiple features i.e., on a set of pixels.

IMAGE ANALYSIS USING MATLAB

For image analysis the de facto standard could be the Image Processing Toolbox of MATLAB. Images can be classified into four types:

1. **Intensity Image:** Consists of only single data matrix where each element of the matrix denotes the intensity of the corresponding pixel.
2. **Indexed Image:** Have a data matrix and a colormap matrix. The colormap matrix is an m-by-3 array of class double containing floating point value.
3. **Binary Image -** Is represented as a logical array and each element of that array has one of two values, and is represented by a byte.
4. **Color Image:** Is a true color RGB image and represented as an m- by –n by -3 data array that are the representation of red, green, and blue color.

Different functions used in MatLab and their utility are described below.

Superimposing a Binary Image on a Gray-Level Image

It is often necessary to display a gray-level image overlaid with its processed version. The function overlays binary image, the second input argument, onto the gray-level image gimg, the first input argument with a color of choice

```
%function J=mipimoverlay(gimg,bimg,c)
%c=1:red, 2:green, 3:blue, 4:white
function J=mipimoverlay(gimg,bimg,c)
Mx=max(gimg(:));
gimg(bimg==1)=0;
J=cat(3,gimg,gimg,gimg);
if Mx<255
        gimg(bimg==1)=255;
else
        gimg(bimg==1)=65535;
end
J(:,:,c)=gimg;
if c==4
        J=cat(3,gimg,gimg,gimg);
else
J(:,:,c)=gimg;
end
```

Region of Interest

A *region of interest* (ROI) is a portion of an image that are subjected to filter or other operation. A binary mask operation is performed with ROI that generates a binary image of the same size as the original image that we want to process. In the mask image, all pixels in ROI are set to 1 while all pixels in the outside of ROI are set to 0. Sometimes more than one ROI is set within an image. Sometimes ROI is set with polygons to encompass contiguous pixels, or by a range of intensities. Pixels are not necessarily contiguous in the latter operation. With an indexed or intensity image application of Roicolor selects a ROI and that in turn, returns a binary image. Image masking with filtering uses roifilt2.

Volume of Interest (VOI)

VOI is applicable for 3-dimensional images having one or multiple slices and represented by a dataset. Once an object is segmented and defined by a VOI, statistics of the volume can be calculated. The isoline contours of multiple slices will specify the VOL in 3-D.

To demonstrate this on the PET image of a phantom consisting of small spheres filled with activity of higher concentration compared to its background region. These small spheres are meant to simulate small lesions in a human body. The following script computes the VOI for one such small sphere cropped from the original image.

```
for i=1:size(oimg,3)
        Img(:,:,i)=imresize(oimg(:,:,i),2,'bilinear');
end
p=0.4;
maxIntensity=max(Img(:));
simg=zeros(size(Img));
for i=1:size(Img,3)
c=contourc(Img(:,:,i), maxIntensity*[P,P]);
tt=mipdecomposeContourCurves(C);
if ~isempty(tt)
        simg(:,:,i)=roipoly(Img(:,:,i),[tt.x],[tt.y]);
        imshow(Img(:,:,i),[]);hold on;
        plot([tt.x],[tt.y],'b','linewidth',2);
end
clear C
end
```

As seen in the script, we first upsample each slice 2:1 to improve the definition of the ROIs. The script plots the contour lines on the gray-level image for display purposes.

Changing Image Intensities

In MATLAB, this subject is generally discussed under the title of indexing. We will demonstrate through examples how image intensities can be changed using what is known as the logical indexing method. We can change all zero intensities to one using

```
Img(Img==0) = 1;
```

This can also be carried out using a for loop, in which we visit every element sequentially, but this would be inefficient. Using the aforementioned technique, one can use Img>200 to change all the intensities greater than 200 in the image. We can change the numbers greater than 10 and less than and equal to 50 in an image by

```
Img(Img>10 & Img<=50) = 20;
```

An alternative method of changing the elements of an image matrix is the use of the *find* function. This function locates the intensities specified by an expression. The following script finds the intensities larger than I1 and replaces them with I2:

```
INDEX = find(Img>I1);
Img(INDEX) = I2;
```

This function can accept any expression that usually consist of some variables or smaller expressions having also some variables that are joined with relational operation (e.g., lower limit<Img<upper limit). The image matrix can have two or more dimensions. INDEX is a column vector including the location of those intensities specified by the expression.

Replacing Infs and Nans

As a result of an image division (element-by-element) operation in which the divisor image has zero elements, we may have *nan* and *inf*, at the end of the image arithmetic. The following function replaces the *infs* and *nans* in a matrix with zero.

```
Function Img=mipremoveundefinedNums(X)
sizeX=size(X);
X=X(:);
X(isnan(X))=0;
X(isinf(X))=0;
Img=reshape(X,sizeX);.
```

Concatenating Images

It may be necessary to concatenate images, for instance, to display multiple images together horizontally in a row or vertically in a column format. Images can be concatenated horizontally:

```
ImgH=[Img1, Img2, Img3,.....];
```

or vertically

```
ImgV=[Img1, Img2, Img3,.....];
```

The image can be displayed using the code

```
Imagesc(ImgH); or Imagesc(ImgV);
```

The cat function can be used to concatenate images as well. To concatenate horizontally or along the second dimension, we use

```
ImgH=cat(2,Img1, Img2, Img3,.....);

ImgV=cat(1,Img1, Img2, Img3,.....);
```

The *cat* function can also be used to form 3-D volume images from 2-D slices:

```
Newimage=cat(3,Img1, Img2, Img3,.....);
```

Resizing Images

Resizing images may be required for processing, analysis, or display purposes. There are two functions, *imresize* and *interp2*, available in MATLAB for resizing 2-D images. To interpolate (or resize) 3-D images in the 3-D image space, the *interp3* function can be used.

Alternatively, 3-D images can be resized slice-by-slice if the slice thickness is to be retained. We create an 11 ´ 11 image of a 2-D Gaussian function with s=2 using *fspecial*, and then upsample it with a ratio of 4:1.

```
Img=fspecial('gauss',[11 11],2);
[r,c]=size(Img);
Img1=imresize(Img,4,'bilinear');
```

Images can be resampled at some new x and y grid points using interp2 function as shown in the following code:

```
[xnew,ynew]=meshgrid(0.25:0.25:r-0.25,0.25:0.25:c-0.25);
[xold,yold]=meshgrid(0.5:r-0.5,0.5:c-0.5);
Img2=interp2(xold,yold,Img,xnew,ynew);
```

Image Padding

Zero padding or, padding images with any number, may be necessary in spatial filtering operations to correctly handle edge pixels. While processing the border regions, extra row and columns around an image must be added so that the sliding kernel neighborhood extends beyond the boundary of the image. The paddarray function has three modes: *circular, replicate,* and *symmetric*. The padding size can also be entered as an input argument. The symmetric mode is commonly used to pad a mirror image. The *paddarray* function can operate on two-or multidimensional images.

Image Histogram

An intensity histogram represents the frequency of occurrence of intensities in an image. It is the approximation of the probability distribution function that intensities follow. Image histograms can be computed in several ways. For instance, the following statement:

```
[h,cbins]=hist(Img(:),nbins);
```

Creates an image histogram in which nbins is the desired number of bins, and cbins denotes their centers (Demirkaya et al, 2009).

AUTOMATED COMPUTATIONAL DIGITAL IMAGE PROCESSING

The automated cancer diagnosis from histological images follows three main computational algorithmic steps: preprocessing, feature extraction, and diagnosis. The preprocessing step improve the image quality by eliminating background noises and thus helps in determining the ROI of an image. This step also performs operation for nucleus/cell segmentation. The detailing steps are already described. The diagnosis step distinguishes between benignity and malignancy and if malignancy exist then level of malignancy is made with the extracted features. With the extracted features, this step uses either statistical analysis or machine learning algorithms to reach a decision. An overview of these three steps is schematically shown in Table 1 (Demir and Yener, 2016). In the following sections, these steps are elaborated in detail.

Thresholding technique is useful to highlight foreground from the background. With the selection of an adequate threshold value T, the gray level image can be converted to binary image. However, due to such process the binary image should not lose any essential information like the position and shape of the objects of interest (foreground). Such conversion reduces the data complexity and helps in recognition and classification. With the application of a single threshold value (T), all the gray level values below the specified T will be classified as black (0), and above the specified T will be white (1) (Al-amri et al, 2010). Otsu's algorithm based on statistical criteria uses gray thresh function performs global image threshold. This criteria considers minimization of the weighted sum of within-class variances of the object and background pixels thus, establishes an optimum threshold. It is needless to mention here that minimization of within-class variances is equivalent to maximization of between-class variance. This method provides a very competent output for bimodal histogram images (Sudha and Jayashree, 2012).

Marker-Controlled Watershed Segmentation

In Marker-based watershed segmentation markers are used. A marker is a connected component of the image. Two types of markers are used - the internal markers, associated with objects of interest; and the external markers, associated with the background. Handling of separated but touching objects in an image is a difficult operations in image processing. Hence, watershed transform algorithm is readily applied to handle this situation. The marker based watershed segmentation can produce unique boundaries within an image. Though over-segmentation problem can be handled through this but it provides a unique solution for a particular image (Kaur and Jindal, 2011). The other advantages of this algorithm are – computation is performed on the gradient of the original image; it is a simple, fast and intuitive

Table 1. Basic steps for automated image processing.

Processing & Segmentation	Feature Extraction & Selection	Disease Detection, Classification & Post Processing
• Color illumination Normalization • Smoothing • Denoising • Thresoholding • Edege based • Active Contour • Clustering	• Morphometry • Color • Textural • Intensity based • Morphological • Linear, Non Linear Feature Reduction	• Supervised • Unsupervised • Neural network • k-nearest neighbourhood • Fuzzy system • Morphological Functions

method; and if image contrast is poor then it gives output with a complete division of the image in separated regions. This algorithm successfully applied to Dicom image for detection of lung cancer (Shanti et al, 2013).

Extraction of Features

After segmentation features are extracted from the region of interest on the basis of some preset rules. Working with lung cancer it is shown that preset rules in the process of segmentation are helpful in the elimination of the false detection of cancer nodules and thus provides better diagnosis. Generally rules are set on the basis of diagnostic indicators that are available in medical literature (Sharma and Jindal, 2011).

Binarization Approach

Binarization approach is a method of counting black pixels vis-à-vis white pixels in both normal as well as in cancer tissue, and thus threshold is selected. This is has been successfully implemented for diagnosis of lung cancer. In normal lung tissue number of black pixels is much more compared to white, so first average is determined by counting the black pixels in both normal and abnormal images and this average is generally be used to determine the threshold. If the number of the black pixels of a new image is greater that the threshold, then it indicates that the image is normal, otherwise, if the number of the black pixels is less than the threshold, it indicates that the image is cancerous (Ada and Kaur, 2013).

Masking Approach

Inside ROI either white or black linked areas appear as masses that in turn, expressed as percentage. In lung cancer percent of white linked areas are increased.

ADVANCED ANALYTICAL METHODS USED IN ONCOLOGY

Different advanced statistical techniques and/or machine learning methods are used to analyze data of the extracted features of an image to classify and thus helps to make a diagnostic decision support system. Applications of some of the popular methods in analyzing histopathological images in oncology are discussed here.

K-Means Algorithm

The Lloyd's algorithm or k-means algorithm, is used to solve problem through clustering. The characteristics of k-means algorithm are:

- It is simple and easily implementable method,
- It can be applied to unstructured data set,
- The K-means algorithm can apply to any clustering problem,
- It is based on centroid hence, determination of clusters or partitions is important,
- Vector-space model from data points can be formulated,
- This measures a similarity/distance between the feature vectors,

##

The basics steps of algorithm is as follows:

Step 1: Selection of K points in initial centroids
Step 2: Repeat
Step 3: Form K cluster by assigning each point to its closest centroid
Step 4: Recomputed the centroid of each cluster until centroid does not change (Rajgire et al, 2017).

The algorithm is just a heuristic, eventually converges to a point or local minima, the local minima would not necessarily be the minimum of the sum of squares. It is used for knowledge extraction, reveal insights by analyzing data and predict future from the data (Kumar et al, 2015). K-nearest neighborhood method is applied to distinguish images into normal and cancerous through its performance on the basis of comparison.

Principle Component Analysis (PCA)

Principal component analysis (PCA) is a statistical technique that can handle multiple variables. This mathematical algorithm reduces the data dimensionality but retains the variation in a data set. This reduction is accomplished by identifying directions, called principal components, along which the variation in the data is maximal. Instead of using values of multiple variables, a few components are used, so that each sample can be represented by relatively few numbers. Samples are then be plotted, so it is possible make comparison between them easily through visual assessment. This is helpful in determination of similarities and differences between samples and thus may be helpful to make decision whether or not the samples can be grouped (Ringnér 2008).

##

Algorithm for PCA

Step 1: Mean center of the data (optional)
Step 2: Computation of the covariance matrix of the dimensions
Step 3: Determination of eigenvectors of covariance matrix
Step 4: Sorting of eigenvectors along with the descending order of eigenvalues
Step 5: Projection of eigenvectors according to the order

Hidden Markov Model

Markov Model and Hidden Markov Model (HMM) both are very powerful classifying technique based on probability over time, have widely used methods to detect cancer with CT and MRI images i.e., at organ level (Vincey and Saravana, 2013), however there is almost no published report regarding its use in analyzing histopathological images. The reason may be that histopathological image processing and analysis is more difficult issues compared to radiological image processing and analysis, as the former images have "exceptionally muddled structure" compared to later type of images (Aswathy and Jagannath, 2017).

Particle Swarm Optimization

Kennedy and Eberhart 1995 first introduced the Particle Swarm Optimization (PSO). It is a simple heuristic technique used for global optimization problem. PSO algorithm is now being widely used for cell detection and separation from histopathology and MRI images in an automated way. From histopathological biospsy image of breast cancer, it is used to differentiate between mitotic and non-mitosis cells and thereby the non-mitosis cells will be deleted. From such extracted features, SVM is applied to classify the mitotic cells (Nateghi et al, 2014). This search technique is inspired by swarm intelligence. Like swarm intelligence, particles in PSO system behaves as a swarm of individuals, fly through the search space looking for target, thus make solution for optimization. To reach optimum result, each particles (swarm) continuously update their position (global best, personal best) and velocity. Each particle looks for its own personal best position (*pbest*) based on previous visits by its own. On the other hand, global best (*gbest*) is calculated from the entire swarm (particles) by selecting each of the *pbest* (Shi and Eberhart, 1998). During each iteration velocity of a particle's is updated by following relation:

$$v_i(t+1) = v_i(\mathrm{t}) + (c_1 \times rand() \times (p_i^{best} - p_i(t))) + (c_2 \times rand() \times (p_{gbest} - p_i(t))),$$

where $v_i(t+1)$ denote new velocity for the *i-th* particle; c_1 and c_2 represent the weighting coefficients for the *pbest* and *gbest* positions respectively, $p_i(t)$ is the *i-th* particle's position at time t, $p_i^{best}$is the *i-th* particle's best known position, and p_{gbest} is the global best position known to the swarm. The *rand*() function generates a uniformly random variable. A particle's position in local neighborhood is updated based on its velocity by the following relation:

$$p_i(t+1) = p_i(t) + v_i(t)$$

Algorithm for cancer cell detection (segmentation) by PSO can be followed as below.

##

Algorithm of Single Object particle swarm optimization

Step 1: Parameter setting for defining population size, boundary selection for optimal solution and initialization of swarm (population)
Step 2: Evaluate fitness value for each particle of swarm (i.e., by determination of *gbest* for all particles), thus *pbest* is selected (If fitness value is better than *pbest* value, then that fitness value become *pbest* value)
Step 3: Next each particle update its velocity and position using above equations
Step 4: Exit if iteration reaches max, else go to step 2.

Support Vector Machine

A Support Vector Machine (SVM) is a supervised learning model that analyzes image data for both classification and regression (Thai, 2012); and different biological problems (Noble, 2004; Noble, 2006). SVM is a discriminative classifier in two dimensional space where a line dividing a plane in two parts such a way that each class lay in either side. The main drawback of SVM algorithm is that, it handles problems through only binary classification; however, it can solve optimization problem for large data sets very quickly. It is used in many Geo- and Environmental Sciences, content based image retrieval, Facial expression classification, Texture Classification, text classification, Image Clustering and Protein Structure Prediction.

##

Algorithm of SVM

Step 1: Select minimum and maximum value from given range of inputs.
Step 2: Scaled the data value using following formula:

New value (after scaling) = (current value - Min value) / (Max value-Min value)

Step 3: Determined new values are transformed to binary form i.e., either 0 or 1.
Step 4: These data value can be used as an input to the neural network for training and testing based on preset vigilance parameter, training parameter and testing parameter.

Genetic Algorithm

Due to poor image contrast or difuse cell/organ/tissue boundaries, segmentation of medical images become a challenge. Genetic algorithm is widely used for automatic segmentation and classification of different type of images like CT/ MRI images. But Genetic algorithm-based techniques sometime suffer from the problem of premature convergence. This problem arises when some individuals in a population are more fit than the other, and are selected for generation of future progeny.

The genetic algorithm (GAs) are derivative free stochastic optimization heuristic methods based on basic operations such as selection, crossover, mutation and also use some given fitness function. The selection operator is used to choose chromosomes from a population for mating. Hence, parents from highest fitness values are considered. A score is assigned for fitness function to each chromosome in the current population, and fitness of each chromosome is dependent to the closeness of the chromosome to the solution of the problem. The crossover function is the sharing of information between two chromosomes. The mutation operator changes allele values in the chromosome thereby structural variability in chromosome is increased. The evaluation of the new candidate solutions comprises the calculation of the fitness values. The algorithm terminates with the reaching of preselected optimum solution or other predefined termination criteria. GA is applied in breast cancer histopathological images for segmentation of elements and classification of extracted features from medical images (Wang et al, 2016). Other applications are in various fields, like automated control of industrial equipment, in the field of Bioinformatics (RNA structure prediction), clustering and optimizing a wide range of different fit-functions, and Quality control.

##

Algorithm of GA

Step 1: [Initialize (population)] The initial population is generated randomly where the parent nodes are represented in binary sequence. The population size is dependent on the solution to the problem.
Step 2: [Evaluate (population)] In this step the fitness function F(x) for each of the population is calculated and stored.
Step 3: [New (Population)] In this step a new population is created by applying the following steps.
Step 3.1: [Selection (Population)] In this selection two of the parent node is selected from the population according to their fitness (the better fitness, the bigger chance to be selected).
Step 3.2: [Crossover (population)] In this step with a crossover probability the cross over is performed between parent to form a new offspring (children). If no crossover was performed, offspring is an exact copy of parents.
Step 3.3: [Mutate (population)] In this step, with a mutation probability the mutation is performed to mutate new offspring at a particular locus (position in chromosome).
Step 3.4: [Accepting (population)] In this step the new offspring are placed in a new population.
Step 4: [Replace (Population)] In this step the old population is replaced by the newly generated population.
Step 5: [Test] In this step check is done to find out if the stopping condition is satisfied or not. If the stopping condition is satisfied, then stop, and return the best solution in current population. Otherwise go to step 2.

From histopathological images nuclei is segmented first followed by feature extraction analysis by GA (Wang et al, 2016). The algorithm is applied in the following manner:

Step 1: Digital RGB image as input
Step 2: Contrast enhancement between nuclei and background by top-bottom hat transform
Step 3: ROI is extracted with Harr wavelet transformation where objects with different pre-defined radius R and threshold T is extracted.

Step 4: Overlapping nuclei are separated based on predefined circularity (R) and area (A). If the calculated R is greater than certain value, ROI is segmented out, thus non-overlapping ROI is saved.

Step 5: Overlapping cells are identified with concavity and morphological erotion followed by reconstruction of cells by morphological dilatation of eroded cells. Both the methods are applied by choosing the appropriate structuring element in an adaptive way. The whole process is termed as 'Improved Morphological Operation'.

Step 6: If any portion is not segmented with the step 4, then curvature scale space (CSS) is applied for further segmentation. With this, corner pairs are linearized, and if all corner pairs are lined then it is segmented and result is saved.

Step 7: Cellular features like area, perimeter, roundness, eccentricity and textual features of spatial are extracted.

Random Forests

The random forests algorithm is a supervised learning algorithm which is generally being used for classification of images and generation of continuous variables. This algorithm is simple and can be used for both classification and regression problem. In regression problems, the dependent variable is continuous on the other hand classification problems is categorical. Random forests is an ensemble model that means it analyzes results that are from other models and thus recalculate to generate a finer result. Hence, it is expected that it provide a better result than results out of single individual models (Dahinden 2009). In this model, several decision trees are created and the result is calculated based on the output result of all the decision trees (Horning 2010).

##

Algorithm of Random Forest

Step 1: In the training set, N number of cases are considered at random - but with replacement, from the original data. So the training set sample will be the growing tree.

Step 2: If there are M input variables, a number mM is specified such that at each node, m variables are selected at random out of the M and the best split on these m is used to split the node. The value of m is held constant during the forest growing.

Step 3: Each tree is grown to the largest extent possible. There is no pruning.

Artificial Neural Networks

An artificial neuron network (ANN) is a computational model. It is based on functions and structure of neural networks. The structure of ANN may be affected for information that flows through network. ANN is a non-linear statistical data modeling tools. It takes data samples rather than whole data sets to get solution, which saves both time and money. This mathematical models use to enhance existing data analysis technologies.

##

Algorithm of ANN

Step1: Multiply that input by its weight for every input.
Step2: Sum all of the weighted inputs are calculated.
Step3: Next the output of the perceptron based on that sum passed through an activation function is computed along with the sign of the sum.

AUTOMATED CANCER CELL DETECTION

The automated system analyzes morphological features like, cell shape for detection and classify cells as cancerous or non-cancerous (Jain et al, 2014). The stages of the entire process is divided into a number of stages, namely, Image Pre-processing, Image Segmentation, Feature Extraction and Classification. Each of the steps follows the steps as mentioned earlier. The major challenge of automated image analysis is the clustered, joined and overlapping cells in an image. With the extracted features there are numerous supervised and unsupervised methods are available for the classification and/or clustering of elements. Followings are most commonly used techniques for biomedical image analysis: K-means, Fuzzy c-means, Super Vector Machine (SVM), Neural Networks, Decision trees, Bayesian classifiers, and NN classifiers and are shown in Figure 1. Algorithm of each of the process is described early. Here a summary of the application of algorithm for histopathological image analysis is presented (Table 2).

Figure 1. Different processes for automated image analysis.

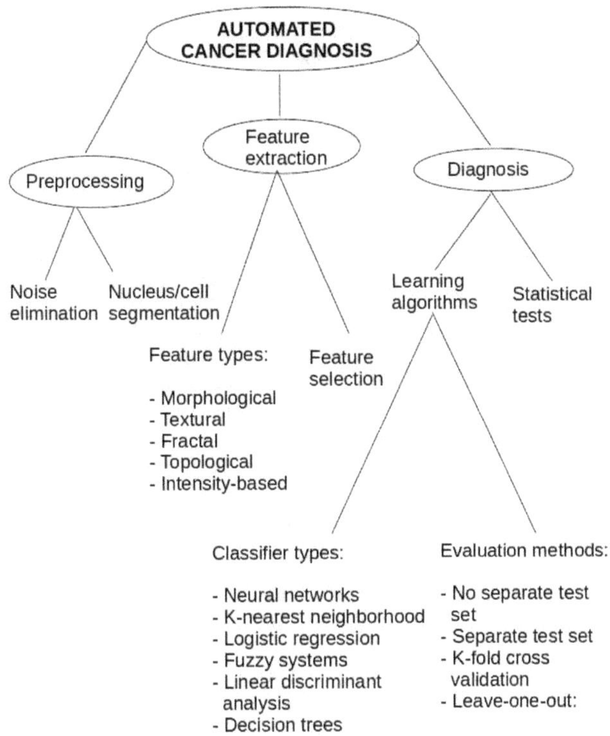

BIOMEDICAL OPEN ACCESS DATA RESOURCE

Conventionally clinical data are collected through case report forms (CRF) in hard copy, therefore it requires further data entry into a relational database. In recent time such data collection can be done through Electronic Data Capture (EDC) an intriguing alternative. The major advantages of EDC would be the reduction of time and faster analysis of data in with online validation checks in real-time (Walther et al 2011). There are two types of data sources viz., primary and secondary. The primary data are those which are collected afresh for the first time by the researcher. The secondary data are those which have already been collected by someone else and which have already been passed through the statistical process and researcher further reanalyze that data to make inference further. So development of web base data collection is now becoming a growing trend in the field of different medical informatics research. This can also be extended towards collection of image data. Presently several online open access image data resources are available. Below is the list of such resources.

Table 2. Comparison of the application of different advanced technique for histopathological image analysis.

Reference	Cancer	Image Size	Number of Images	Comment
Ali et al, 2008	Prostate	500 × 324 pixels	129 images	Development of Computer aided diagnosis (CAD) system for automatic grading of histological images of prostate cancer tissue. This CAD system is based on Support Vector Machines (SVM) with accuracy of 92.24%.
Nateghi et al, 2014	Breast	40x magnification	236 images from 35 image database	Automatic mitotic cell detection using PSO & classify them using SVM with the F-measure 78.57%.
Kumar et al, 2015	Cancer	Different magnifications – 5x, 10x, 20x and 40x	2828 images	For segmentation of background cells, K-means segmentation algorithm is used also -nearest neighborhood method is used for classification of images with an accuracy of 92%.
Spanhol et al, 2016	Breast	Different magnifications - 40×, 100×, 200×, and 400× acquired from a single slide of breast tissue	7909 images from http://web.inf.ufpr.br/vri/breast-cancer-database	Using Convolution Neural Network, accuracy is 87% at 100x magnification.
Wang et al, 2016	Breast	40x magnification	68 images	Genetic algorithm is used to classify between normal and malignant with an accuracy of 96.19%.
Araujo et al, 2017	Breast	40x magnification	70 images	Using Convolution Neural Network classify different types of breast cancer (benign, in-situ, invasive) with an accuracy of 77.8% and malignant non-malignant with an accuracy 95.6%.

- Cell Image Library (url: www.cellimagelibrary.org/pages/contribute)
- The National Center for Biomedical Ontology (url: www.alpha.bioontology.org)
- DAML Ontology Library (url: www.daml.org/ontologies)
- The Cancer Genome Atlas (TCGA)

IMAGE ANALYSIS FOR EARLY DETECTION OF CANCER

Mathematical morphology and image processing methods have used for early detection of cancer. Cachexia is a prevalent condition occur in all types of cancer. Considering leukemia, it has been hypothesized that RBCs are affected under the condition and morphological alterations in both intact RBC and its membrane was noted by high resolution ultrastructural images (Majumder et al, 2006). As such observations are confirmed in both hypoplastic anemia and myelodysplastic syndrome, so it is hypothesized that such features may be the representative of early sign of leukemia. Mathematical morphology and image processing techniques are utilized to get the quantitative changes in the ultrastructural images of RBCs (Das et al, 2015). The same algorithm for mathematical morphology and image processing have utilized to detect changes in light microscopic images (Das and Majumder, 2016).

CONCLUSION

Though histopathological image analysis is more difficult compared to radiological image analysis, but recent attempts are more promising and encouraging (Aswathy and Jagannath, 2017). It is becoming very powerful method for not only cancer detection, but also may be utilized to detect pre-cancerous state. Morphological alteration in red blood cells (RBCs) could be an indicator of cancer cachexia. Such alterations are also noted in hypoplastic anemia and myelodysplasia. These disease conditions are considered as the pre-leukemic state. Though such changes can readily be validated through ultra-structural images, but high resolution ultra-structural image acquisition may not be possible for ordinary clinical settings. Recent work suggests that image analysis techniques with light microscopic images reflect the ultra-structural changes in red blood cells (Das and Majumder, 2016). Interestingly this can be performed with few blood drops of peripheral blood. So it can be inferred that image analysis techniques are powerful tool for diagnosis of pre-leukemic state. However, there is no image database of peripheral blood of different cancers. With the availability of histological images of peripheral blood, this can be tested to validate whether or not image analysis of RBCs could show any sign for the early stage of other cancers. Different machine learning tools and statistical analysis could be the necessary aid in this direction.

Due to the steady increase of the amount of medical image data, fast procedures are needed for feature extraction. This will help in narrowing the gap between the numerical nature of features and the semantic meaning of images. Though several computational methods are being applied for analyzing medical images, but those methods are being applied for few cases of histopathological images of cancer and moreover, in most scientific works scientists are concerned with a specific technique and on a specific case, therefore at present it is difficult to make a comparative analysis about the performance of different techniques. Future works are needed to make a comparison of different algorithms on different types and cases of cancer with respect to histopathological image data analysis.

Several symptoms based qualitative information still be important criteria in medical diagnostic. Hence, combining image content with natural language-based access to medical case records will provide advanced case-based reasoning methodology for medical diagnostics as well as treatment. Therefore, interfacing image processing with automatic text analysis could be the subsequent challenge in computer assisted diagnostics (Scholl et al 2011). Such combination has suggested by Middle-out Rational Approach (MORA) of Systems Biology for transforming qualitative information into quantitative statement (Majumder et al, 2017). Hence, such amalgamation has further importance in the diagnosis of pre-cancerous state.

REFERENCES

Ada & Kaur, R. (2013). Feature extraction and principal component analysis for lung cancer detection in CT images. *International Journal of Advanced Research in Computer Science and Software Engineering*, *3*(3), 187–190.

Al-amri, S. S., Kalyankar, N. V., & Khamitkar, S. D. (2010). Image Segmentation by using Thresholding Technique. *Journal of Computers*, *2*(5), 83–86.

Ali, U., Shaukat, A., Hussain, M., Ali, J., Khan, K., Khan, M. B., & Shah, M. A. (2016). Automatic Cancerous Tissue Classification using Discrete Wavelet Transformation and Support Vector Machine. *Journal of Basic and Applied Scientific Research*, *6*(7), 15–23.

Andrion, A., Magnani, C., Betta, P. G., Donna, A., Mollo, F., Scelsi, M., ... Terracini, B. (1995). Malignant mesothelioma of the pleura: Inter-observer variability. *Journal of Clinical Pathology*, *48*(9), 856–860. doi:10.1136/jcp.48.9.856 PMID:7490321

Araújo, T., Aresta, G., Castro, E., Rouco, J., Aguiar, P., Eloy, C., ... Campilho, A. (2017). Classification of breast cancer histology images using Convolutional. *Neural Networks*, *12*(6), e0177544. doi:10.1371/journal.pone.0177544 PMID:28570557

Aswathy, M. A., & Jagannath, M. (2017). Detection of breast cancer on digital histopathology images: Present status and future possibilities. *Informatics in Medicine Unlocked*, *8*, 74–79. doi:10.1016/j.imu.2016.11.001

Basavanhallya, A., Yu, E., Xu, J., Ganesan, S., Feldman, M., Tomaszewski, J., Madabhushi, A. (2011). Incorporating Domain Knowledge for tubule detection in breast histopathology using O'Callaghan neighborhoods, *SPIE Medical Imaging, 7963: 796310.*

Chatap, N., & Shibu, S. (2014). Analysis of blood samples for counting leukemia cells using Support vector machine and nearest neighbour. *IOSR Journal of Computer Engineering*, *16*(5), 79–87. doi:10.9790/0661-16537987

Dahinden, C. (2009). *An improved random forests approach with application to the performance prediction challenge datasets*. Zurich, Switzerland: Seminar fur Statistik. pp. 1-6

Das, M., Das, B., Das, A., Chatterjee, I., & Majumder, D. (2015). Computational analysis of ultrastructural images of red blood cells. *Journal of Oncology Translational Research*, *1*, 104. doi:10.4172/jotr.1000104

Das, M., & Majumder, D. (2016). An analytical approach for leukemia diagnosis from light microscopic images of RBCs. *Proceedings of 2nd International Conference of Next Generation Computing Technology*, 21-24. doi: 10.1109/NGCT.2016.7877383

Demir, C., & Yener, B. (2005). Automated cancer diagnosis based on histopathological images: A systematic survey. *Technical Report, Rensselaer Polytechnic Institute, Department of Computer Science, TR 05-09*, 1–16.

Demir, C., & Yener, B. (2016). Automated cancer diagnosis based on histopathological images A systematic survey. *Technical Report, TR 05-09*, 1–16.

Demirkaya, O., Aysali, M. H., & Sahoo, P. K. (2009). Image processing with MATLAB applications in medicine and biology (pp. 53). London: CRC Press.

Di Ruberto, C., Dempster, A., Khan, S., & Jarra, B. (2000). Segmentation of blood images using morphological operators. *Proceedings of 15th International Conference on Pattern Recognition*, 3, 397 –400. 10.1109/ICPR.2000.903568

Di Ruberto, C., Dempster, A., Khan, S., & Jarra, B. (2002). Analysis of infected blood cell images using morphological operators. *Image and Vision Computing*, *20*(2), 133–146. doi:10.1016/S0262-8856(01)00092-0

Gillibert, L., & Jeulin, D. (1994). Stochastic multiscale segmentation constrained by image content, In J. Serra & P. Soille (Eds.), Mathematical morphology and its applications to image processing (pp. 132-138). Kluwer Academic Publishers.

Gonzalez, R. C., Woods, R. E., & Eddins, S. L. (2009). Introduction. In *Digital Image Processing Using MATLAB* (3rd ed.; pp. 2–3). Knoxville, TN: Pearson.

Gurcan, M. N., Boucheron, L., Can, A., Madabhushi, A., Rajpoot, N., & Yener, B. (2009). Histopatological Image Analysis: A Review. *IEEE Reviews in Biomedical Engineering*, *2*, 147–171. doi:10.1109/RBME.2009.2034865 PMID:20671804

Gurcan, M. N., Pan, T., Shimada, H., & Saltz, J. (2006). Image analysis for neuroblastoma classification: Segmentation of cell nuclei. *Proceedings of IEEE International Conference on Engineering in Medicine and Biology Society*, *1*, 4844-4847. 10.1109/IEMBS.2006.260837

Horning, N. (2010). Random forests: an algorithm for image classification and generation of continuous fields data sets. *Proceedings of International Conference on Geo-informatics for Spatial Infrastructure Development in Earth and Allied Science*, 1-6.

Ismail, S. M., Colclough, A. B., Dinnen, J. S., Eakins, D., Evans, D. M., Gradwell, E., ... Newcombe, R. G. (1989). Observer variation in histopathological diagnosis and grading of cervical intraepithelial neoplasia. *British Medical Journal*, *298*(6675), 707–710. doi:10.1136/bmj.298.6675.707 PMID:2496816

Jain, A., Atey, S., Vinayak, S., & Srivastava, V. (2014). Cancerous cell detection using histopathological image analysis. *International Journal of Innovative Research in Computer and Communication Engineering*, *2*(12), 7419–7426. doi:10.15680/IJIRCCE.2014.0212026

Kadachha, S. L., & Patel, P. J. (2013). Cancer detection using modified watershed. *International Journal of Engineering Research & Technology*, *2*(5), 2161–2164.

Kaur, S., & Jindal, G. (2011). Watershed segmentation of lung ct scan images for early diagnosis of cancer. *International Journal of Computer and Electrical Engineering*, *3*, 850–855. doi:10.7763/IJCEE.2011.V3.431

Kennedy, J., & Eberhart, R. C. (1995). Particle swarm optimization. In *Proceedings of the IEEE International Conference on Neural Networks, IV* (pp. 1942–1948). Piscataway, NJ: IEEE Service Center. 10.1109/ICNN.1995.488968

Kennedy, J., & Eberhart, R. C. (1997), A discrete binary version of the particle swarm algorithm, *Proceedings 1997 Conference on Systems, Man, and Cybernetics* (pp. 4104–4109). Piscataway, NJ: IEEE Service Center. 10.1109/ICSMC.1997.637339

Khan, A. (2016). Content based image retrieval using genetic algorithm. *International Journal Engineering Science and Computing*, *6*(7), 8144–8148.

Kumar, R., Srivastava, R., & Srivastava, S. (2015). Detection and classification of cancer from microscopic biopsy images using clinically significant and biologically interpretable features. *Journal of Medical Engineering* 457906: 1-14. doi: 10.1155/2015/457906

Ledda, A., Quintelier, J., Samyn, P., Baets, P. D., & Philips, W. (2000). Quantitative image analysis with mathematical morphology. *Proceeding of ProRISC2003*, (pp. 399-406), Veldhoven, Netherlands.

Magota, K., Kubo, N., Kuge, Y., Nishijima, K., Zhao, S., & Tamaki, N. (2011). Performance characterization of the Inveon preclinical small-animal PET/SPECT/CT system for multimodality imaging. *European Journal of Nuclear Medicine and Molecular Imaging*, *38*(4), 742–752. doi:10.100700259-010-1683-y PMID:21153410

Majumder, D., Banerjee, D., Chandra, S., Banerjee, S., & Chakrabarti, A. (2006). Red cell morphology in leukemia, hypoplastic anemia and myelodysplastic syndrome. *Pathophysiology*, *13*(4), 217–225. doi:10.1016/j.pathophys.2006.06.002 PMID:16876391

Majumder, D., Ray, D. K., Chatterjee, I., & Dhar, P. K. (2017). Translation of middle out rational approach (MORA) in an understanding of therapeutic outcome of cancer: Experience from India. *Journal of Translational Research*, *1*(1), 4–7.

Mankoff, D. (2007). A definition of molecular imaging. *Journal of Nuclear Medicine*, *48*(6), 18N–21N. PMID:17536102

Nateghi, R., Danyali, H., Helfroush, M. S., & Tashk, A. (2014). Mitosis detection from breast cancer histology slide images using particle swarm optimization and support vector machine. *International Journal of Sciences: Basic and Applied Research*, *16*(2), 164–177.

Noble, W. S. (2004). Support vector machine applications in computational biology. In *Kernel Methods in Computational Biology* (pp. 71–92). Cambridge, MA: MIT Press.

Noble, W. S. (2006). What is a support vector machine? *Nature Biotechnology*, *24*(12), 1565–1567. doi:10.1038/nbt1206-1565 PMID:17160063

Omran, M. (2005). *Particle swarm optimization methods for pattern recognition and image processing* (Ph.D. Thesis Computer Science). University of Pretoria.

Pichler, B., Kolb, A., Nagele, T., & Schlemmer, H. (2010). PET/MRI: Paving the way for the next generation of clinical multimodality imaging applications. *Journal of Nuclear Medicine*, *51*(3), 333–336. doi:10.2967/jnumed.109.061853 PMID:20150252

Rajgire, B., Khobragade, P., Haygune, B. K., & Dhoke, G. (2017). Formation of clusters with K –Means algorithm using tumor classification. *Proceedings of the International Conference on Recent Trends in Engineering Science and Technology*, *5*(1), 199-201.

Renato, K. (2000). A morphological view on traditional signal processing. In *Mathematical morphology & its applications to image & signal processing, Computational imaging & vision series* (Vol. 18, pp. 3–12). Springer.

Ringnér, M. (2008). What is principal component analysis? *Nature Biotechnology, 26*(3), 303–304. doi:10.1038/nbt0308-303 PMID:18327243

Scholl, I., Aach, T., Deserno, T. M., & Kuhlen, T. (2011). Challenges of medical image processing. *Computer Science Research & Development, 26*(1-2), 5–13. doi:10.100700450-010-0146-9

Sertel, O., Catalyurek, U. V., Shimada, H., & Gurcan, M. N. (2009). Computer-aided prognosis of neuroblastoma: Detection of mitosis and karyorrhexis cells in digitized histological images. In *Proceedings of IEEE Engineering in Medicine and Biology Society* (pp. 1433-1436). IEEE. 10.1109/IEMBS.2009.5332910

Sharma, D., & Jindal, G. (2011). Identifying lung cancer using image processing technique. *Proceedings of International Conference Computation Technique Artificial Intelligence*, 115-120.

Shi, Y., & Eberhart, R. C. (1998a). Parameter selection in particle swarm optimization, In *Evolutionary Programming VII: Proc. EP98* (pp. 591-600). New York: Springer-Verlag.

Shi, Y., & Eberhart, R. C. (1998b). A Modified Particle Swarm Optimizer. In *IEEE International Conference on Evolutionary Computation* (pp. 69-73). Anchorage, AK: IEEE.

Spanhol, F. A., Oliveira, L. S., Petitjean, C., & Heutte, L. (2016). Breast cancer histopathological image classification using convolutional neural networks. *Proceedings of the International Joint Conference of Neural Networks (IJCNN 2016)*, 2560-2567. 10.1109/IJCNN.2016.7727519

Sudha, V., & Jayashree, P. (2012). Lung nodule detection in CT images using thresholding and morphological operations. *International Journal of Emerging Science & Engineering, 1*, 17–21.

Thai, L. H., Hai, T. S., & Thuy, N. T. (2012). Image classification using support vector machine and artificial neural network. *International Journal of Information Technology and Computer Science, 5*(5), 32–38. doi:10.5815/ijitcs.2012.05.05

Tolxdorff, T., Deserno, T. M., Handels, H., & Meinzer, H. P. (2004). Advances in biomedical image analysis past, present and future challenges. *Methods of Information in Medicine, 43*(4), 308–314. doi:10.1055-0038-1633873 PMID:15472739

Townsend, D., Carney, J., Yap, J., & Hall, N. (2004). PET/CT today and tomorrow. *Journal of Nuclear Medicine*, *45*(1), 4S–14S. PMID:14736831

Vincey, J. M. V., & Saravana, K. E. (2013). Computer aided diagnosis for liver cancer using statistical model. *International Journal of Research in Engineering & Technology*, *2*(12), 84–89. doi:10.15623/ijret.2013.0212014

Waheed, S., Moffitt, R. A., Chaudry, Q., Young, A. N., & Wang, M. D. (2007). Computer aided histopathological classification of cancer subtypes. *Proceedings of the 7th IEEE International Conference on Bioinformatics and Bioengineering*, 503-508. 10.1109/BIBE.2007.4375608

Walther, B., Hossin, S., Townend, J., Abernethy, N., Parker, D., & Jeffries, D. (2011). Comparison of electronic data capture (EDC) with the standard data capture method for clinical trial data. *PLoS One*, *6*(9), 1–11. doi:10.1371/journal.pone.0025348 PMID:21966505

Wang, P., Hu, X., Li, Y., Liu, Q., & Zhu, X. (2016). Automatic cell nuclei segmentation and classification of breast cancer histopathology images. *Signal Processing*, *122*, 1–13. doi:10.1016/j.sigpro.2015.11.011

Xu, J., Janowczyk, A., Chandran, S., & Madabhushi, A. (2010). A weighted mean shift, normalized cuts initialized color gradient based geodesic active contour model: Applications to histopathology image segmentation. *Proceeding SPIE Digital Library*, *7623*(76230Y), 1-12. Retrieved from http://spiedl.org/terms

Yu, K-H., Zhang, C., Berry, G.J., Altman, R.B., Re,´C., Rubin, D.L., & Snyder, M. (2016). Predicting non-small cell lung cancer prognosis by fully automated microscopic pathology image features. *Nature Communications*, *7*. doi: 10.1038/ncomms12474

ADDITIONAL READING

Chakraborty, S., Chatterjee, S., Ashour, A. S., Mali, K., & Dey, N. (2017). *Intelligent Computing in Medical Imaging: A Study* (p. 143). Advancements in Applied Metaheuristic Computing.

Chakraborty, S., Chatterjee, S., Dey, N., Ashour, A. S., Ashour, A. S., Shi, F., & Mali, K. (2017). Modified cuckoo search algorithm in microscopic image segmentation of hippocampus. *Microscopy Research and Technique*, *80*(10), 1051–1072. doi:10.1002/jemt.22900 PMID:28557041

Das, H., Jena, A. K., Nayak, J., Naik, B., & Behera, H. S. (2015). A novel PSO based back propagation learning-MLP (PSO-BP-MLP) for classification. In *Computational Intelligence in Data Mining-Volume 2* (pp. 461–471). New Delhi: Springer. doi:10.1007/978-81-322-2208-8_42

Das, M., Das, B., Das, A., Chatterjee, I., & Majumder, D. (2015). Computational analysis of ultrastructural images of red blood cells. *Journal of Oncology Translational Research*, *1*, 104. doi:10.4172/jotr.1000104

Das, M., & Majumder, D. (2016). An analytical approach for leukemia diagnosis from light microscopic images of RBCs, In *Proceedings of 2nd International Conference of Next Generation Computing Technology*, pp. 21-24, doi: 10.1109/NGCT.2016.7877383

Dey, N., & Ashour, A. S. "Computing in Medical Image Analysis." In Soft Computing Based Medical Image Analysis, pp. 3-11. 2018. doi:10.1016/B978-0-12-813087-2.00025-7

Kamal, S., Dey, N., Nimmy, S. F., Ripon, S. H., Ali, N. Y., Ashour, A. S., ... Shi, F. (2018). Evolutionary framework for coding area selection from cancer data. *Neural Computing & Applications*, *29*(4), 1015–1037. doi:10.100700521-016-2513-3

Rajinikanth, V. (2018). Suresh Chandra Satapathy, Nilanjan Dey, and R. Vijayarajan. "DWT-PCA Image Fusion Technique to Improve Segmentation Accuracy in Brain Tumor Analysis. In *Microelectronics, Electromagnetics and Telecommunications* (pp. 453–462). Singapore: Springer. doi:10.1007/978-981-10-7329-8_46

Thanki, R., Borra, S., Dey, N., & Ashour, A. S. (2018). Medical Imaging and Its Objective Quality Assessment: An Introduction. In *Classification in BioApps* (pp. 3–32). Cham: Springer. doi:10.1007/978-3-319-65981-7_1

Chapter 5 Multi-Criteria Decision-Making Techniques for Histopathological Image Classification

Revathi T.
Mepco Schlenk Engineering College, India

Saroja S.
Mepco Schlenk Engineering College, India

Haseena S.
Mepco Schlenk Engineering College, India

Blessa Binolin Pepsi M.
Mepco Schlenk Engineering College, India

ABSTRACT

This chapter presents an overview of methods that have been proposed for analysis of histopathological images. Diagnosing and detecting abnormalities in medical images helps the pathologist in making better decisions. Different machine learning algorithms such as k-nearest neighbor, random forest, support vector machine, ensemble learning, multilayer perceptron, and convolutional neural network are incorporated for carrying out the analysis process. Further, multi-criteria decision-making (MCDM) methods such as SAW, WPM, and TOPSIS are used to improve the efficiency of the decision-making process.

DOI: 10.4018/978-1-5225-6316-7.ch005

INTRODUCTION

Over past decades, determination of diseased histopathological image has become a difficult task for radiologists. Image analysis with computer aided analytical approaches for diagnosis play a major rule in present era (Barik, Dubey, Misra, Borthakur, Constant, Sasane, & Mankodiya, 2018). Histopathology refers a minute identification of a tissue in order to learn the symptom of a disease which is being carried out from biopsy examination or by a surgical specimen. The process highly depends on radiologist or pathologist's opinion which becomes a hectic issue in some preliminary cases. To add up with manual result, a computational environment is recommended for working in digitized tissue histopathological images. As microscopic images have a momentous role for visualizing and interpreting the cells and tissues, image analysis is opted in this chapter with new machine learning techniques and decision making algorithms incorporated together for disease detection, diagnosis and prognosis prediction which can aid the physician's opinion. In addition, this chapter also deals quantitative characterization and analysis of pathological imagery which is important for clinical and research application to reduce variations in diagnosis and to comprehend the biological mechanism of disease. This chapter mainly focuses on method to identify the categories by classification into favorable or unfavorable tissue morphology and multicriteria decision making method assists with it to correctly diagnose the diseased tissue for further treatment planning. This chapter also includes experimental analysis results of various classification algorithms with multicriteria decision making techniques to determine class labels with high accuracy (Blessa Binolin Pepsi & Bargavi, 2017). Overall design of this chapter is presented in Figure 1.

BACKGROUND

Automated histopathological image data analysis is a research to complement the pathological diagnosis process thereby to relieve their workload. Once preprocessing has been performed, data analytics is carried out to the histopathological image which is one of challenge that is discussed in detail in this chapter (Panigrahi, Tiwary, Pati, & Das, 2016: Sarkhel, Das & Vashishtha, 2017). The techniques are applied on training samples to classify the images which are facilitated by machine learning approaches. Further the pre trained model can be made accurate using decision making algorithms. The performance of the algorithms is measured using experimental analysis. The results define the efficiency and effectiveness of the multi criteria decision making approach for histopathological image classification.

Figure 1. Overall design

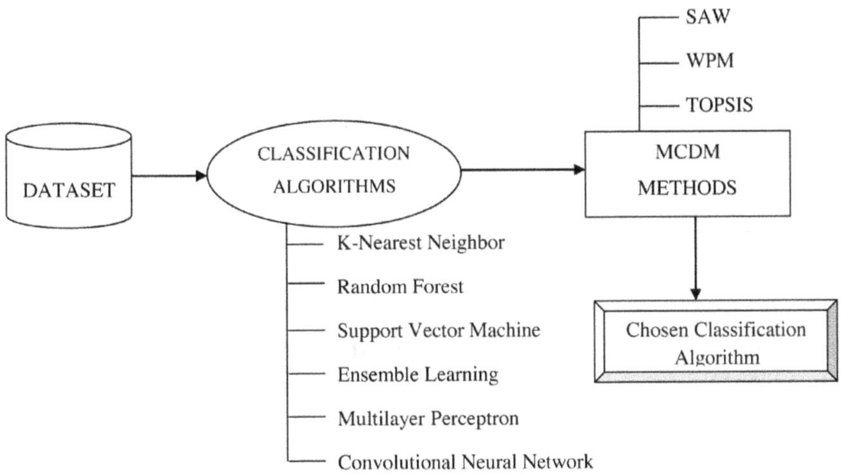

MAIN FOCUS OF THE CHAPTER

This chapter presents machine learning techniques for image analysis and multicriteria decision making techniques for quantitative characterization and analysis of classification algorithms (Thanki, Rohit, Surekha, Nilanjan, & Amira, 2018).

Issues, Controversies, Problems

Conventional histopathological image analysis includes biopsy examination or by means of surgical specimen. Accuracy of this method is in the hands of radiologist or pathologist decision, it may be error prone. Moreover, this method is invasive; it incurs time, pain and discomfort.

IMAGE ANALYSIS BY CLASSIFICATION

Classification is one of the broad areas of decisions making approaches to distinguish the images (Haseena, 2015). The algorithms used for classification depicts the decision of classes based on one or more features. The value of features is assigned based on pixel values in the image. The classes can be specified prior by an analyst with the number of categories needed to divide. Image classification normally relies on numerical values of features to be organized into classes. In general, classification being a supervised approach (i.e. learning process forms a mapping between data to another set of variable information classes) is divided into training and testing phase (Reddy, Das & Roy, 2017). In training, based on image features classification category are assigned. Hence, based on category the training phase and the testing phase classify the new features. The main idea here is to learn the relationship between the data and categorized classes. Image classification can include two or more classes based on the process. The classification methods are explained as follows.

Instance Based Learning

In machine learning, instance based learning is group of algorithms applied on training instances stored thereby improving the performance (Ripon, Shamim, Linkon, Amira & Nilanjan, 2018). This builds a hypothesis for the training instances mapping to a class label. From the store of built hypothesis on training set, the system can predict the class for new test instance based on computation of distance or similarities between the observed training instances. This being a supervised learning task involves learning from examples. Each instance in the data includes attribute-value pairs. The attributes given in an n-dimensional space corresponds to multiple predictor attributes with one category attribute. The values in the category attribute are disjoint. The prime output of this Instance Based Learning (IBL) algorithm is concept description that is a function used for mapping instances to categories on a set of stored instances based on past performance during classification (Sahani, Rout, Badajena, Jena, & Das, 2018).

The three main components of IBL algorithm are similarity function, classification function and concept description updater. Similarity function identifies the similarity measure between instance and concept description at a particular time. Classification function use the similarity values, instances in the concept description and determines the class labels Concept Description Updater maintains a record of classification performance values to include instances in the concept description.

In general, IBL algorithm classifies similar category for similar instances i.e. based on most similar neighbors rather than prior knowledge.

This IBL algorithm focuses on 3 steps of classification based on updated concept description, limited storage and noise tolerance. In the initial step of concept description, the similarity function is calculated

$$Similarity\left(x,y\right)=-\sqrt{\sum_{i=1}^{n}f\left(x_i,y_i\right)} \tag{1}$$

where n represents the number of attributes.

$$f\left(x_i, y_i\right) = \left(x_i - y_i\right)^2 \tag{2}$$

In case of missing values $f\left(x_i, y_i\right)$ is considered to be 1. This algorithm works similar to nearest neighbor algorithm but it normalizes the attribute ranges processing the instances incrementally. The concept description in IBL algorithm changes over time. Hence an extensional concept description is evolved from the set of saved instances to identify the classes.

In the second step, the collections of majority of misclassified instances are found to be near boundary instances that are located in c-neighborhood and outside the c-core of the target concept (for any small c). The instance away from concept boundary doesn't matter a lot. This is approximated by reducing the storage requirement i.e. not necessary to store all the instances to classify the test instance. The storage requirement is sensitive to noise and also the reduced instances should provide good accuracy. The third step is to check for noise tolerance in a reduced data with updated concept description. If instances in dataset are noise tolerant, then on misclassified instances, the probability of attribute value of each instance in test set can be modified with randomly selected value from the same attribute domain. A classification record is maintained to save the performance of training instances so that it performs well in near future. In addition, this IBL algorithm uses an implication to conclude which instances are good classifiers and which are noisy. The previous one can assist to classify the subsequent instances and latter can be discarded from the concept description

The overall flow of IBL algorithm can be given as,

```
Concept Description (CD) = NULL
for each instance in training set do
        for each y ∈ Concept Description do
                Sim[y] = Similarity(x,y)
        If  {y ∈ CD | acceptable(y)}
              then y_max = some acceptable y ∈ Concept
Description with maximal sim[y]
        else
              i = random value between [1, |CD|]
                      y_max  = some y ∈ CD that is the i^th most
similar instance to x
                    if class(x) ≠ class(y_max)
                      then classification <- correct
                else
```

```
                classification <- incorrect
                  CD = CD U {x}
                  for each y in CD do
                  if sim[y] >= sim [ymax  ]
                  then
                         update y's classification
record
                         if y's record is
significantly poor
                              Then CD = C - {y}
```

Advantage of the IBL algorithm is that it's simple and has the ability to adapt its model to formerly unobserved data instance. This simply stores a new instance or just throws away old instance. Simple example of an IBL algorithm is k nearest neighbor which stores a subset of the training instances to predict the class of new instance by computing the distances or similarity function values.

K Nearest Neighbor

K-NN is a simple machine learning algorithm that classifies the input based on K nearest neighbors to it. This is a non parametric method since the hypothesis is not made based on probability distribution of the input. It's a lazy learning method as it generalizes in testing phase and not training phase. K-NN has no model to be built i.e. model is dependent only on test instance, just stores the entire dataset to look up for the matching pattern, hence no learning is required. The outlier and erroneous data can be removed to maintain consistency in the entire data.

Predictions are made for a new test instance (y) by identifying the K most similar instances (neighbor) for y and define the output variable i.e. class label. High accuracy can be obtained for models at each instance level.

In order to find out the similarity for K instances given in training set to a new test instance, distance measure is used. For input variables, the most popular used distance measurement is Euclidean Distance. This Euclidean Distance given by the equation,

$$Euclidean\,Distance = \sqrt{\sum_{i=1}^{n}(x_i - y_i)^2} \tag{3}$$

Figure 2. An example of K-nn Classification

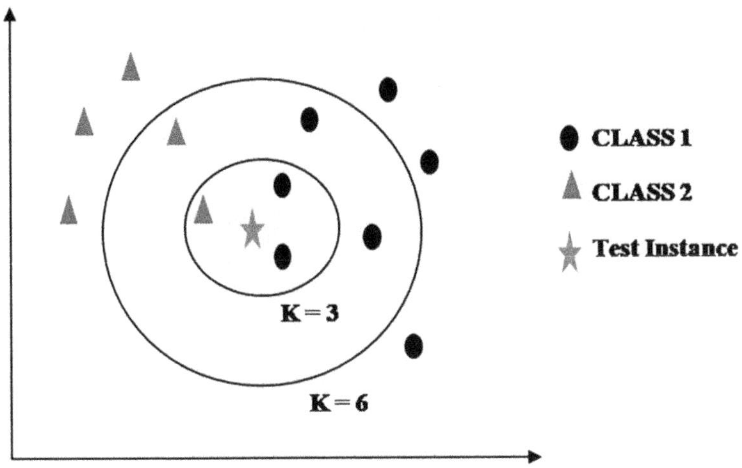

The other popular distance measures are Manhattan, Minkowski, Hamming, Jaccord, and Cosine distance etc. The distance metric can be chosen in relation to their properties i.e. real vector, binary vector etc. Hence in KNN the output classification result is based on highest frequency obtained by the K most similar instances.

The simple method choice of K on training instances can be framed by algorithm tuning which tries many values of K to identify the appropriate K for the given instance. The main conflict in the KNN is the curse of dimensionality. It works the best on low dimension but as the dimension increases, input volume space raises the exponential rate. Points that are similar may have large distances being far way from each other. So, in order to overcome the drawbacks of KNN and to maintain consistency of training data, it's better to perform dimensionality reduction, replace or delete missing values and standardize the data.

Random Forest

Random forest is ensembling of large number of decision trees during the training phase and identifies the output of the class label using the mode of resultant classes. Decision tree include a tree like graph structure to make decisions with the attributes as leaves or nodes and edges represent the conditional attribute values i.e the internal nodes tests an attribute, branch specifies the outcome of test and final leaf node represents class label. The pathway from root node to leaf node expresses the built

Figure 3. Overall flow of the k-nn algorithm

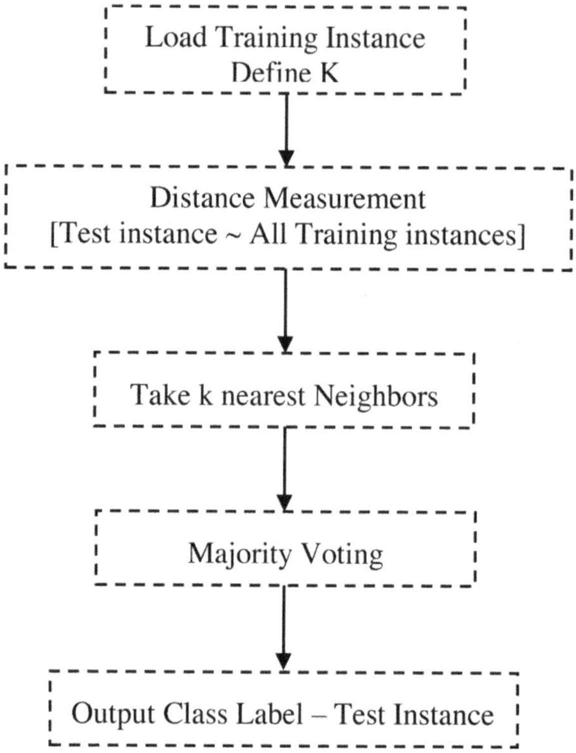

classification rules. They over fit their training sets with low bias but high variance. A simple example for binary classification decision tree problem is shown in Figure 4, where X1 and X2 represent the attributes given as nodes, the edges refer to the conditional values for identifying the class labels. The attribute value in X1 if ≥ 0.5 can be directly labeled as class 1 but if less than proceeds for the next level of node to check the value of X2. This example illustrates the working of decision tree model built with the predictions using training instances. Using this data tree model classification is done for the given set of test instances in testing phase.

Random forest works in such a way that it comprises the decision analysis based on different decision trees built on various sets of the same training set in order to reduce the variance value. This enhances the performance of the model. The bagging algorithm on a tree takes a set of training instances $A= a_1,a_2,\ldots a_n$ with output class labels as $B = b_1, b_2\ldots b_n$, then a random set of training samples are taken as input for training phase. Once trained, the classification results are attained for the given test set. This process is repeated for many set of repeated random training samples. Finally

Figure 4. Sample binary classification decision tree

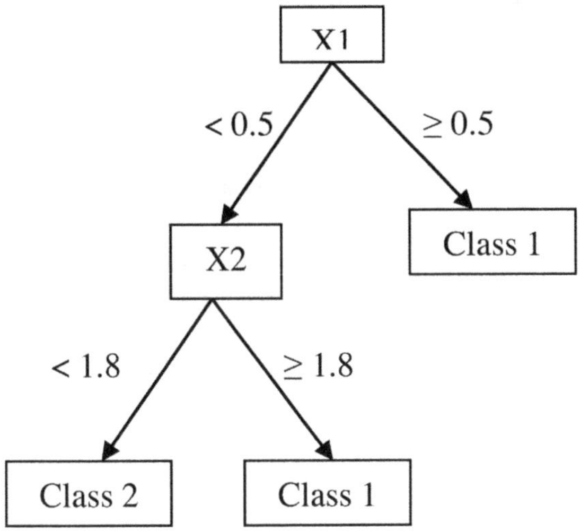

the prediction is made by identifying the mode of class responses from different trees thereby decreasing the variance of the model by not raising the bias value. This method can be further modified by pruning the attribute set. The correlation of attribute values with output class label can be noted. Those instances can be retained as a priority sample and made as subset of features for classification. Hence if less number of features has strong correlation over response then it's enough to choose these attributes alone for multiple decision tree models built.

Support Vector Machine (SVM)

Support vector machine a supervised technique to analyze the data for classification that maps the given points in an n-dimensional space (Wang, Yu, Fuqian, Luying, Nilanjan, Qun, Amira, Simon, Rajinikanth, & Lijun, 2018). The points are mapped in such a way that the categories are separated by a clear gap between them. When test instances arrive, they are mapped into the same space to predict the category of instances into which side they fall. SVM perform classification on a linear and non linear data. The non linear data input is converted to higher dimensional space using kernel functions.

The input data form an n-dimensional space i.e. data with 2 input variables define 2-dimensional space. In the space, a linear optimal decision boundary is identified known a hyper plane to separate the input variable space based on categories or classes.

Figure 5. A & B Two possible hyperplanes separating class 1 and class 2. Best linear optimal hyperplane – B with maximum margin.

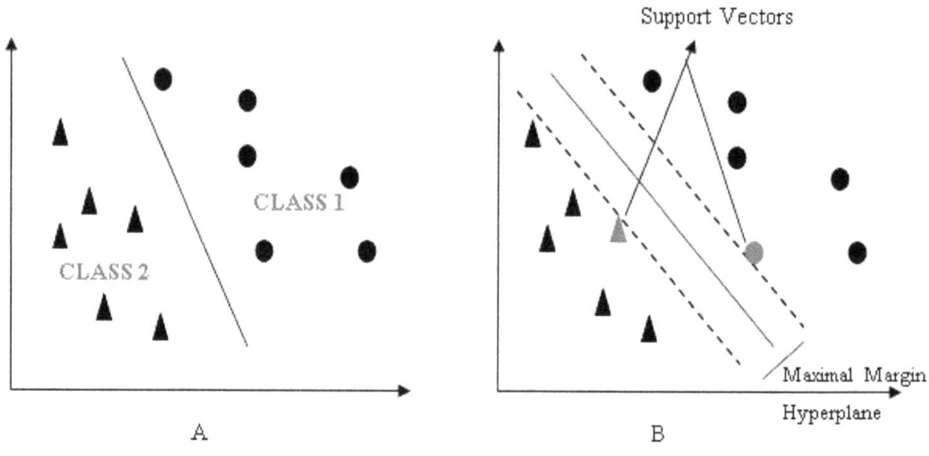

The hyper plane is chosen based on the support vector (training tuples) and margins (defined by support vectors). There is a possibility to have multiple lines separating the two classes but the best one is to be identifies which obtains a minimum classification error. Hence it spots out the hyperplane with maximal margin given as maximal margin hyperplane. Normally the less number of support vector have good generalization.

Linear SVM

In case of two class problem which are linearly separable on a given data set D given as (X_1, y_1), (X_2,y_2)...... (X_n,y_n) where X_i includes the set of training instances and yi refers to class values i.e. either 0 or 1. The hyperplane that separates the group of points in X vector with class 0 and class 1 is to be identified with maximal margin known as Maximal Margin Hyperplane(MMH). The maximal margin hyperplane is determined the X vector which lies very nearest to it. These are known as support vectors.

A separating hyperplane can be given as

$$W.X + b = 0 \tag{4}$$

W is a weight vector(w_1, w_2, ...w_n), n is the number of attributes and b is a scalar. If the given training tuples are two dimensional X= $(x_1,x_2)$with the values of attributes as A1 an A2, then equation to separate hyperplane can be rewritten as,

$$w_1x_1+w_2x_2+b=0 \quad (5)$$

The distance from a separating hyperplane to any point on Hyperplane1 and Hyperplane2 is $\frac{1}{\|W\|}$ where $(\|W\|)$ the Euclidean norm of W that is $\sqrt{W.W^2}$. Hence maximal margin i.e. distance between two hyperplanes is $\frac{2}{\|W\|}$ with minimized $(\|W\|)$. The constraints state that $w_1x_1+b >=1$, if $y_i=1$ else $w_1x_1+b<1$ if $y_i=0$ showing that the data points lie on right side of margin. In order to attain an optimization problem, minimize $(\|W\|)$ subject to $y_i\ (w.x_i-b) >=1$ for i=1,2 ….n.

Non Linear SVM

In case if the given data is linearly inseparable, there is a need to identify the non linear decision boundaries in input space. For the non linear approach two steps are involved. The one is to transform the original input space into higher dimension space using non linear mapping. Then the second step move towards examining the linear optimal line to separate the classes as a maximal margin hyperplane. This works similar to linear SVM.

Figure 6. Linear SVM – Maximal margin hyperplane

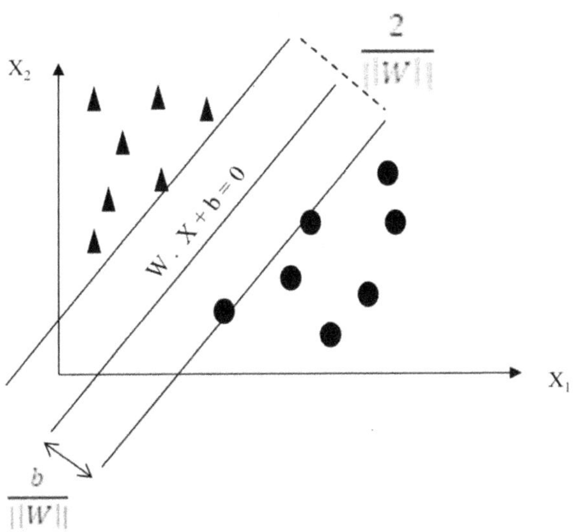

Note: A sample non linear transformation on 6D space for a given 3D vector X={x1,x2,x3} using the Kernel mapping Φ1(X)=x1, Φ2(X)=x2, Φ3(x3)=x3, Φ4(X)=$(x1)^2$, Φ5(X) =(x1x2), Φ6(X)=(x1x3). So, the linear decision hyperplane in the new space corresponds to,

$$d\left(Z\right) = w_1 x_1 + w_2 x_2 + w_3 x_3 + w_4 x_1^{\ 2} + w_5 x_1 x_2 + w_6 x_1 x_3 + b \tag{6}$$

This computation is costly since given a test tuple its necessary to compute dot product with every one of the other support vectors. Similarly during training phase there is a need to compute dot product several times to calculate maximal margin hyperplane. Instead of this is a Kernel function K ($x_{i},_{xj}$) applied on training data. Then kernel trick is applied to maximize the margin hyperplanes. The dot product can be replaced by a non linear kernel function. This aids to fit the data into a given transformed feature space. The kernel is related to the transform Φ(Xi) with the equation K(xi,xj)= Φ(xi). Φ(xj).

Some of the kernel functions are,

- Polynomial of power d: $K(\mathbf{x}_i,\mathbf{x}_j)= (1+ \mathbf{x}_i^{\ T}\mathbf{x}_j)d$
- Gaussian (radial-basis function network):

$$K(\mathbf{x}_i, \mathbf{x}_j) = \exp(-\frac{\left\| \mathbf{x}_i - \mathbf{x}_j \right\|^2}{2\sigma^2}) \tag{7}$$

Figure 7. Kernel Function on non linear SVM

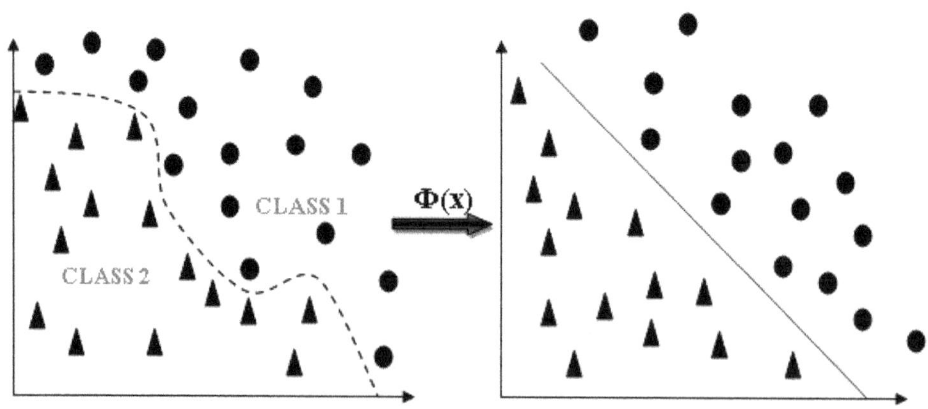

- Sigmoid: $K(\mathbf{x}_i,\mathbf{x}_j)= \tanh(\beta_0\mathbf{x}_i{}^T\mathbf{x}_j + \beta_1)$ for some $\beta_0 > 0$ and $\beta_1 < 0$

Ensemble Learning

Ensemble learning encompasses multiple learning algorithms together to produce better results than using a single algorithm. An ensemble is supervised learning algorithm as they are trained to make decisions. There are two classes of ensemble methods that include sequential and parallel ensemble methods. An ensemble contains a number of learners called base learners. The sequential methods exploit the dependence between the base learners. On the other hand parallel methods exploit the independence between the base learners. Most common methods in ensemble learning are bagging, boosting and stacking.

Bagging is abbreviated as bootstrap aggregation (Chatterjee, Sankhadeep, Nilanjan, Fuqian, Amira, Simon, & Soumya, 2017). It trains the base learners from a different bootstrap sample by calling a base learning algorithm. A bootstrap sample can be obtained by sub sampling the training data set with replacement. The size of a sample is as the same as that of the training data set. Once base learners are obtained bagging combines with majority voting and finds the highly-voted class. Random Forest method is one of the widely used ensemble methods.

Boosting refers to a collection of algorithms which are capable of converting weak learners to strong learners. It incrementally builds a new model to determine the training instances that are misclassified in the previous stage. More weight can be given to the misclassified samples. Though boosting gives higher accuracy than bagging, it may sometimes overfit the data. The main principle of boosting is to fit a sequence of weak learners– models that are only slightly better than random guessing, such as small decision trees– to weighted versions of the data. More weight is given to examples that were misclassified by earlier rounds. Ada Boost is one of the widely used boosting methods.

Stacking is one of the ensemble learning techniques also called as stacked generalizations, combines multiple classification or regression models using a meta-classifier or a meta-regressor. All the algorithms are trained on the entire training data and then the combiner carries out the prediction task. It can be used on both supervised and unsupervised learning models.

Thus when the histopathological breast cancer images are sent as input to the ensemble learning algorithms it predicts the classes as either malignant or benign. Experimental results are carried out to shows accuracy of this method.

Multi-Layer Perceptron

The idea of Artificial Neural Network (ANN) was inspired from the working of biological neuron networks process in the human brain (Pattnaik, Rautaray, Das, & Nayak, 2018). Human brain is composed of collection of biological neurons that are connected together by axon. Likewise, ANN is composed of collection of artificial neurons called nodes with a weight associated with it and the output of each node is called activation. ANN receives input, say x(N) where N=1,2…n with the weight w(N) associated. Let Z represent the computational unit with the following computation,

$$Z = \sum_{i=1}^{n} \left(\mathrm{x}_i w_i + \mathrm{b}\right) \tag{8}$$

where b represents bias, which helps in producing non-zero output incase weighted sum becomes zero. The value of bias is set to 1 in most cases. The output of the upper limit is infinity and to avoid this, a threshold is set called as activation function. An activation function is the one that helps in achieving desired output. There are number of activation functions available among which the commonly used activation function includes binary, bipolar, sigmoidal, logistic etc., Figure 8 shows the artificial neural network with the nodes connected with other and an activation function applied to the input to obtain the output.

Artificial Neural Network architecture consists of three different layers that include input layer, hidden layer and output layer as shown in figure 9. The input layer receives input from the outside world and passes it to the hidden layer. The hidden layer performs computation between input and output layer. The output layer responds in the format required by the user.

Artificial Neural Networks consists of two different structures that include the following

1. Feedforward
2. Feedback.

The feedforward neural network is the simplest artificial neural network that contains multiple nodes arranged in the form of layers. The connections between the nodes at adjacent layers are unidirectional with the weight associated with them. The information flows forward and there is no loops in the network with fixed input and output. Figure 10 shows the Feedforward neural network.

Figure 8. Artificial Neural Network

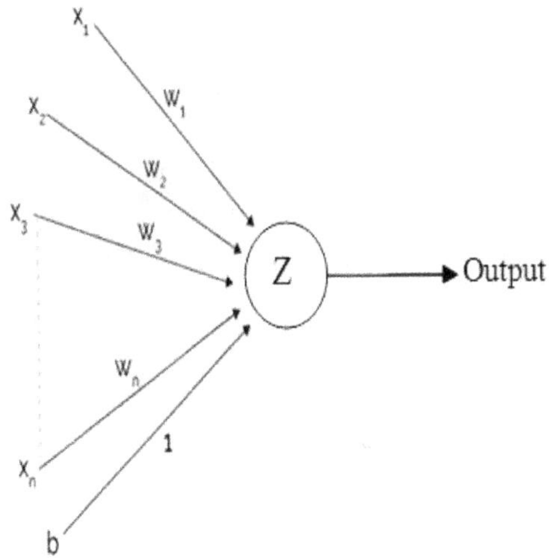

Figure 9. Architecture of ANN

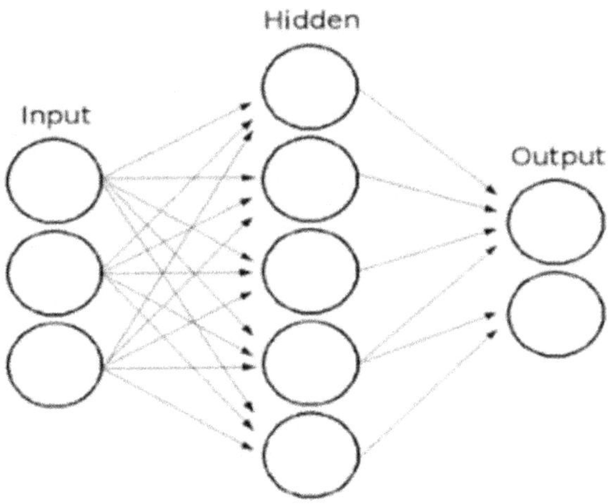

Another type of artificial neural network is Feedback neural networks which consist of signals travelling in both directions with loops in the network. These networks are called dynamic networks as state of the network changes dynamically till equilibrium is reached. Nodes from adjacent layers have connections or edges between them. All these connections have weights associated with them. Figure 11 shows the Feedback neural network with the loop in it.

Figure 10. Feedforward neural network

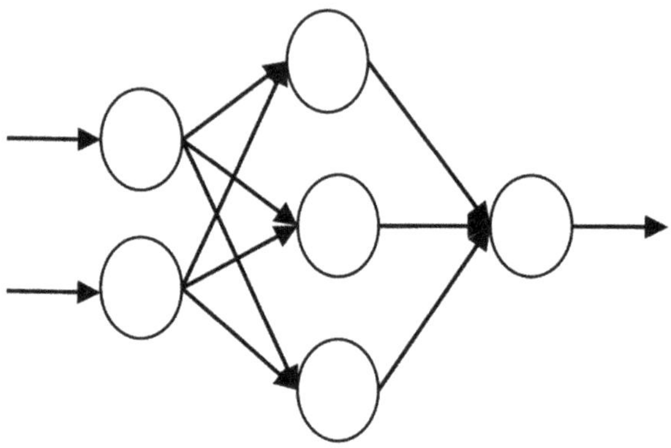

Figure 11. Feedback neural network

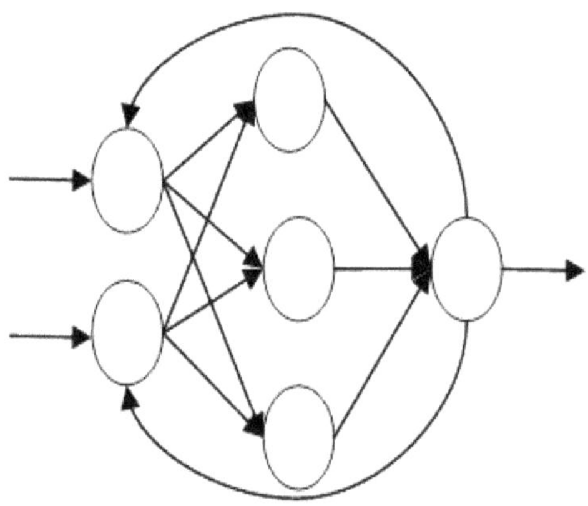

A multilayer perceptron (MLP) is a type of feedforward artificial neural network with one or multiple layers between input and output layer (Das, Jena, Nayak, Naik, & Behera, 2015). Unlike multilayer perceptrons, single layer perceptrons network has input and output layer without any hidden layers in it. A multilayer perceptron has at least three layers that include input layer, hidden layer and output layer. Non-linear activation function can be applied to all layers except the input layer. This network uses back propagation algorithm for training. Multilayer perceptron is used for training histopathological image features to produce different classes of output for predicting whether it is benign or malignant. Figure 12 shows the architecture of multilayer perceptron containing more than one hidden layer.

Perceptron learning algorithm discovered by Rosenblatt is discussed below:

Figure 12. Multilayer perceptron

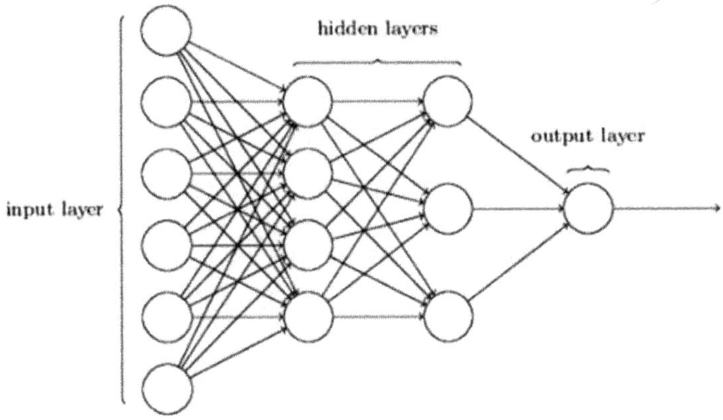

Step 0: Initialization: bias = 0, Weight $w_i = 0$ where i = 1 to n
Step 1: Continue till stopping condition is false; Repeat steps 2-5
Step 2: For each training sample s:t repeat steps 3 -5
Step 3: Input $(x_i) := s_i$, i = 1 to n
Step 4: Compute output, y= f(Yin)
Step 5: If y != target(t)
Step 6: Weight and Bias updation,
$w_i(new) := w_i(old) + ax_it$, i = 1 to n
b(new):= b(old) + at

If a MLP constitutes one hidden layer, then the function becomes $func : R^{in} \rightarrow R^{out}$ where in and out are the size of input and output vector respectively. The matrix notation is expressed as,

$$f\left(x\right) = A1(b^{(2)} + w^{(2)}(A2\left(b^{(1)} + w^{(1)}x\right))) \tag{9}$$

where b^1,b^2 represents bias, w^1,w^2 represents weight and A1, A2 represents activation function respectively.

The hidden layer is represented using the vector h(x) as,

$$h\left(x\right) = A2\left(b^{(1)} + w^{(1)}\mathrm{x}\right) \tag{10}$$

The weight associated with the input vector to the hidden layer is represented as,

$$w^{(1)} \quad R^{in*in_h} \tag{11}$$

The output vector is represented as,

$$o\left(x\right) = A1\left(b^{(2)} + w^{(2)}\mathrm{h}\left(\mathrm{x}\right)\right) \tag{12}$$

Thus the MLP network contains one or many hidden layer based on the application. Time and complexity increases when hidden layer increases.

Convolutional Neural Networks (CNN)

Convolutional Neural Network is a feed forward neural network that is made of neurons that consists of learnable weight and bias. Similar to a neural network, CNN consist of input, output and multiple hidden layers. These hidden layers include convolutional layers, pooling layers, fully connected layers and classification layer. A CNN may include number of convolutional and subsampling layers possibly followed by fully connected layers.

The input of the convolution layer is the histopathological breast cancer images. The output from this network is the classification result that determines whether the image is malignant/benign or finding the probability of classes that best describes the input image (Das, Naik, & Behera, 2018). The input to the CNN is an image which is arranged in 3 dimensions that include width, height and depth. The third dimension depth represents the total number of layers or RGB image in the network. If the input is [48x48x3] the image width is 48, height is 48, and with three color channels R,G,B.

The first layer in Convolutional Neural Network is the convolutional layer that has a number of filters that applies the convolution operation to the input image. It

Figure 13. Convolutional neural network architecture

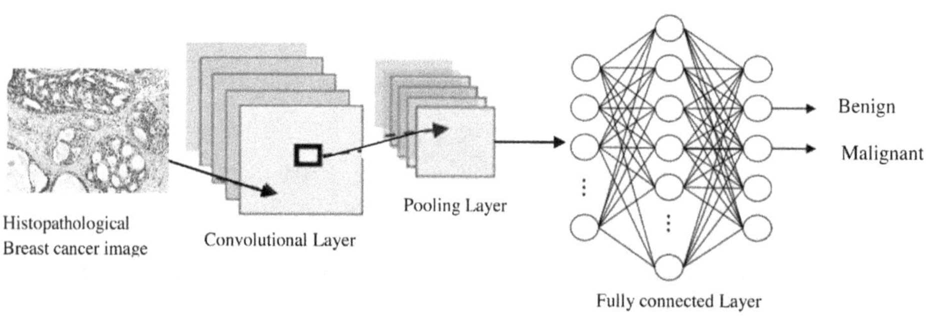

will compute the output of neurons which are linked to local regions in the input, each computing a dot product between their weights and a small region they are connected to in the input volume. There are three different factors that control the size of the output volume are the depth, stride and zero-padding. Depth is the number of filters used, zero padding can be used for controlling the spatial size and the stride is the way of sliding the filter in the input image. If the stride size is one, then it is moved one pixel at a time. When the size of the input image becomes larger, each neuron is connected only to a local region of the input image which is called as the receptive field (equal to filter size). Figure 14 shows the convolution operation applied to an image 6x6 with filters and stride one to obtain feature map.

The spatial size of the output volume can be determined as follows,

$$\left(\frac{W - F + 2P}{S} + 1\right) \tag{13}$$

where w is the input size, F is the receptive field, S is the stride and P is the zero padding of filters that does convolutional operation.

The pooling layer lies between the successive convolutional layers. The main advantage of using a pooling layer is to reduce the computation, reduce the parameters and to avoid overfitting problem. It operates individually on the depth of the input image and thus reduces the spatial size. The pooling operations include max pooling, min pooling, average pooling, L2 norm pooling etc. Figure 15 shows the max pooling operation applied to the convolution layer thus producing sub-sampled image.

After performing pooling operation the image size is reduced this is shown in Figure 16. Sub-sampling the pixel will reduce the size of the image to get fewer parameters to characterize the image.

Rectified Linear Units(ReLU) is a non-saturating activation function that increases the nonlinear properties of the decision function and of the overall network. It does not affect the receptive fields of the convolution layer.

Figure 14. Convolution operation for an image

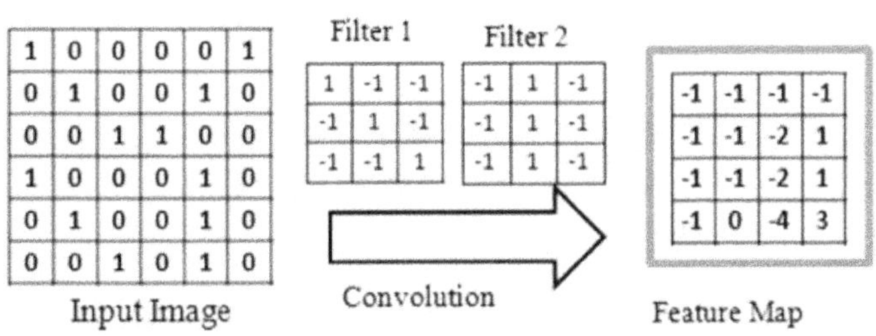

Figure 15. Pooling operation using Max pooling

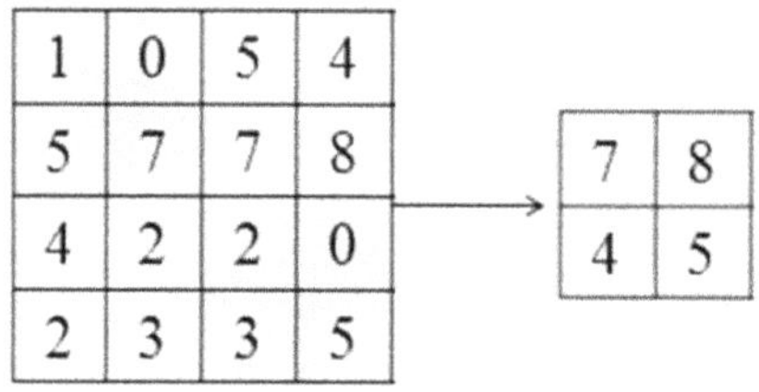

Figure 16. Sub-sampling the image

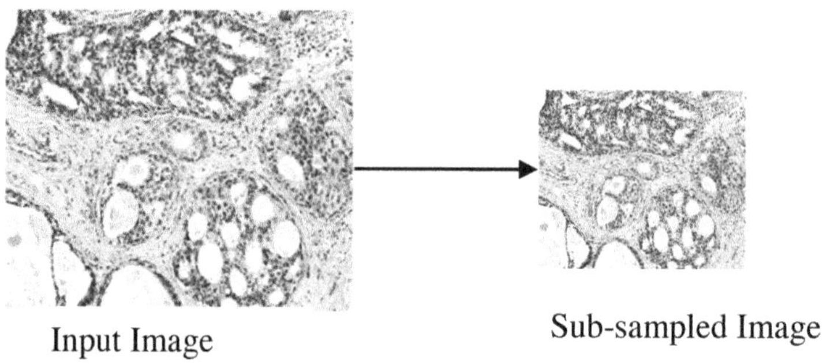

Fully connected layer is the next layer in the network following many convolutional and max pooling layers. The fully connected layer has connections with all activations present in previous layer. The classification layer is the last layer present in the CNN that classifies the histopathological breast cancer image as malignant/ benign which helps the pathologist in making better decisions (Dey, Nilanjan, Amira, & Surekha, 2017). Based on the application and requirement the number of convolution and pooling layers can be set.

Experimental Analysis on Classification Algorithms

A dataset of 569 histopathological breast cancer images was taken for analysis. The data includes benign and malignant as two classes to predict the diseased images. Images were preprocessed and 30 features were extracted from it. The ten real valued features are radius, texture, perimeter, area, smoothness, compactness, concavity, concave points, symmetry, fractal dimension. With each feature including three information - mean, standard error, mean of the three largest values are computed. As a whole of 30 features, based on which 357 instances are found to be benign and 212 are malignant on analysis.

Among these 569 instances, 70% of the data was taken as training samples and 30% as test instances. The analysis results was measured based on the results of accuracy, root mean squared error, precision and recall (Das, Jena, Badajena, Pradhan, & Barik, 2018). The diverse measures estimated analysis are stated using confusion Matrix (Table 1).

Furthermore the time take for the execution was measured to calculate the performance. These varied results of image classification are provided as input to decision making methods to determine the best method in terms of accuracy and performance. The decision making methods are explained in the next section.

MULTICRITERIA DECISION MAKING TECHNIQUES

This section deals with three different Multiple Criteria Decision Making (MCDM) methods and explains how they are used in classification of histopathological tissue images (Madavan, Sujatha, Saroja, 2017: Mishra, Das, Dehuri, & Jagadev, 2018: Dey, & Amira, 2018). Employing MCDM methods in classification of histopathological tissue images will improve the classification accuracy.

MCDM methods help decision maker in selection of the best decision from a set of alternatives, each of which is evaluated against multiple criteria. There exists a number of MCDM techniques including SAW (Simple Additive Weighting), WPM (Weighted Product Model), TOPSIS (Technique for Order Preference by Similarity to the Ideal Solution), PROMETHEE (Preference Ranking Organization METHod for Enrichment Evaluation), AHP (Analytical Hierarchy Process), SMART (The Simple Multi Attribute Rating Technique) and ANP (Analytic network process). The methods are selected based on the requirement of the problem domain. This chapter proposes the first three methods in classification of histopathological tissue images (Kar, Parida, & Das 2016: Nayak, Naik, Jena, Barik, & Das, 2018).

Steps involved in MCDM technique are as follows:

- Define the problem

Table 1. Confusion Matrix

		Predicted Class	
		POSTIVE	NEGATIVE
Actual Class	POSITIVE	True Positive	False Negatives
	NEGATIVE	False Positive	True Negative

Table 2. Classification Results for Breast Cancer Wisconsin Diagnosis Dataset

Breast Cancer Wisconsin Diagnosis Dataset						
Total Instances: 569						
Training Phase: 70% [399 Instances] Testing Phase: 30% [170 Instances]						
Classes: **Benign & Malignant**						
Classification Algorithm	**Accuracy**	**Time**	**Wrongly classified Instances**	**Root Mean Squared Error**	**Precision**	**Recall**
Instance Based Learning(Knn)	93.53	0.14	11	0.2537	0.935	0.935
Random Forest	92.94	0.07	12	0.2088	0.930	0.929
Support Vector Machine	95.29	0.25	8	0.2169	0.956	0.953
Ensemble (Adaboost)	95.29	0.32	8	0.1934	0.953	0.953
Ensemble (Bagging)	93.53	0.18	11	0.1958	0.935	0.935
Multi Layer Perceptron	96.47	0.12	6	0.146	0.965	0.965
Deep Learning	97.14	0.23	5	0.124	0.97	0.964

- ◦ Identify the problem statement describing the initial and desired conditions of the problem in concise, crisp and unambiguous manner.
- Determine the requirements
    - Identify constraints involved in the problem and state them in quantitative form.
- Establish the goals of the problem
    - Identify the objectives and state them in quantitative form.
- Determine the various alternatives involved in the problem.
    - Identify the various alternatives; alternatives change the initial condition in to desired condition.
- Identify the relevant criteria for evaluating the alternatives.
    - Represent a goal with at least one criterion, complex goals can be represented by more than one criterion.
    - Criteria should be able to discriminate among the alternatives.
    - Criteria should support the comparison of the performance of the alternatives.
    - Criteria should be less in number.
    - Criteria can be either of benefit type (positive) or of cost type (negative).
- Select a decision making tool.
- Evaluate alternatives against criteria.

    - Used to rank the alternatives or to choose the promising alternatives.
    - Decision makers can pick the best alternative based on its rank.
- Validate solutions against problem statement.
    - Make sure that generated solutions are correct.
    - Inform the decisions to stakeholders.

Simple Additive Weighting (SAW)

SAW method is also called as weighted linear combination method; this method calculates the score of the alternatives based on the weighted average. It is done by summing up the product of weight (importance) of the criteria by the normalized value of the criteria pertaining to the given alternative. This result is called weighted average or score or rank of the alternative. Mathematically, weighted average of a particular alternative can be expressed as follows:

$$R_i = \sum_{j=1}^{j=n} x_{ij} * w_j \tag{14}$$

where,

R^i denotes the rank or score of the ith alternative
w_j denotes weight of the jth criterion (j=1,2,…,m)
x_{ij} denotes the normalized performance value of ith alternative for j^{th} criterion
'm' denotes the number of alternatives and
'n' denotes the number of criteria

The alternative with highest score will be chosen as the best alternative.

Histopathological Image Classification Using SAW

Here, the classification algorithms are alternatives; SAW selects the best classification algorithm based on the criteria including classification accuracy, execution time and root mean squared error. Here classification accuracy is the benefit criteria and other two are cost criteria. Hence, it is necessary to normalize them in to benefit criteria. If we assign the weight values for the criteria as w1=0.85(accuracy), w2=0.05 (execution time) and w3=0.1 (root mean squared error), then the results of SAW for chosen weight factor is given in Table 3.

Table 3. Performance measures by SAW

Classification Algorithm	Score	Rank
Instance Based Learning(Knn)	80.25181	6
Random Forest	80.19221	7
Support Vector Machine	81.65754	4
Ensemble (Adaboost)	81.66981	3
Ensemble (Bagging)	80.289	5
Multi Layer Perceptron	83.1011	2
Deep Learning	83.59284	1

From this SAW method, we can conclude that Deep learning and MultiLayer Perceptron are the two different best classification techniques for histopathological images.

Weighted Product Model (WPM)

Weighted Product Model was introduced in the year 1995 by Yoon and Hwang. In this method normalization step is not necessary hence it is also called as dimensionless analysis, this makes this method as unique when compared to other MCDM methods.

Criteria can be of two types: benefit criteria (higher value denotes betterment) and cost criteria (lower value denotes betterment). Weights become exponents, for benefit criteria, positive power weight will be used, and for cost criteria, negative power weight will be used. Due to this exponent property, performance values of alternatives for different criteria should be greater than one. If we want to compare the two alternatives (A_1 & A_2) using weighted product model then calculate: $P\left({}^{A_1}\!/\!{}_{A_2}\right)$. If it is greater than one, it indicates that alternative A_1 is better than alternative A_2; else A_2 is better than A_1.

$$P\left({}^{A_1}\!/\!{}_{A_2}\right) = \prod_{j=1}^{j=n} \left(x_{1j} / x_{2j}\right)^{w_j} \tag{15}$$

By following the above calculation, we can sort the alternatives based on the performance scores.

Histopathological Image Classification Using WPM

Here, the classification algorithms are alternatives, WPM selects the best classification algorithm based on the criteria including classification accuracy, and execution time and root mean squared error. Here classification accuracy is the benefit criteria and other two are cost criteria. Hence, negative power weight will be used for cost criteria. If we assign the weight values for the criteria as w1=0.85(accuracy), w2=0.05 (execution time) and w3=0.1 (root mean squared error), then the results of WPM for chosen weight factor is given in Table 4.

From this WPM method, we can conclude that Deep learning and MultiLayer Perceptron are the two different best classification techniques for histopathological images.

Technique for Order Preference by Similarity to the Ideal Solution (TOPSIS)

TOPSIS ranks the alternative based on the distance to positive ideal solution and the distance to negative ideal alternative. Positive ideal solution is the one which has the best value for all the considered criteria. Negative ideal solution is the one, which has the worst value for all the considered criteria. If we have 'm' alternatives and 'n' criteria then x_{ij} denotes the performance value of ith alternative for j^{th} criterion. Let J be the set of benefit criteria (more is better) and J' be the set of negative criteria (less is better)

The steps involved in TOPSIS method are as follows:

1. Construct normalized matrix.

Table 4. Performance measures by WPM

Classification Algorithm	Rank
P(A1/A2)	0.952413
P(A2/A3)	1.047314
P(A3/A4)	1.000876
P(A4/A5)	0.988379
P(A5/A6)	0.926882
P(A6/A7)	1.010367
P(A1/A4)	0.998349
P(A1/A6)	0.914599
P(A1/A7)	0.924081

This method transforms criteria values of alternatives in to normalized form.

This method is needed, since the performance values of alternatives for different criteria will have incongruous dimensions. Normalization can be done in two different ways: Linear normalization and Vector normalization. The vector method of normalization is given as follows:

$$r_{ij} = \frac{x_{ij}}{\sqrt{\sum_{i=1}^{i=n} x_{ij}^{2}}}, i = 1,2,\ldots,m \, and \, j = 1,2,\ldots,n \quad (16)$$

2. Construct weight vector.

Decide the relative importance (*i.e.,*weights) of different criteria with respect to the objective. A set of weights w_j is framed (for j=1, 2,.., n) such that

$$\sum_{j=1}^{j=n} w_j = 1 \quad (17)$$

3. Construct weighted normalized decision matrix.

This step involves the construction of weight vector for each criteria and it is denoted as $w_{j.}$ Then multiply each column of the normalized decision matrix by its associated weight. Weighted normalized decision matrix is calculated as follows:

$$v_{ij} = w_j * norm_{ij} \quad (18)$$

4. Determine the positive ideal and negative ideal solutions.

Positive ideal solution and negative ideal solution can be determined with the help of the following equations.

Positive ideal solution:

$$V^{+} = \left\{ (\max V_{ij} | j = J), \left(\min V_{ij} \; | j = J'\right) \right\} \forall i = 1,2,..,m \quad (19)$$

$$V^{+} = \left\{V_1^{+}, V_2^{+}, \ldots, V_M^{+}\right\} \tag{20}$$

Negative ideal solution:

$$V^{-} = \left\{\left(\min V_{ij} \mid j = J\right), \left(\max V_{ij} \mid j = J'\right)\right\} \forall i = 1, 2, \ldots, m \tag{21}$$

$$V^{-} = \left\{V_1^{-}, V_2^{-}, \ldots, V_M^{-}\right\}. \tag{22}$$

5. Calculate the separation measure for each alternative.

This step calculates the separation measure of an alternative from positive ideal solution and also from negative ideal solution.

Separation measure from positive ideal solution is calculated as follows:

$$S_i^{+} = \sqrt{\sum_{j=1}^{j=n} \left(V_j^{+} - V_{ij}\right)^2} \quad \forall \text{ i=1, 2, ..., m} \tag{23}$$

Separation measure from negative ideal solution is calculated as follows:

$$S_i^{-} = \sqrt{\sum_{j=1}^{j=n} \left(V_j^{-} - V_{ij}\right)^2} \quad \forall \text{ i=1, 2, ..., m} \tag{24}$$

6. Calculate the relative closeness coefficient of each alternative.

This step calculates the similarity of the alternatives by considering positive ideal solution and negative ideal solution. Relative closeness coefficient value is calculated as follows:

$$C_i^{*} = S_i^{-} / \left(S_i^{+} + S_i^{-}\right) \tag{25}$$

Select the alternative with high relative closeness coefficient C_i^{*} value.

Histopathological Image Classification Using TOPSIS

Here, the classification algorithms are alternatives, TOPSIS selects the best classification algorithm based on the criteria including classification accuracy, and execution time and root mean squared error. Here classification accuracy is the benefit criteria and other two are cost criteria. If we assign the weight values for the criteria as w1=0.85(accuracy), w2=0.05 (execution time) and w3=0.1 (root mean squared error), then the results of TOPSIS for chosen weight factor is given in Table 5.

From this TOPSIS method, we can conclude that Deep learning and MultiLayer Perceptron are the two different best classification techniques for histopathological images.

FUTURE RESEARCH DIRECTIONS

This work can be further extended to large scale image analysis using big data. This can be implemented using cloud environment for incorporating storage as a service. Privacy preserving security challenges can be solved.

CONCLUSION

The diseased histopathological image diagnosis using computer aided analytical approach is proposed and exhaustive approach is stated in the chapter using various multicriteria decision making methods on different classification algorithms. The methods proposed for image analysis was tested on breast cancer Wisconsin dataset. The experimental results and analysis on the three decision making methods SAW,

Table 5. Performance measures by TOPSIS

Classification Algorithm	Relative closeness coefficient	Rank
Instance Based Learning(Knn)	0.370587	5
Random Forest	0.533555	3
Support Vector Machine	0.33038	7
Ensemble (Adaboost)	0.338669	6
Ensemble (Bagging)	0.450044	4
Multi Layer Perceptron	0.818469	1
Deep Learning	0.668376	2

WPM and TOPSIS evolves the final conclusion stating that MultiLayer Perceptron are the best classification algorithms for diagnosing the diseases in histopathological images in terms of accuracy and performance.

ACKNOWLEDGMENT

Authors thank lord almighty for his benevolence grace and blessings through every stage of this work. Authors would like to thank the management and principal of Mepco Schlenk Engineering College for providing the needful resources and allowing us to perform this fruitful work. Last but not least, we would like to thank family members and friends for supporting us with their encouraging words and helping hands to make this chapter a success.

REFERENCES

Barik, R. K., Dubey, H., Misra, C., Borthakur, D., Constant, N., Sasane, S. A., & Mankodiya, K. (2018). Fog Assisted Cloud Computing in Era of Big Data and Internet-of-Things: Systems, Architectures, and Applications. In *Cloud Computing for Optimization: Foundations, Applications, and Challenges* (pp. 367–394). Cham: Springer. doi:10.1007/978-3-319-73676-1_14

Blessa Binolin Pepsi, M., & Bargavi, G. (2017). Analysis of Accuracy and Performance of Big Data using Data Mining Techniques in Hadoop Mapreduce. In *Advances and Applied Sciences* (Vol. 11). AENSI Publisher.

Chakraborty, S., Chatterjee, S., Ashour, A. S., Mali, K., & Dey, N. (2017). *Intelligent Computing in Medical Imaging: A Study*. Advancements in Applied Metaheuristic Computing.

Chatterjee, S., Dey, N., Shi, F., Ashour, A. S., Fong, S. J., & Sen, S. (2017). Clinical application of modified bag-of-features coupled with hybrid neural-based classifier in dengue fever classification using gene expression data. *Medical & Biological Engineering & Computing*, 1–12. PMID:28891000

Das, H., Jena, A. K., Badajena, J. C., Pradhan, C., & Barik, R. K. (2018). Resource Allocation in Cooperative Cloud Environments. In Progress in Computing, Analytics and Networking (pp. 825-841). Springer. doi:10.1007/978-981-10-7871-2_79

Das, H., Jena, A. K., Nayak, J., Naik, B., & Behera, H. S. (2015). A novel PSO based back propagation learning-MLP (PSO-BP-MLP) for classification. In *Computational Intelligence in Data Mining-Volume 2* (pp. 461–471). New Delhi: Springer. doi:10.1007/978-81-322-2208-8_42

Das, H., Naik, B., & Behera, H. S. (2018). Classification of Diabetes Mellitus Disease (DMD): A Data Mining (DM) Approach. In Progress in Computing, Analytics and Networking (pp. 539-549). Springer.

Dey, N., & Ashour, A. S. (2018). Computing in Medical Image Analysis. *Soft Computing Based Medical Image Analysis*, 3–11.

Dey, N., Ashour, A. S., & Borra, S. (Eds.). (2017). *Classification in BioApps: Automation of Decision Making* (Vol. 26). Springer.

Haseena, S. (2015). Segmentation of Optic Disc and Hard Exudates. In *International Journal of Applied Engineering Research* (Vol. 10). Research India Publications.

Madavan, R., Balaraman, S., & Saroja, S. (2017). Multi-Criteria Decision Making Methods for Grading High-Performance Transformer Oil with Antioxidants Under Accelerated Ageing Conditions. In IET Generation, Transmission and Distribution (Vol. 11). IET Publisher.

Mishra, B. S. P., Das, H., Dehuri, S., & Jagadev, A. K. (2018). *Cloud Computing for Optimization: Foundations, Applications, and Challenges* (Vol. 39). Springer. doi:10.1007/978-3-319-73676-1

Panigrahi, C. R., Tiwary, M., Pati, B., & Das, H. (2016). Big Data and Cyber Foraging: Future Scope and Challenges. In *Techniques and Environments for Big Data Analysis* (pp. 75–100). Cham: Springer. doi:10.1007/978-3-319-27520-8_5

P. K. Pattnaik, S. S. Rautaray, H. Das, & J. Nayak (Eds.). (2018). Progress in Computing, Analytics and Networking*: Proceedings of ICCAN 2017* (Vol. 710). Springer.

Reddy, K. H. K., Das, H., & Roy, D. S. (2017). *A Data Aware Scheme for Scheduling Big-Data Applications with SAVANNA Hadoop. Futures of Network.* CRC Press.

Ripon, S., Chowdhury, L., Ashour, A. S., & Dey, N. (2018). Machine-Learning Approach for Ribonucleic Acid Primary and Secondary Structure Prediction from Images. *Soft Computing Based Medical Image Analysis*, 203–221.

Sahani, R., Rout, C., Badajena, J. C., Jena, A. K., & Das, H. (2018). Classification of Intrusion Detection Using Data Mining Techniques. In Progress in Computing, Analytics and Networking (pp. 753-764). Springer. doi:10.1007/978-981-10-7871-2_72

Sarkhel, P., Das, H., & Vashishtha, L. K. (2017). Task-Scheduling Algorithms in Cloud Environment. In *Computational Intelligence in Data Mining* (pp. 553–562). Singapore: Springer. doi:10.1007/978-981-10-3874-7_52

Thanki, R., Borra, S., Dey, N., & Ashour, A. S. (2018). Medical Imaging and Its Objective Quality Assessment: An Introduction. In *Classification in BioApps* (pp. 3–32). Cham: Springer. doi:10.1007/978-3-319-65981-7_1

Wang, Yu., Shi, F., & Cao, L. (2018). Morphological segmentation analysis and texture-based support vector machines classification on mice liver fibrosis microscopic images. *Current Bioinformatics.*

ADDITIONAL READING

AlShahrani. (2018). Alaa M., Manal A. Al-Abadi, Areej S. Al-Malki, Amira S. Ashour, and Nilanjan Dey. "Automated system for crops recognition and classification. In *Computer Vision: Concepts, Methodologies, Tools, and Applications* (pp. 1208–1223). IGI Global.

Amar, Y. B., Trabelsi, I., Dey, N., Shi, F., Satapathy, S. C., & Bouhlel, M. S. (2017). Robust watermarking of polygonal meshes based on vertex norms variance distortion. [JGIM]. *Journal of Global Information Management, 25*(4), 46–60. doi:10.4018/JGIM.2017100104

Banerjee, S., Nath, S. S., Dey, N., & Eto, H. (2018). Global medical tourism: A review. In *Medical Tourism: Breakthroughs in Research and Practice* (pp. 1–19). IGI Global. doi:10.4018/978-1-5225-3920-9.ch001

Barik, R. K., Dubey, H., Misra, C., Borthakur, D., Constant, N., Sasane, S. A., & Mankodiya, K. (2018). Fog Assisted Cloud Computing in Era of Big Data and Internet-of-Things: Systems, Architectures, and Applications. In *Cloud Computing for Optimization: Foundations, Applications, and Challenges* (pp. 367–394). Cham: Springer. doi:10.1007/978-3-319-73676-1_14

Barik, R. K., Tripathi, A., Dubey, H., Lenka, R. K., Pratik, T., Sharma, S., . . . Das, H. (2018). Mistgis: Optimizing geospatial data analysis using mist computing. In Progress in Computing, Analytics and Networking (pp. 733-742). Springer, Singapore.

Borra, S., Thanki, R., Dey, N., & Borisagar, K. (2018). *Secure transmission and integrity verification of color radiological images using fast discrete curvelet transform and compressive sensing*. Smart Health.

Chakraborty, S., Chatterjee, S., Dey, N., Ashour, A. S., Ashour, A. S., Shi, F., & Mali, K. (2017). Modified cuckoo search algorithm in microscopic image segmentation of hippocampus. *Microscopy Research and Technique*, *80*(10), 1051–1072. doi:10.1002/jemt.22900 PMID:28557041

Chakraborty, S., Chatterjee, S., Dey, N., Ashour, A. S., & Shi, F. "Gradient approximation in retinal blood vessel segmentation." In Electrical, Computer and Electronics (UPCON), 2017 4th IEEE Uttar Pradesh Section International Conference on, pp. 618-623. IEEE, 2017. 10.1109/UPCON.2017.8251120

Cheriguene, S., Azizi, N., Dey, N., Ashour, A. S., & Ziani, A. (2018). A new hybrid classifier selection model based on mRMR method and diversity measures. *International Journal of Machine Learning and Cybernetics*, 1–16.

Das, H., Jena, A. K., Rath, P. K., Muduli, B., & Das, S. R. (2015). Grid computing-based performance analysis of power system: a graph theoretic approach. In *Intelligent Computing, Communication and Devices* (pp. 259–266). New Delhi: Springer. doi:10.1007/978-81-322-2009-1_30

Das, H., Mishra, S. K., & Roy, D. S. (2013). The topological structure of the Odisha power grid: a complex network analysis. IJMCA, 1(1), 012-016.

Das, H., Naik, B., Pati, B., & Panigrahi, C. R. (2014). A survey on virtual sensor networks framework. *International Journal of Grid and Distributed Computing*, *7*(5), 121–130. doi:10.14257/ijgdc.2014.7.5.11

Das, H., & Roy, D. S. (2013). A grid computing service for power system monitoring. *International Journal of Computers and Applications*, *62*(20).

Deb, S., Tian, Z., Fong, S., Tang, R., Wong, R., & Dey, N. (2018). Solving permutation flow-shop scheduling problem by rhinoceros search algorithm. *Soft Computing*, 1–10.

Dey, N., & Ashour, A. S. (2017). *Meta-Heuristic Algorithms in Medical Image Segmentation: A Review* (p. 185). Advancements in Applied Metaheuristic Computing.

Dey, N., Ashour, A. S., & Hassanien, A. E. (2018). Feature detectors and descriptors generations with numerous images and video applications: a recap. In *Computer Vision: Concepts, Methodologies, Tools, and Applications* (pp. 571–600). IGI Global. doi:10.4018/978-1-5225-5204-8.ch022

Dey, N., Ashour, A. S., Shi, F., Fong, S. J., & Simon Sherratt, R. (2017). Developing residential wireless sensor networks for ECG healthcare monitoring. *IEEE Transactions on Consumer Electronics*, *63*(4), 442–449. doi:10.1109/TCE.2017.015063

Dey, N., Hassanien, A. E., Bhatt, C., Ashour, A., & Satapathy, S. C. (Eds.). (2018). *Internet of Things and Big Data Analytics Toward Next-Generation Intelligence*. Springer. doi:10.1007/978-3-319-60435-0

Dey, N., Rajinikanth, V., Ashour, A., & Tavares, J. M. (2018). Dey, Nilanjan, Venkatesan Rajinikanth, Amira S. Ashour, and João Manuel RS Tavares. "Social Group Optimization Supported Segmentation and Evaluation of Skin Melanoma Images. *Symmetry*, *10*(2), 51. doi:10.3390ym10020051

(2018). Dey, Nilanjan, Amira S. Ashour, Fuqian Shi, Simon James Fong, and João Manuel RS Tavares. "Medical cyber-physical systems: A survey. *Journal of Medical Systems*, *42*(4), 74. PMID:29525900

Elhayatmy, G. (2018). Nilanjan Dey, and Amira S. Ashour. "Internet of Things Based Wireless Body Area Network in Healthcare. In *Internet of Things and Big Data Analytics Toward Next-Generation Intelligence* (pp. 3–20). Cham: Springer. doi:10.1007/978-3-319-60435-0_1

Fong, S., Li, J., Song, W., Tian, Y., Wong, R. K., & Dey, N. (2018). Predicting unusual energy consumption events from smart home sensor network by data stream mining with misclassified recall. *Journal of Ambient Intelligence and Humanized Computing*, 1–25.

Hore, S., Chatterjee, S., Shaw, R. K., Dey, N., & Virmani, J. (2018). Detection of Chronic Kidney Disease: A NN-GA-Based Approach. In *Nature Inspired Computing* (pp. 109–115). Singapore: Springer. doi:10.1007/978-981-10-6747-1_13

Kamal, S., Dey, N., Nimmy, S. F., Ripon, S. H., Ali, N. Y., Ashour, A. S., ... Shi, F. (2018). Evolutionary framework for coding area selection from cancer data. *Neural Computing & Applications*, *29*(4), 1015–1037. doi:10.100700521-016-2513-3

Kar, I., & Das, H. (2016). Energy Aware Task Scheduling Using Genetic Algorithm in Cloud Datacentres. *International Journal of Computer Science and Information Technology Research*, *4*(1), 106–111.

Kar, I., Parida, R. R., & Das, H. (2016, March). Energy aware scheduling using genetic algorithm in cloud data centers. In Electrical, Electronics, and Optimization Techniques (ICEEOT), International Conference on (pp. 3545-3550). IEEE. 10.1109/ICEEOT.2016.7755364

Le, D.-N., Nguyen, G. N., Chung, L. V., & Dey, N. (2017). MMAS Algorithm for Features Selection using 1D-DWT for Video-based Face Recognition in the Online Video Contextual Advertisement User-Oriented System. *Journal of Global Information Management*, *25*(4), 103–124. doi:10.4018/JGIM.2017100107

Li, J., Fong, S., Hu, S., Chu, V. W., Wong, R. K., Mohammed, S., & Dey, N. "Rare Event Prediction Using Similarity Majority Under-Sampling Technique." In *International Conference on Soft Computing in Data Science*, pp. 23-39. Springer, Singapore, 2017. 10.1007/978-981-10-7242-0_3

Mishra, BB, S Dehuri, BK Panigrahi, AK Nayak, BSP Mishra, and Himansu Das, "Computational Intelligence in Sensor Networks", vol. 776, Studies in Computational Intelligence, Springer, 2018

Moraru, L., Moldovanu, S., Culea-Florescu, A.-L., Bibicu, D., Dey, N., Ashour, A. S., & Sherratt, S. (2018). Texture spectrum coupled with entropy and homogeneity image features for myocardium muscle characterization. *Current Bioinformatics*.

Moraru, L., Obreja, C. D., Dey, N., & Ashour, A. S. (2018). "Dempster-Shafer Fusion for Effective Retinal Vessels' Diameter Measurement." In Soft Computing Based. *Medical Image Analysis*, 149–160.

Nayak, J., Naik, B., Jena, A. K., Barik, R. K., & Das, H. (2018). Nature Inspired Optimizations in Cloud Computing: Applications and Challenges. In *Cloud Computing for Optimization: Foundations, Applications, and Challenges* (pp. 1–26). Cham: Springer. doi:10.1007/978-3-319-73676-1_1

Panigrahi, C. R., Sarkar, J. L., Pati, B., & Das, H. (2015, December). S2S: a novel approach for source to sink node communication in wireless sensor networks. In *International Conference on Mining Intelligence and Knowledge Exploration* (pp. 406-414). Springer, Cham. 10.1007/978-3-319-26832-3_38

Parah, S. A., Sheikh, J. A., Dey, N., & Bhat, G. M. (2017). Realization of a New Robust and Secure Watermarking Technique Using DC Coefficient Modification in Pixel Domain and Chaotic Encryption. *Journal of Global Information Management*, *25*(4), 80–102. doi:10.4018/JGIM.2017100106

Pradhan, C., Das, H., Naik, B., & Dey, N. (2018). *Handbook of Research on Information Security in Biomedical Signal Processing* (pp. 1–414). Hershey, PA: IGI Global; doi:10.4018/978-1-5225-5152-2

Rajinikanth, V. (2018). Suresh Chandra Satapathy, Nilanjan Dey, and R. Vijayarajan. "DWT-PCA Image Fusion Technique to Improve Segmentation Accuracy in Brain Tumor Analysis. In *Microelectronics, Electromagnetics and Telecommunications* (pp. 453–462). Singapore: Springer. doi:10.1007/978-981-10-7329-8_46

Rajinikanth, V., Dey, N., Satapathy, S. C., & Ashour, A. S. (2018). Nilanjan Dey, Suresh Chandra Satapathy, and Amira S. Ashour. "An approach to examine magnetic resonance angiography based on Tsallis entropy and deformable snake model. *Future Generation Computer Systems*, *85*, 160–172. doi:10.1016/j.future.2018.03.025

Sahoo, A. K., & Das, H. (2016). Energy Efficient Scheduling Using DVFS Technique in Cloud Datacenters. *International Journal of Computer Science and Information Technology Research*, *4*(1), 59–66.

Sarkar, J. L., Panigrahi, C. R., Pati, B., & Das, H. (2016). A novel approach for real-time data management in wireless sensor networks. In *Proceedings of 3rd International Conference on Advanced Computing, Networking and Informatics* (pp. 599-607). Springer, New Delhi. 10.1007/978-81-322-2529-4_62

Shriranjani, D., Tebby, S. G., Satapathy, S. C., Dey, N., & Rajinikanth, V. (2018). Kapur's Entropy and Active Contour-Based Segmentation and Analysis of Retinal Optic Disc. In *Computational Signal Processing and Analysis* (pp. 287–295). Singapore: Springer. doi:10.1007/978-981-10-8354-9_26

Tuan, T. M., Fujita, H., Dey, N., Ashour, A. S., Vo, T. N. N., & Chu, D.-T. (2018). Dental diagnosis from X-Ray images: An expert system based on fuzzy computing. *Biomedical Signal Processing and Control*, *39*, 64–73. doi:10.1016/j.bspc.2017.07.005

Wang, D., He, T., Li, Z., Cao, L., Dey, N., Ashour, A. S., ... Shi, F. (2018). Image feature-based affective retrieval employing improved parameter and structure identification of adaptive neuro-fuzzy inference system. *Neural Computing & Applications*, *29*(4), 1087–1102. doi:10.100700521-016-2512-4

Yadav, P., Sharma, S., Tiwari, P., Dey, N., Ashour, A. S., & Nguyen, G. N. (2018). A Modified Hybrid Structure for Next Generation Super High Speed Communication Using TDLTE and Wi-Max. In *Internet of Things and Big Data Analytics Toward Next-Generation Intelligence* (pp. 525–549). Cham: Springer. doi:10.1007/978-3-319-60435-0_21

KEY TERMS AND DEFINITIONS

Computer-Aided Diagnosis: Use of computer systems to aid in medical image diagnosis to improve the quality of treatment.

Digital Pathology: Provides an image-based environment which includes acquisition, diagnosis, and interpretation from the generated digitized data.

Histopathology: Includes study of changes in diseased tissues.

Image Analysis: Process of extracting meaningful information from images.

Machine Learning: A field of information technology that has the ability to learn data insights by using statistical techniques.

Multi-Criteria Decision Making: A field of operation research that evaluates multiple conflicting criteria in decision making.

Root Mean Squared Error: A measure to evaluate the differences between predicted model values to the observed values.

Chapter 6
Histopathological Image Analysis in Medical Decision Making:
Classification of Histopathological Images Based on Deep Learning Model

R. Meena Prakash
Sethu Institute of Technology, India

Shantha Selva Kumari R.
Mepco Schlenk Engineering College, India

ABSTRACT

Digital pathology is one of the significant methods in the medicine field to diagnose and treat cancer. The cell morphology and architecture distribution of biopsies are analyzed to diagnose the spread and severity of the disease. Manual analyses are time-consuming and subjected to intra- and inter-observer variability. Digital pathology and computer-aided analysis aids in enormous applications including nuclei detection, segmentation, and classification. The major challenges in nuclei segmentation are high variability in images due to differences in preparation of slides, heterogeneous structure, overlapping clusters, artifacts, and noise. The structure of the proposed chapter is as follows. First, an introduction about digital pathology and significance of digital pathology techniques in cancer diagnosis based on literature survey is given. Then, the method of classification of histopathological images using deep learning for different datasets is proposed with experimental results.

DOI: 10.4018/978-1-5225-6316-7.ch006

INTRODUCTION

Digital pathology means the investigation of a biopsy or surgical specimen at microscopic level. The tissues are chemically processed and sectioned onto glass slides to study cellular morphology for cancer diagnosis and prognosis. For the tissue components to be visualized under the microscope, the sections are dyed with one or more stains including Hematoxylin-Eosin (H&E) and Immunohistochemical (IHC). The nuclei regions are stained in dark blue colour by Hematoxylin and the other structures like cytoplasm, stroma etc., are stained with pink colour. IHC is used to determine the cancer stage whether it is benign or malignant based on the presence or absence of proteins. After the process of staining, digital images are generated using fast slide scanners which contain one or multiple lenses to magnify the images at X20 or X40 magnification. Uniform light spectrum is used to illuminate the tissue slide. The slide scanners are provided with standard packages for corrections in spectral and spatial illumination variation.

Figure 1 shows the different types of nuclei (Irshad et al, 2014). Lymphocyte is the white blood cell which plays major role in immune system of the body. Epithelial tissues line the outer surfaces of organs, blood vessels and inner surfaces of cavities of human body. Lymphocyte Nuclei have regular shape and are smaller in size than Epithelial nuclei. EN's in high grade cancer tissues are larger in size and have clearly visible nucleoli. Also, they show heterogeneous chromatin distribution and irregular boundaries called nuclear plemorphism.

The problems associated with detection, segmentation and classification of nuclei are due to variation in slides preparation, image acquisition like artifacts caused during image compression, noise etc., and also the overlapping clusters of nuclei. The aspect of nuclei plays a major role in evaluating the existence of cancer and its severity. For example, in breast cancer prediction, the infiltration of LN is related to patient survival and death. Similarly, nuclear plemorphism aids in cancer grading. Mitotic count is an important prognostic parameter in breast cancer grading.

Figure 1. Different types of nuclei (a) LN (b) EN (c) EN in cancer tissue

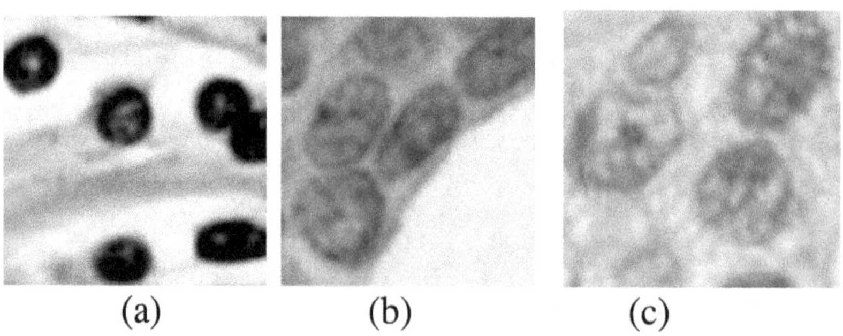

In the conventional cancer diagnosis, pathologists analyze the cell morphology and architecture in biopsies of patients to make diagnostic and prognostic assessments. The images of histopathological specimen can now be digitized and stored in the form of digital images. CAD algorithms are used now-a-days which perform disease detection, diagnosis and prognosis. They assist pathologists to make informed decisions. Pathological images give details such as progression of cancer while radiographs give coarse information such as classification of lesions. The histological subtypes of cancer can also be determined which is not possible with radiological data. A number of cancer detecting and grading applications have been proposed for different organs including brain, breast, cervix, liver, lung and prostate. Segmentation of histopathological tissues is more difficult since they are part of tissues with complex and irregular shapes.

The two problems associated with histopathological image segmentation and classification are that the images are very large in size and only a small number of training data is available. For such larger size images, the parameters to be estimated, required computational power and memory also increase. Hence, the images have to be resized to smaller images which results in loss of information at cellular level and there will be decrease of identification accuracy. Therefore the entire Whole Slide Image (WSI) is divided into partial regions called patches and each patch is analyzed independently. For increased patch sizes, the accuracy increases (Irshad et al, 2014; Komura et al, 2018).

Computer Aided Diagnosis (CAD) of digital histopathology images assist pathologists in diagnostic process. The classification accuracy is improved by the CAD analysis and also the variability in disease interpretations is greatly reduced. The time is significantly reduced compared to manual analysis. The histopathological images exhibit high level of diversity and complexity and in such cases, deep learning techniques for segmentation and classification provide high accuracy. The objective of the work is to propose an automated method of classification of benign or malignant tumours in histopathology images. The contribution of the work includes, a custom-made CNN is proposed for classification of histopathological images. The rest of the chapter is organized as follows. A background on the segmentation and classification of the histopathology images which describes the recent methods in literature is given. The detailed description on Convolutional Neural Network is given. The method of Gabor feature extraction and Support Vector Machine (SVM) classification is presented. Then, the experimental results are given with performance comparison. Subsequently, the concluding remarks are presented.

BACKGROUND

Al-Kofahi et al (2010) proposed improved automatic detection and segmentation of cell nuclei in which the image foreground is extracted using a graph cuts based binarization. The nuclear seed points are detected by mulit scale Laplacian of Gaussian filtering and graph cuts based algorithm is used for segmentation. The method achieves an overall accuracy exceeding 86%. Han et al (2017) proposed automated breast cancer multi-classification from histopathological images using structured deep learning model. The method classifies subordinate classes of breast cancer which include Ductal carcinorma, Fibroadenoma, Lobular Carcinoma etc. Jia et al (2017) proposed a weakly supervised learning algorithm to segment cancerous regions in histopathological images. An end-to-end learning system that segments cancerous regions with Fully Convolutional Networks (FCN) is proposed and constraints are introduced to the neural networks to assist the learning process. Kumar et al (2017) compared the methods of Local Binary Patterns (LBP), Bag-of-Visual (BOV) words, and deep features for the classification of histopathological images. They introduced a new dataset, KIMIA Path960, that contains 960 histopathological images belonging to 20 different tissue types and they demonstrated an highest accuracy of 94.72% for deep features. Pan et al (2017) proposed an automatic nuclei segmentation for H&E stained breast cancer histopathology images. First, the sparse reconstruction method is employed to remove the background and accentuate the nuclei of pathological images. Then multi-layer convolution networks are employed to segment the cell nuclei form the background which are trained using gradient descent techniques. Then, morphological operations and some prior knowledge are employed to improve the segmentation performance. The method is tested on 58 H&E images of breast tissue with 32 benign and 26 malignant images and an accuracy of 92.45% is achieved. Mitosis detection is one of the important factors of cancer prognosis and is necessary for cancer grading. Saha et al (2018) proposed a supervised model using deep learning for detection of mitosis signature from histopathological images. There are five convolution layers, four max-pooling layers, four rectified linear units (ReLu), and two fully connected layers in the proposed architecture. Handcrafted features consisting of morphological, textural and intensity features are incorporated. The method provides an efficient second opinion for breast cancer grading from whole slide images.

Sirinukunwattana et al. (2016) proposed a Spatially Constrained Convolutional Neural Networks (SC-CNN) for nucleus detection. A Neighboring Ensemble Predictor (NEP) is used along with CNN to classify the detected cell nuclei. The method is tested on a large dataset of colorectal adenocarcinoma images and classified into 4 classes. Xu et al. (2016) proposed a deep convolutional neural network for segmentation and classification of epithelial and stromal regions in histopathological images which is essential for analyzing the tumour. Stromal tissue includes the fatty and fibrous connective tissues surrounding the blood vessels, ducts and lobules, and lymphatic vessels. The spatial arrangement of stromal cell in tumors is a prognostic factor in breast cancer. The method employed two alternating convolutional layers, max pooling layers, two full connection layers, and a final classification layer. Xu et al. (2013) proposed multi-label classification for Colon Cancer in which four kinds of features – Color Histogram, Gray-Level Co-occurrence Matrix (GLCM), Histogram of Oriented Gradients (HOG), and Euler Number are introduced in the feature set. The four different classes are well and moderately differentiated tubular adenocarcinoma (HM), moderately and poorly differentiated tubular adenocarcinoma (LM), Signet-ring carcinoma (LR) and mucinous adenocarcinoma (RMu). Yonekura et al (2017) proposed a deep convolutional network for classification of glioma histopathological images of brain tumours and demonstrated an accuracy of 87.2%. Zheng et al (2017) proposed nucleus-guided feature extraction framework based on convolutional neural network for classification of histopathological images. The nuclei are first detected from images and then used to train the CNN. The dataset used in the method comprised of 2 class dataset with malignant and benign breast tumours and 15-class dataset with 13 sub categories of breast tumours.

METHODS

GLCM Feature Extraction and SVM

Feature extraction is the process of dimensionality reduction in which the input data of large size is transformed into representative features of reduced size. The features of interest are color, shape, texture, etc., Grey Level Co-occurrence Matrices (GLCM) introduced by Haralick describes texture by statistically sampling how certain grey levels occur in relation to other grey levels (Haralick et al, 1973). The GLCM features used in the method are defined as follows.

1. **Correlation:** Correlation is defined as the dependency of the gray level intensities on that of the neighboring pixels.

$$Correlation = \sum_{i=0}^{l-1}\sum_{j=0}^{L-1} G\left(i;j\right)\frac{\left(i-\mu_i\right)\left(j-\mu_j\right)}{\sigma_i \sigma_j} \quad (1)$$

G represents the gray level value of the image of each pixel. μ and σ represent the mean and standard deviation.

2. **Entropy:** Entropy represents the randomness present in the image or it is a measure of the degree of disorder. If all the elements in co-occurrence matrix are same, the value of entropy is large and vice-versa.

$$Entropy = -\sum_{i=0}^{L-1}\sum_{j=0}^{L-1} G(i;j) ln\, G\left(i;j\right) \tag{2}$$

3. **Contrast:** Contrast is a measure of the intensity variations between the reference pixel and its neighboring pixels. The higher value of contrast indicates larger the structural variations in the image. It is given by

$$Contrast = \sum_{i=0}^{L-1}\sum_{j=0}^{L-1}\left(i-j\right)^2 G\left(i;j\right) \tag{3}$$

4. **Variance:** Variance is the deviation of the intensity values of the pixels from the mean and is a measure of the contrast in the image.

$$Variance = \sum_{i=0}^{L-1}\sum_{j=0}^{L-1}\left(i-\mu\right)^2 G\left(i;j\right) \tag{4}$$

Support Vector Machine (SVM) is one of the supervised linear classification methods and serves as an important tool for applications including medical diagnosis, pattern recognition, and bioinformatics etc., For linearly separable patterns, SVM finds the optimal hyperplane that separates the patterns. For patterns that are not linearly separable, the data are transformed into kernel function and the hyperplane is constructed. On each side of the hyperplane separating the data, two parallel hyperplanes are constructed and larger the margin between these parallel hyperplanes, better the classification performance. The margin is maximized in an optimum way with the reduction in the number of non-zero weights, considering only important features called support vectors that decide the separating hyperplane.

Convolutional Neural Network

The basic processing element of the neural network is the neuron which receives an input, processes it, and generates an output which is sent to other neurons and further processed or it is the final output. The inputs to the neuron are multiplied by weights and these weights are updated during the training process. Another linear component bias is added to the result of input-weight product. Then a nonlinear function called activation function is applied to the linear combination of inputs to obtain the final output. The commonly used activation functions are sigmoid functions, Rectified Linear Units, Softmax etc., Neural networks are the backbone of deep learning and they are formed by numerous interconnected neurons. The input layer is the first layer of the neural network which receives the input. The hidden layers perform specific tasks on the input data and pass the output to the next layer. The output layer is the final layer of the network. There will be multiple neurons present in each layer and all the neurons in each layer are connected to all the neurons in the next layer. It is called Multi Layer Perceptron (MLP) and the networks are called Fully Connected Layers (Belsare, 2012; Chatterjee et al, 2017; Das et al, 2014).

The accuracy of the network is measured using cost or loss function, for example, mean squared error and the learning process strives to minimize the cost. The optimization algorithm used to minimize the cost is Gradient Descent method. The rate at which the network descends towards the minima of the cost function is called the learning rate. The selection of learning rate should be optimal since a too large learning rate will result in missing of the optimal solution and if the learning rate is too small, it will be difficult for the network to converge. In a neural network, initially random weights and bias values are assigned to the nodes. As the output is received after first iteration, the network error is calculated and is fed back to the network along with the gradient of the cost unction. The weights are then updated such as to minimize the error in the subsequent iterations and this is called back propagation. During the training of neural network, the input is divided into several batches of equal size randomly. A single training iteration of all the batches in both forward and back propagation is called an epoch. Increasing the number of epoch will increase the accuracy, but setting too high will take longer time to converge and the network might be over-fit. During the training process, a certain number of neurons is randomly dropped to prevent over-fitting of the network which is called dropout. Also, the data is normalized at each layer before passing it to the next layer which is called batch normalization to ensure that distribution of data remains unchanged.

In the convolutional layers of Convolutional Neural Networks, the input images are convolved with filters to give 2-dimensional activation map. These activation maps are stacked along the depth dimension to produce the output volume. Pooling layers are periodically introduced in between the convolution layers to reduce the number of parameters and over-fitting. The most commonly used operation of pooling layer is MAX operation which takes the maximum of each 4x4 matrix of the original image. For matching the sizes of input and output after the filtering operation, padding is done, that is, extra layer of zeros is added. If the output of neuron is sent back to the input, it is called recurrent neuron whose advantage is that it give more generalized output. For sequential data, the previous output is used to predict the value of next output and such networks have loops within them. These networks are called Recurrent Neural Network (RNN) (Dey, N., & Ashour, 2018; Vieira et al, 2017).

Convolutional neural networks are feed forward neural networks in which the images are directly given as inputs instead of the features extracted from the images given as inputs. The three layers of CNN are convolutional layer, pooling layer and fully connected layer. As the depth of CNN increases, more abstract features are derived, for example, from low level features like lines, to edges, to eyes and then to face. Let the Convolutional Network be denoted by 'f' consisting of 'l' layers $(f_1, f_2, f_3, \ldots f_l)$. Let '$x$' denotes the input vector, 'y' denotes the output vector, 'v_l' denotes the weight and bias vector for the lth layer. The equation for output vector can be written as

$$y = f\left(x; v_1, v_2, \ldots . v_l\right) = f_1\left(\cdot; x_1\right) ¿ f_2\left(\cdot; x_2\right) ¿ \ldots \ldots . f_{l-1}\left(\cdot; x_{l-1}\right) ¿ f_l ¿ \left(\cdot; x_l\right) \tag{5}$$

f_l is used to perform convolution with filter banks, pooling and non-linear activation.

With the gradient descent method, the optimized weight vector is calculated by

$$Opt\left(v_1, v_2, \ldots . v_l\right) = \frac{1}{M}\sum_{i=1}^{M}\Omega(f(x^i; v_1, v_2, \ldots . v_l), y^i) \tag{6}$$

'Ω' denotes the loss function, 'M' is the number of data.

EXPERIMENTAL SET UP

Dataset

Two datasets are used in the experiment. The KIMIA Path960 dataset comprises of images from 20 scans of muscle, epithelial and connective tissue with different texture and pattern types. From each scan, 48 regions of interest are selected and downsampled to 308x168 patches. Hence, the whole dataset consists of 960 images. Figure 2 shows the sample images from first 9 scans of the dataset. It is assessed that though large texture variability exists between the classes, some inter-class similarities exist which may affect the classification. Also, intra class variability exists in the dataset images.

The UCSB Bio-Segmentation Benchmark dataset consists of 58 breast cancer histopathological images categorized as 36 beningn tumour cells and 28 malignant tumour cells (Gelasca et al, 2008). Figure 3 shows the sample images of UCBS dataset.

Top row - beningn tumor images and bottom row - malignant tumour images

Implementation of DCNN and SVM

The Deep Convolutional Neural Network employed in the proposed work comprises of three convolutional layers, three batch normalization layers, three rectified linear unit layers, two max pooling layers, one fully connected layer, softmax layer and a final classification layer. The convolutional and the pooling layers produce feature

Figure 2. Sample images from 9 classes of the Kimia Path960 dataset

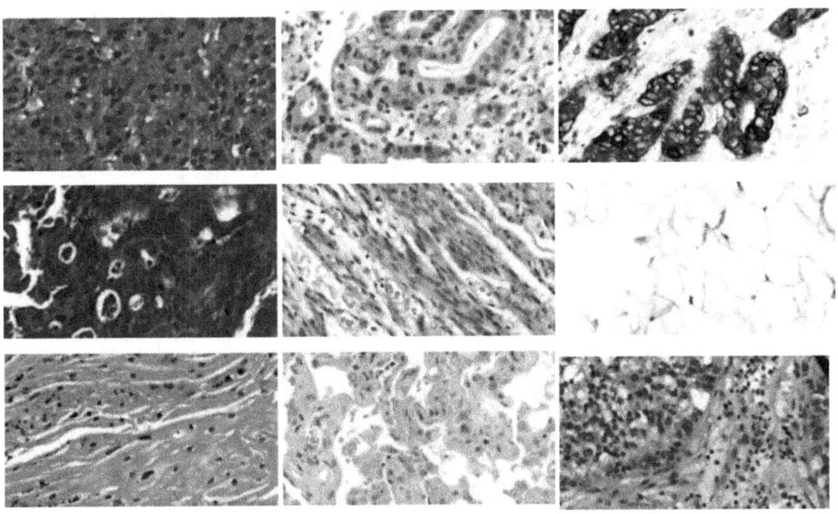

Figure 3. Sample images from UCBS Breast cancer dataset

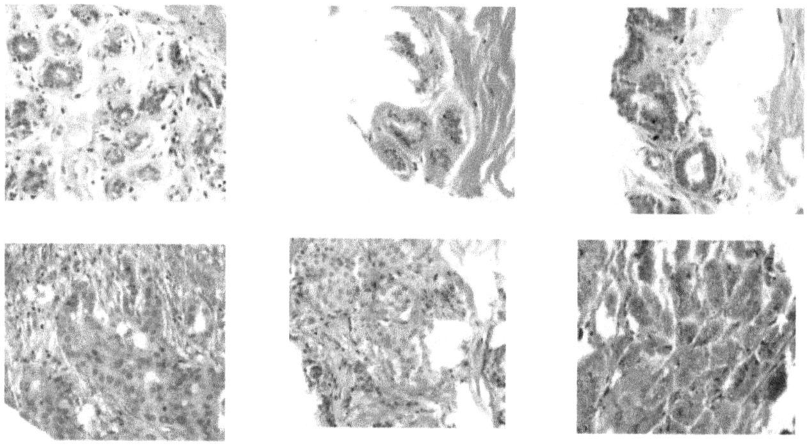

maps through successive convolution and max-pooling operations. These feature maps extract a set of image features from the training dataset. The number of iterations is selected as 15. For the Convolutional layer (C) and the pooling layer (P), 3x3 convolutional and 2x2 pooling kernel are used.

The representative GLCM features – Contrast, Correlation, Entropy and variance are extracted from the input images and fed to SVM classifier and trained. Then, classification is done using SVM.

EXPERIMENTAL RESULTS

The performance of CNN is evaluated by training the CNN with 80% of the input data and 20% of the input data is used for testing. The input color images of size 308x168 are converted to gray scale images and down sampled to half the size (154x84) and fed as input to CNN. The downsampled gray scale images are shown in Figure 4. Table 1 shows the classification accuracy obtained on KimiaPath960 dataset.

Table 1 illustrates the results obtained for the classification of images of "Kimia Path960" dataset. Figure 5 illustrates the training and classification stages of CNN.

The results are compared with that of the segmentation accuracy obtained with Support Vector Machine classifier subsequent to GLCM feature extraction. The GLCM features – Correlation, Contrast, Entropy and variance are extracted from the input gray scale images and used for training and classification using SVM. Figure 6 illustrates the classification using SVM.

Figure 4. Downsampled Gray scale images

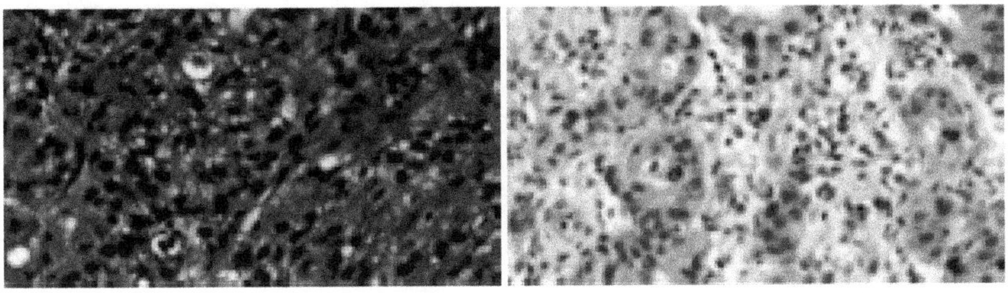

Figure 5. Illustration of CNN training and classification

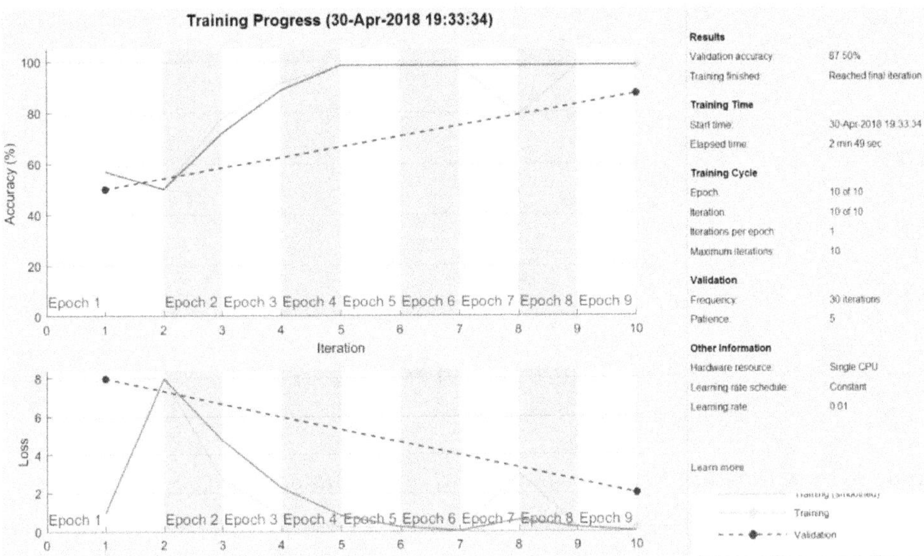

The classification results obtained using KimiaPath960 dataset is shown in Table 1. The result indicate that though there exists inter class and intra class variability among the images of the different classes, it gives better classification accuracy. Table 2 depicts the performance comparison of the CNN with SVM and it shows that CNN method gives more promising results compared to SVM. Table 3 depicts the comparison of accuracy obtained on the classification of benign and malignant breast cancer tumors of the histopathological images from UCBS dataset. It is evident from the experiments that the proposed custom-made CNN gives better classification accuracy and can be better employed for medical diagnosis applications.

Figure 6. Illustration of SVM classification

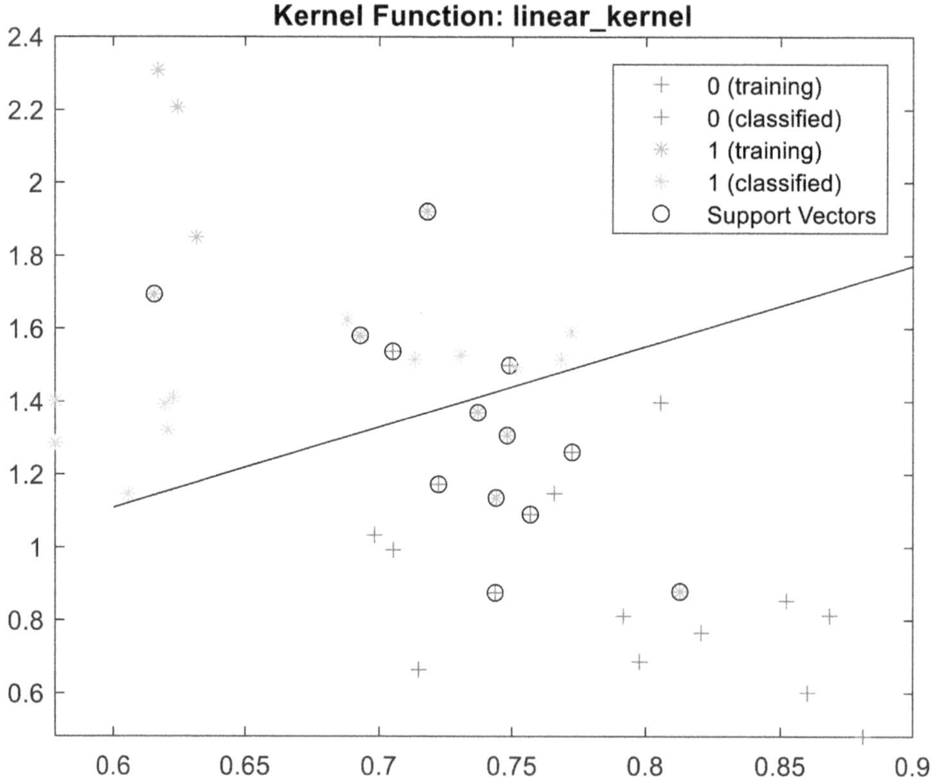

Table 1. Classification Results of the KimiaPath960 dataset images using CNN

No. of images	Dataset used	No. of classes	Accuracy
192	1-4	4	92.10%
192	5-8	4	81.25%
192	9-12	4	93.75%
192	13-16	4	89.58%
192	17-20	3	97.20%

Table 2. Comparison of Results of the KimiaPath960 dataset – CNN and SVM

No. of images	Dataset used	No. of classes	Accuracy	
			CNN	SVM
96	1,2	2	95.8%	81.4%
96	3,4	2	87.5%	75.0%

Table 3. Comparison of results for Breast cancer histo dataset - CNN and SVM

No. of images		Accuracy	
Beningn	Malignant	CNN	SVM
32	26	81.2%	65.0%

CONCLUSION

The significance of digital pathology techniques in cancer diagnosis is analyzed based on the recent research papers in nuclei detection and classification methods. Then, the method of classification using deep learning is proposed and the method is tested on images from two publicly available histopathology dataset. The results achieved show that CNN classifier performs better in classification of histopathological images compared to SVM. Also, if pre trained networks are used, the training time reduces and also it leads to better classification accuracy. New methods are in research focus for optimization of the CNN. The deep convolutional networks are better suited for automated classification problems in histopathological images and aid in automatic diagnosis and prognosis of different types of cancer in different organs of the human body.

REFERENCES

Al-Kofahi, Y., Lassoued, W., Lee, W., & Roysam, B. (2010). Improved Automatic Detection and Segmentation of Cell Nuclei in Histopathology Images. *IEEE Transactions on Biomedical Engineering*, *57*(4), 841–852. doi:10.1109/TBME.2009.2035102 PMID:19884070

Belsare, A. (2012). Histopathological Image Analysis Using Image Processing Techniques: An Overview. *Signal and Image Processing: an International Journal*, *3*(4), 23–36. doi:10.5121ipij.2012.3403

Chatterjee, S., Dey, N., Shi, F., Ashour, A. S., Fong, S. J., & Sen, S. (2017). Clinical application of modified bag-of-features coupled with hybrid neural-based classifier in dengue fever classification using gene expression data. *Medical & Biological Engineering & Computing*, *56*(4), 709–720. doi:10.100711517-017-1722-y PMID:28891000

Das, H., Jena, A. K., Nayak, J., Naik, B., & Behera, H. S. (2014). *A Novel PSO Based Back Propagation Learning-MLP (PSO-BP-MLP) for Classification. In Computational Intelligence in Data Mining* (Vol. 2, pp. 461–471). Smart Innovation, Systems and Technologies.

Dey, N., & Ashour, A. S. (2018). Computing in Medical Image Analysis. *Soft Computing Based Medical Image Analysis,* 3-11.

Gelasca, E. D., Byun, J., Obara, B., & Manjunath, B. (2008). Evaluation and benchmark for biological image segmentation. *2008 15th IEEE International Conference on Image Processing.*

Han, Z., Wei, B., Zheng, Y., Yin, Y., Li, K., & Li, S. (2017). Breast Cancer Multi-classification from Histopathological Images with Structured Deep Learning Model. *Scientific Reports*, *7*(1). PMID:28646155

Haralick, R. M., Shanmugam, K., & Dinstein, I. (1973). Textural Features for Image Classification. *IEEE Transactions on Systems, Man, and Cybernetics*, *SMC-3*(6), 610–621. doi:10.1109/TSMC.1973.4309314

Irshad, H., Veillard, A., Roux, L., & Racoceanu, D. (2014). Methods for Nuclei Detection, Segmentation, and Classification in Digital Histopathology: A Review—Current Status and Future Potential. *IEEE Reviews in Biomedical Engineering*, *7*, 97–114. doi:10.1109/RBME.2013.2295804 PMID:24802905

Jia, Z., Huang, X., Chang, E. I., & Xu, Y. (2017). Constrained Deep Weak Supervision for Histopathology Image Segmentation. *IEEE Transactions on Medical Imaging*, *36*(11), 2376–2388. doi:10.1109/TMI.2017.2724070 PMID:28692971

Komura, D., & Ishikawa, S. (2018). Machine Learning Methods for Histopathological Image Analysis. *Computational and Structural Biotechnology Journal*, *16*, 34–42. doi:10.1016/j.csbj.2018.01.001

Kumar, M. D., Babaie, M., Zhu, S., Kalra, S., & Tizhoosh, H. R. (2017). A comparative study of CNN, BoVW and LBP for classification of histopathological images. *2017 IEEE Symposium Series on Computational Intelligence (SSCI)*. 10.1109/SSCI.2017.8285162

Pan, X., Li, L., Yang, H., Liu, Z., Yang, J., Zhao, L., & Fan, Y. (2017). Accurate segmentation of nuclei in pathological images via sparse reconstruction and deep convolutional networks. *Neurocomputing*, *229*, 88–99. doi:10.1016/j.neucom.2016.08.103

Saha, M., Chakraborty, C., & Racoceanu, D. (2018). Efficient deep learning model for mitosis detection using breast histopathology images. *Computerized Medical Imaging and Graphics*, *64*, 29–40. doi:10.1016/j.compmedimag.2017.12.001 PMID:29409716

Sirinukunwattana, K., Raza, S. E., Tsang, Y., Snead, D. R., Cree, I. A., & Rajpoot, N. M. (2016). Locality Sensitive Deep Learning for Detection and Classification of Nuclei in Routine Colon Cancer Histology Images. *IEEE Transactions on Medical Imaging*, *35*(5), 1196–1206. doi:10.1109/TMI.2016.2525803 PMID:26863654

Vieira, S., Pinaya, W. H., & Mechelli, A. (2017). Using deep learning to investigate the neuroimaging correlates of psychiatric and neurological disorders: Methods and applications. *Neuroscience and Biobehavioral Reviews*, *74*, 58–75. doi:10.1016/j.neubiorev.2017.01.002 PMID:28087243

Xu, J., Luo, X., Wang, G., Gilmore, H., & Madabhushi, A. (2016). A Deep Convolutional Neural Network for segmenting and classifying epithelial and stromal regions in histopathological images. *Neurocomputing*, *191*, 214–223. doi:10.1016/j.neucom.2016.01.034 PMID:28154470

Xu, Y., Jiao, L., Wang, S., Wei, J., Fan, Y., Lai, M., & Chang, E. I. (2013). Multi-label classification for colon cancer using histopathological images. *Microscopy Research and Technique*, *76*(12), 1266–1277. doi:10.1002/jemt.22294 PMID:24123468

Yonekura, A., Kawanaka, H., Prasath, V. B., Aronow, B. J., & Takase, H. (2017). Improving the generalization of disease stage classification with deep CNN for Glioma histopathological images. *2017 IEEE International Conference on Bioinformatics and Biomedicine (BIBM)*. 10.1109/BIBM.2017.8217831

Zheng, Y., Jiang, Z., Xie, F., Zhang, H., Ma, Y., Shi, H., & Zhao, Y. (2017). Feature extraction from histopathological images based on nucleus-guided convolutional neural network for breast lesion classification. *Pattern Recognition*, *71*, 14–25. doi:10.1016/j.patcog.2017.05.010

Chapter 7
A Novel Approach of K-SVD-Based Algorithm for Image Denoising

Madhu Golla
VNR Vignana Jyothi Institute and Engineering and Technology, India

Sudipta Rudra
VNR Vignana Jyothi Institute and Engineering and Technology, India

ABSTRACT

In recent years, denoising has played an important role in medical image analysis. Image denoising is still accepted as a challenge for researchers and image application developers in medical image applications. The idea is to denoise a microscopic image through over-complete dictionary learning using a k-means algorithm and singular value decomposition (K-SVD) based on pursuit methods. This approach is good in performance on the quality improvement of the medical images, but it has low computational speed with high computational complexity. In view of the above limitations, this chapter proposes a novel strategy for denoising insight phenomena of the K-SVD algorithm. In addition, the authors utilize the technology of improved dictionary learning of the image patches using heap sort mechanism followed by dictionary updating process. The experimental results validate that the proposed approach successfully reduced noise levels on various test image datasets. This has been found to be more accurate than the best in class denoising approaches.

DOI: 10.4018/978-1-5225-6316-7.ch007

INTRODUCTION

In recent developments of modern digital image analysis, denoising assumes a key part of image processing. Denoising is an elementary issue of signal improvement in image processing then it requires moderating the noise levels of the detected images while stabilizing the texture features, corner features and edge particulars of the original image (Wang, Wang, & Liu, 2017). Image denoising is the method of reducing the noise levels, which makes imaging analysis easier (de FontesGuillermo, Pierrick Coupé, & Hellie, 2011). The aim of denoising method is to reduce the noise levels homogeneous regions while stabilizing the image forms and reconstruct the original image form (de FontesGuillermo, Pierrick Coupé, & Hellie, 2011; Guo, Zhang, Zhang, & Liu, 2016). In recent decades, numerous researchers have proposed distinctive sorts of image denoising algorithms to enhance the quality and decrease the noise in images (Wang, Wang, & Liu, 2017). Because such noise could affect the major applications such as medical image analysis (Han, Xu, Baciu, & Li, 2015; Liang & Weller, 2016; Wu, Huang, & Shi, 2015; Gu, Tao, Qiao, & Lin, 2018; Hung & Siu, 2012), signal processing and video processing (Mairal, Sapiro, & Elad, 2008), and others (Aharon, Elad, & Bruckstein, 2006), suggested K- means based SVD algorithm for single-scale dictionary learning and sparse representation of grayscale image related patches. In the literature, K-SVD algorithm has represented dictionary learning for sparsity representation (Yang, Bouzerdoum, & Phung, 2009). Similarly, K-SVD has several issues in dealing with higher dimensional signals. A major limitation of K-SVD is to choose suitable dictionary learning for the dataset, which is a non-convex problem then it works by an iterative update passion that does not an assurance to find the global optimum. In addition, another disadvantage of K-SVD is that it is relatively slow in time complexity with every iteration of decomposition. Still, interesting sparse representation technique has been verified fruitful for Gaussian and impulse noise elimination. This research, motivated by earlier research works highlight on impulse noise elimination and sparse representation. Keeping these issues, we suggested an efficient three-stage patch-based denoising method. That is to combine the heap sorting technique (Hwang & Haddad, 1995; Ko & Lee, 1991) with a competent dictionary learning approach and improved images abnormal by Gaussian and impulse noise (Hwang & Haddad, 1995; Aharon, Elad, & Bruckstein, 2006). The first stage, we use the dictionary initialization method to detect the overlapping patches. In the second stage, we follow the sparse coding with the help of orthogonal matching pursuit (OMP) in this stage, the denoising phenomenon applied through heap sort technique. Finally, the dictionaries are updated in such a way that image reconstruction occurs through the noise-based image. The objective of this research is a dual sparsity-based methodology for Gaussian noise and impulse noise elimination using both heap sort and SVD based approximations.

To overcome the above challenges, we proposed the sparse representations and redundant representations of trained dictionaries on the grayscale image using heap sort technique. This approach is utilized to reduce the computational space. The two stages and K-SVD motivate the proposed method; we developed a three-stage method for denoising with dictionary learning. In starting stage, the authors utilize the dictionary initialization procedure to detect the overlapping patches. In the second stage, the authors follow the sparse coding with the help of orthogonal matching pursuit (OMP) applied through heap sort technique to the denoising phenomenon. In the third stage, the dictionaries are updated in such a way that the image reconstruction occurs through the noised image.

The rest of the chapter organized as follows. Section 2 briefly discussed the related works of the denoising methods. Section 3 presents the categorization of proposed denoising method and its mathematical descriptions in detail with stage wise. Section 4 presents experimentations and results in order to validate the suggested denoising method on medical image datasets and Section 5 concludes the chapter.

RELATED WORKS

This related works shortly reviewed denoising methods about image denoising and its applications. The up-to-date denoising methods adopt different approaches to address the denoising issues. In the literature, many researchers have been concentrating on processing the image in the spatial methods, due to the simplicity of such methods (Tomasi & Manduchi, 1998; Dai, Lu, Wang, Wang, & Xia, 2017; Buades, Coll, & Morel, 2005). Michal Aharon, Michael Elad, and Alfred Bruckstein (2006) proposed a sparse representation of image patches and *k*-means clustering algorithm with SVD to train overcomplete dictionary for denoising as such learning methods are computationally expensive. Kostadin Dabov, Alessandro Foi, Vladimir Katkovnik, and Karen Egiazarian (2007) proposed a well-known hybrid method also known as Block-matching and 3-D filter (BM3D) algorithm that used for image denoising. In addition, BM3D is a robust algorithm that still has room for improvements. The BM3D algorithm performs to improve the sparsity representation of an image by categorization and increasing the noise removal but at the same time, protective image features such as limited details, for example, sharp edges etc. Kostadin Dabov, Alessandro Foi, Vladimir Katkovnik, and Karen Egiazarian. (2009) suggested an enhanced filter also known as BM3D-SAPCA algorithm, this method utilizes the image patches in terms of data-adaptive shape with principal component analysis (PCA) and its disadvantage is very high computational complexity. Lei Zhang, Weisheng Dong, David Zhang, and Guangming Shi (2010) suggested an impressive image denoising method based on principal component analysis with local pixel grouping.

This chapter, noise levels adaptively adjusted and training models selected with a local window through block matching based LPG method. Furthermore, the local search approach may not discover similarity for unusual patches in local surroundings and disadvantage of this approach is its computational cost. Yanmin He, Tao Gan, Wufan Chen, and Houjun Wang (2011) presented adaptive denoising method using SVD also called adaptive singular value decomposition (ASVD), which utilizes the SVD mechanism to training the global subspace test into the structure of local basis selection for representing image patches. Weisheng Dong, Guangming Shi, and Xin Li (2013) presented singular value decomposition based denoising approach also called SAIST that utilize singular value decomposition in terms of sparse coding on image patches which decreases noise levels in the image and repeated retiring the singular values by Bayes Shrink. The chapter compared with the K-SVD, LPG-PCA, BM3D with SAPCA and SAIST using different parameters discussed in section 4.

PROPOSED METHODS

In this chapter, demonstrates that classical image-denoising issue for imaging analysis for which an ideal image Z calculate additive zero-mean white and standardized Gaussian noise W as well as standard deviation σ. The real underlying reason behind adding noise levels for sparse representations or noise modeling is that it is difficult to visually measure the statistical noise levels, biological based molecular interferences present in the microscopic images. So that the notation is represented as follows:

$$Z = W + \sigma \tag{1}$$

Motivated by Michal Aharon, Michael Elad, and Alfred Bruckstein (2006) developed three stages for denoising with dictionary learning where the first stage deals with the spatial and sparse representation of images. The second stage represents the dictionary patches extraction and updating methods whereas in the third stage this represents the denoising methodology using modified K-SVD.

We denote the normal K-SVD for which $\min_{dx}\left\{\left|Y - DX\right|_2^p\right\}$ represents the normal K-SVD for image denoising; Subject to $\forall$ where, $x_i = e_k$ for some k, $\text{minimum}_{dx}\left\{\left|Y - DX\right|_2^p\right\}$; Subject to $\forall$ where, $\left\|z\right\| = 1$. Again, for updating, $\text{minimum}_{dx}\left\{\left|Y - DX\right|_2^p\right\}$: Subject to $\forall$; $N_{X_I} \le n_p$ or $\text{minimum}_{dx} \sum \left\|x_i\right\|$ subject to $\forall_i$, $\left\|Y - DX\right\|_2^F \leq \in$ m. Let D be fixed coefficient matrix that tends to counts to

$$\left\|Y - DX\right\|_2^F = \left\|\sum X_i w_i \otimes \frac{1}{2}\left(X - \mathrm{E}^2\right)\right\| \tag{2}$$

In this chapter, proposed approach restores the dictionary once a batch of training vectors prepared and used in this training vector that iteratively to update the dictionary learning. Karl Skretting and Kjersti Engan (2010) discoursed recursive least squares dictionary-learning algorithm (RLS-DLA) which updates the dictionaries in a constant mode then each training vector is prepared and this can be more efficiently used and executed.

Figure 1 shows the block diagram of the proposed works. Concretely, pursuit algorithm step calculates the coefficient matrix of noise image. Then pixel grouping with patches selection by using Euclidean distance measure. Once patches selection completed estimated the dictionary initialization using K-SVD method. In the sequential algorithm, first fewer atoms of the dictionaries that deeply learned from the input noise image data itself then apply the max heap sort technique to compute the sparse matrices. Finally, dictionary updations process this stage following K-SVD method as it improves the gamma correction rate, which is a very helpful application in color image processing.

Figure 1. Block diagram of the proposed image denoising method

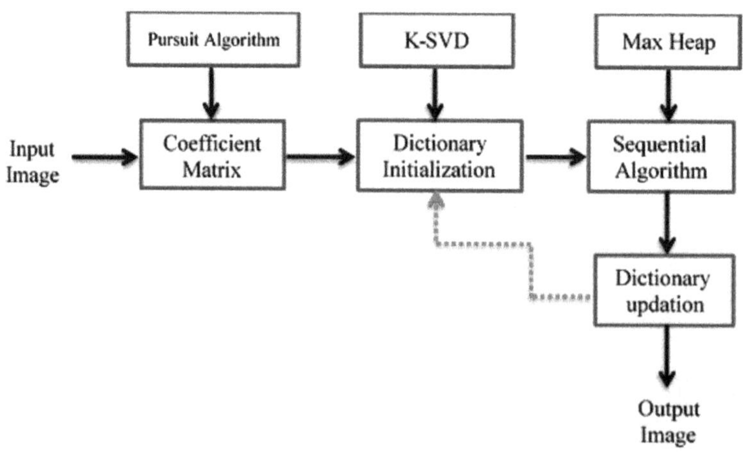

Stage 1

Michal Aharon, Michael Elad, and Alfred Bruckstein (2006) proposed K-SVD algorithm which is one of the popular filters in the field of image denoising, which uses the *k*-means based clustering method. An iterative approach presented which varies in sparse coding stage and this method is to modify and modernize the dictionary atoms effectively. The aim of sparse coding is to discover the greatest coefficient vector x when dictionary **Φ** value specified. Under this stage, simple pursuit algorithms utilize and calculate coefficient matrix. In addition, SVD based decomposition method is used to determine the column vector updation process. The algorithm interchanges between the two stages of sequential algorithm and dictionary learning updating process until best level dictionary is generated. Using this updation dictionary learning instruction and K-SVD converges at a much faster rate and improves more noise based patch elements rather than state-of-the denoising algorithms.

However, during the dictionary updating stage (Mairal, Elad, & Sapiro, 2008), we use the K-SVD objective function represented as follows:

$$\left\| Z - DY_2^F \right\| = \left\| Z - \sum_{M}^{N-1} d_{x2}^{F} \right\| \tag{3}$$

$$= \left\| \left(Z - \sum_{N \neq M} d_x \right) - d_j \right\| \tag{4}$$

$$= \left\| E_K - d_{x2}^{F} \right\| \cdots \tag{5}$$

The kth row in Y being defined as x_t^j which has not been mentioned due to mathematical ambiguity and the d_x is the kth column in dictionary D. Matrix E_K represents the fault matrix where the kth atom is detached. In addition, the group of such similar samples are generated based on atom d_k this atom d_k is well-defined as follows:

$$\delta_k = \{(i) \mid 1 \leq K, x_t^j(i) \neq 0\} \tag{6}$$

Using equation (6), find K-SVD updates with dictionary learning after a group of training vectors has refined and used the training set systematically increase the dictionary learning for patches. In the image, the positions being corrupted by the impulse noises can be represented as μ and let z be the characteristic matrix that represents as follows

$$z = \begin{cases} 1 \; if \left(i, j \in 0 \right) \\ 0, otherwise \end{cases} \tag{7}$$

In addition, the equations (3)-(7) formulated for initializing the dictionary as follows

$$\left\| \lambda \Sigma E_K - d_x \otimes \left(Z - \sum_{N \neq M} d_x \right) \right\|_2^F + \Sigma \left(X - \mathrm{E}^2 \right) + \sum_J^I \mu_{ij} \tag{8}$$

where $\otimes$ represents decision-based multiplication operator between noise matrix and characteristic matrix and Z is being denoted as the matrix of constant term records both 1 and 0 and with similar dimension. The initial expression is a term used for initializing the dictionary from the images, which selects the pixels, which is not disrupted by the noise levels, whereas the second data ε^2 is a fidelity term covering the patch-based atoms. The importance of ε^2 will be the removal of random valued noise levels as well as Gaussian and impulse based noise levels.

From the Algorithm 1, it is being stated that an input noise based image, a patch size of $x \times y$ is being selected and being fixed as a reference with the column vectors

Algorithm 1. Dictionary Initialization

Input: Noise level based image.
Output: Overlapped patches.
Step 1: Let i, j be the image pixels.
Step 2: Fix the patch size(x, y) along with step and iteration.
Step 3: Select the column vectors as patches, $f\left(x, y\right) \in j$
Step 4: Repeat K times (K= no. of iterations)
Step 5: Detect the overlapping patches with initialization of learned dictionaries with the help of ε^2.
Step 6: Stop

as j of the image matrix as the function of image patch size being denoted as $f\left(x,y\right)$. With the repetition of step 1, step 2, and step 3 in the mentioned above algorithm, the overlapped patches in the noise based image are detected with the help of patch-based atoms. This module discusses the dictionary initialization process whereas the second stage mentioned in next section discussed a sequential algorithm (Algorithm 2) that improves the sparse coding process in the normal K-SVD algorithm.

Stage 2

The second stage consists of sparse coding of all signals or patches for which we used orthogonal matching pursuit (OMP) algorithm where the OMP is a step sequence wise forward based selection algorithm and is easy for implementation in denoising applications. A key element of pursuit algorithm is the stopping rule that builds upon the noise structure present in the images.

Algorithm 2. Sequential Algorithm

Input: overlapped patch-based image.

Output: Extraction of patches for reconstruction or denoising.

Step 1: Initialize the noise patches x_0 and select the residual patches as f (x_0) = y. let the iteration count is K=1 as mentioned in algorithm 1 in Step-1.

Step 2: Detect the patches variable y_{t_i}, which resolves the maximization criterion.

$max\left|y_t^{'}x_0 - 1\right|$

add the patches variable y_{t_i} to the residual patches and update.

Step 3: Let $Y_i = f\left(y_{t_i}\right)f\left(y_{t_i}\right)^{'}f\left(y_{t_i}\right)^{-1}$, which denotes the projection into the linear space spanned through the use of patch elements of the noisy image.

Step 4: If the stopping rule is attained then exit the algorithm.

else

Initialize the $I = i+1$ and then go to Step 2.

Step 5: Stop.

Note: Whereas, the stopping criteria represented as given below:

Let the mutual coherence between the noise patches and clean patches be X.

Let T = {I: μ ≠ 0} be the support vector of μ and let X (T) be the set of column vectors (j) of X that corresponds to T.

$$N = maximum_{x \in T/X(T)} \left\{ \left\| X\left(T\right)^{'} * X\left(T\right)^{-1} * X\left(T\right)^{'} * x \right\|^{2} \right\} \ldots \tag{9}$$

The stopping condition will be satisfied when M < 1.

In addition, sparse coding objective is to construct pure representations of given input image data, i.e. the linear form of first fewer atoms of the dictionaries that deeply learned from the input noise image data itself. However, Sparse coding is mainly used behind dictionary learning in such a way that it decomposes the images into two variable matrices that are a sparse matrix and learning value atom matrix, which becomes a satisfying condition to be suitable for denoising method other than LASSO, sparse approximation method.

Given the set of atoms $y = \{ y_1, y_2, y_3, \ldots y_{n,} y_{n+1} \}$. Here, in the sequential algorithm, the sparse coding aims at detecting a dictionary $D = \{ d_1, d_2, d_3, \ldots d_{n,} d_{n+1} \}$, such that each atom $n \in N$ atoms can be well checked by a linear combination of $\left\{ d_J \right\}_{j=1,2\ldots n}^{M}$ such that y = $\sum_{n=1}^{m} a_l b_l$ and such, coefficients a_l are zero or nearest to zero. Then sparse coding can be regionally expressed as the following denoising phenomenon as $\min_{D,c_i,p_{\max}} \sum_{i=1}^{p_{\max}} \frac{3}{4} \left\| y_i - Dc \right\|_i^2 \otimes \tau \left\| c \right\|_{i2}$ subject to $\left\| d_i \right\|$ = 1.0, 1.0 ≤ i ≤ m. Here, dictionary size m is represented as more than the signal dimension n. Usually, this stage works for optimal noise removal such as impulse noise. Therefore, to increase the optimal performance of noise removal we introduced new insertion technique in sparse coding such that learning value α becomes higher. Let the sparse code matrix represented by

$$min_{dx} \left\{ \left\| Y - DX \right\|_2^p \right\} \text{Subject to } \forall \; N_{X_I} \leq n_p \tag{10}$$

This study, we utilized the max-heap property proposed by Svante Carlsson, Jingsen Chen, and Christer Mattsson (1996), which is represented as follows: If Z is an array representation of a heap, then in max-heap is

$$Z\left[Parent\left(i\right)\right] \leq Z\left(i\right) \tag{11}$$

This means that a node cannot have a greater value than its parent can. In a max-heap, the largest element is stored at the root, and the minimum elements are in the leaves. So in order to apply in the sparse coding stage $\min_{dx}\left\{\left|Y - DX\right|_2^p\right\}$ is subjected to Max heap property then it becomes in search maximum value of trained patches, which can be defined as follows

$$W = \begin{cases} 1, \ if\left|Y - DX\right|_2^p \ll N_{X_I} \\ 0, \ if\left|Y - DX\right|_2^p = N_{X_I} \\ -1, \ if\left|Y - DX\right|_2^p \gg N_{X_I} \end{cases} \tag{12}$$

We know that $N_{X_I} \leq n_p$ represented above. So optimal performance the dictionary D such be initialized as

$$\max_{E_K,z/X}\left\|\Sigma E_K - d_x\right\| \otimes \left(\left\|Z - \sum_{N \neq M} d_x\right\|_2\right)^F + \Sigma\left(X - \mathrm{E}^2\right) + \sum_J^I \mu_{ij} \tag{13}$$

where ε^2 should be greater than n_p, such that optimal node selection becomes easier whether it may be trained atoms or extracted noisy patches. Therefore, it solves also the time complexity problem in denoising application. Now on with dictionary initialization, the search initiates with this formula

$$\left.\frac{\max_{E_K,z/X}\Sigma\left\|E_K - d_x\right\| \otimes \left(\left\|Z - \sum_{N \neq M} d_x\right\|_2\right)^F + \Sigma\left(X - \mathrm{E}^2\right) + \sum_J^I \mu_{ij}}{y_i - Dc_i^2}\right/ W \tag{14}$$

Here with search initialization, the higher node or atom selection follows the max heap property as follows:

$$\lim_{n\to\infty}\left(1+\frac{1}{\dfrac{\max_{E_K,z/X}\sum\left\|E_K-d_x\right\|\otimes\left\|\left(Z-\sum_{N\neq M}d_x\right)_2^F\right\|+\sum\left(X-\mathrm{E}^2\right)+\sum_J^I\mu_{ij}}{\left\|y_i-Dc_i^2\right\|}\Big/W}\right)^N \quad (15)$$

Herein, after higher atom selection, the sorting technique starts. So that for heap sort we use minimization problem to compute the sparse matrices. Therefore, with condition W >> 1 the sorting process starts with lower atom selection. Such that the sparse matrix results with the introduction of this methodology in K-SVD (Aharon, Elad, & Bruckstein, 2006) based denoising phenomenon, extreme results with higher peak signal to noise ratio are observed. Therefore, by employing this technique, it cannot learn with the good dictionary from trained levels but it provides much more efficient denoising applications than K-SVD (Aharon, Elad, & Bruckstein, 2006). This methodology is especially being proposed for removal of impulse noises in images.

$$\min_{D,c_i,p_{\max}}\left\|\sum_{i=1}^{p_{\max}}\frac{3}{4}y_i-Dc_i^2\otimes\tau c_{i2}\times\left(Z-\sum_{N\neq M}d_x\right)_2^F+\varphi c_{i2}\right\| \quad (16)$$

Stage 3

In this stage, we present the dictionary updation process. However, this stage following K-SVD method as it improves the gamma correction rate, which is a very helpful application in color image processing. After sparse coding, the entire atom patches through the sequential algorithm from section 3.2. For this stage, fix all the m_{ij} and on behalf of each atom $d_{n,}$, where n $\in$ 1, 2, 3….in dictionary D. Select the patch k^l that is used by this atom notation

$$k^l = \left(m, n\right) \mid m_{ij}\left(l\right) \neq 0 \tag{17}$$

So for each of the patches (i, j) $\in k^l$. Therefore, we compute the residual using the following formula $\forall$ each patches; (i, j) that belongs to k^l

$$e_{ij}^l = d_{ij} u - D m_{ij} + d_J \tag{18}$$

and $\lambda_{ij}^l = D_{ij} \lambda$ is an index vector representing candidate pixels from the patches of small image size $\sqrt{m} \times \sqrt{m}$ from the location coordinate of $\left(i, j\right)$ of the image.

Therefore, now $E_l = (e_{ij}^l)_{i,j \in k^l}$ set, i, j for image patches apply the computation as stated below in the Algorithm 3.

EXPERIMENTAL RESULTS

This study demonstrates the ability of the proposed denoising methodology. This chapter present experimental results about simulations, which has conducted on

Algorithm 3. Dictionary Updation

Input: Patch-based image for reconstruction
Output: Reconstructed image
Step 1: Set $E_l = (e_{ij}^l)_{i,j \in k^l}$, i, j for image patches;
Step 2: Initialize U, S, V for E_l;
Step 3: Apply for all patches to be reconstructed [U, S, V] = svd (E_l) $\forall$ k;
Step 4: Replace coefficient of the atom D_{ij} in the image with the entries of s_1, v_1, d_{ij}.
Step 5: After performing step 4 to checks the stopping condition, if it is satisfied then
Stop.
else
then return to algorithm-2 and again perform sequential based heap sort.
Step 6: To set the final recovered patches as $E_l = \widehat{E_l}$
Step 7: Stop.

four different stages of pathological images of malaria parasite of microscopic blood images as test input images with sizes (512×512), such as Plasmodium *falciparum*, Plasmodium *vivax*, Plasmodium *malaria,* Plasmodium *Ovale*. These test images converted into grayscale images and used to validate the proposed denoising algorithms. The noise levels (σ) is from 10 to 50 and intensity of each pixel value of the given image series from 0 to 255. The grayscale images used for testing of our suggested method are shown in Figure 2.

Evaluation Measures

The performance of the denoising results was evaluated by the denoised imaged from the proposed method. This chapter used three evaluation measures, which are mostly used for a quality measure such as Peak Signal-to-Noise Ratio (PSNR), Structural Similarity Index Measure (SSIM) (Zhou Wang, Alan C. Bovik, Hamid R. Sheikh, & Eero P. Simoncelli. 2004; Kieran G. Larkin.2015) and Entropy measure (Jan Urban. 2016) was adapted to evaluate the experimental results of the proposed denoising method.

- **PSNR:** PSNR is one of the popular image qualities metric in the image analysis. This chapter, PSNR value for the grayscale image are defined by

$$PSNR = 20 * \log_{10}\left(A\right) - 10 * \log_{10}\left(A - \hat{A}\right) / 255 \tag{19}$$

where $\hat{A}$ represent the reconstructed image and A denotes the original malaria blood image throughout the experiments; This chapter set the size of the dictionary as 64×256, as well as image patch size as 7×7. In this study, have fixed the image

Figure 2. Grayscale images are used for testing of proposed methods (i) Plasmodium falciparum (ii) Plasmodium vivax (iii) Plasmodium malaria (iv) Plasmodium ovale

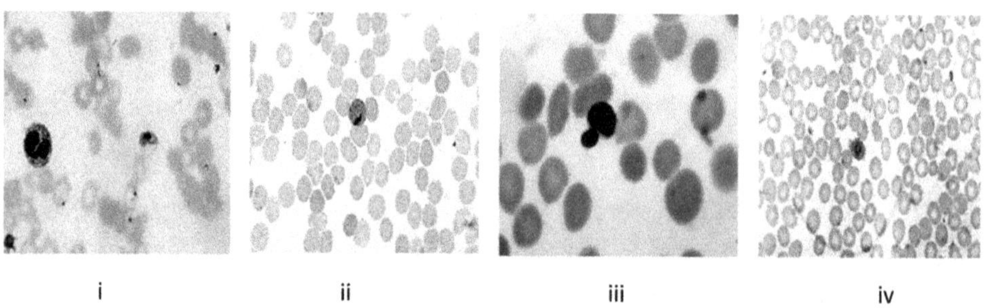

window size as 10 and step size= 20. Note that, sigma (σ) is reassumed to be known or can be roughly estimated.

- **SSIM:** Computing similarity among the images through SSIM. This metric represented as a quality measurement metric between the images. The structural similarity index measure is defined as follows:

$$\text{SSIM}(\text{A}, \hat{A}) = \frac{1}{k}\sum_{J=1}^{k} SSIM_J\left(A, \hat{A}\right) \tag{20}$$

where

$$SSIM_J = \left[\frac{2\sigma_1\sigma_2}{\sigma_1^2 + \sigma_2^2}\right] \times \left[\frac{\sigma_{12}}{\sigma_1\sigma_2}\right] = \frac{2\sigma_{12}}{\sigma_1^2 + \sigma_2^2} \tag{21}$$

Here also, $\hat{A}$ represents the restored image or reconstructed image and if A represents an original image in all the experiments taken into the record; for calculating the SSIM values which are recorded in Table-1.

- **Entropy:** This chapter used the Shannon entropy from information theory with respect to the image analysis. This metric represented as a quality measurement metric between the images. The entropy measure is represented as follows:

$$Entropy\left(S\right) = -\sum_{i} p_i * \log_2\left(p_i\right) \tag{22}$$

Thus, entropy is the sum of the distinct information weighted by the probabilities of their occurrences and for calculating the entropy values are shown in Table 2.

Results

To estimate the performance of the proposed method, we compared with four major image denoising algorithms like a) *K-SVD*; b) *LPG-PCA*; c) *BM3D-SAPCA*; d) *SAIST*. However, above discussed approaches employ the self-similarity of ordinary images to conquer noise. In addition, these procedures consist of few limitations that must tune according to the different levels of noise in the image. In this chapter, we utilize the default parameters, which are advised by the respective authors. The proposed method is implemented in PYTHON because of a good collection of image processing libraries and its simplicity and graphs implemented in MATLAB programming language.

In Table 1 and 2, show the experimental results of all four challenging denoising methods with different metrics on grayscale images of microscopic blood images of malaria parasites with different levels of noise. From the Table 1 and 2, clearly observe that SAIST, which is measured to be one of the up-to-date image denoising methods attains the maximum PSNR value at $\sigma = 50$, and somewhat outperforms proposed method. Therefore, proposed approach achieves high PSNR rate in average then it achieves better outcomes on blood images with high reciting configurations such as *P. falciparum, P. malaria and P. ovale*. However, proposed method adequately does the nonlocal repletion in these microscopic images. In addition, observe that proposed method outperforms with LPG-PCA and SAIST in terms of psnr, ssim and entropy averages shown in Table 1 and 2. However, a proposed technique

Table 1. Test result of the PSNR (dB) and SSIM values with other denoising methods

Test Images	Noise Levels (σ)	K-SVD		LPG-PCA		BM3D-SAPCA		SAIST		Proposed	
		PSNR	SSIM	PSNR	SSIM	PSNR	SSIM	PSNR	SSIM	PSNR	SSIM
Falciparum	10	29.36	0.928	35.84	0.910	26.83	0.928	36.58	0.925	46.87	**0.931**
	20	24.49	0.843	34.98	0.896	24.86	**0.927**	35.43	0.914	43.61	0.926
	30	23.80	0.824	33.67	0.864	23.56	0.856	33.42	0.848	40.56	**0.918**
	40	20.89	0.809	32.09	0.837	23.10	0.716	31.78	0.816	37.87	**0.910**
	50	19.36	0.784	29.16	0.782	21.42	0.705	29.46	0.805	33.54	**0.849**
Vivax	10	33.58	0.878	35.46	**0.935**	34.56	0.926	38.42	**0.932**	43.57	0.928
	20	31.18	0.856	33.78	**0.927**	32.76	0.915	37.57	**0.924**	41.25	0.910
	30	28.39	0.842	31.58	**0.911**	30.45	0.857	33.75	0.895	40.48	0.895
	40	25.78	**0.826**	28.97	**0.856**	28.57	**0.826**	31.38	0.876	38.56	0.824
	50	23.39	**0.814**	28.15	0.829	27.35	0.813	30.17	0.847	36.68	0.801
Malariae	10	30.97	0.925	35.54	0.946	32.31	0.927	40.64	0.926	48.24	**0.948**
	20	28.76	0.910	33.48	0.938	29.47	0.907	40.26	0.891	45.26	**0.939**
	30	25.37	0.868	31.76	**0.922**	28.67	0.854	38.25	0.835	43.25	0.921
	40	22.53	0.851	29.16	0.846	27.43	0.823	37.25	0.802	39.94	**0.901**
	50	20.16	0.826	28.56	0.815	27.15	0.804	35.25	0.795	37.25	**0.856**
Ovale	10	28.76	0.892	34.56	0.916	27.86	0.924	42.56	**0.935**	48.60	0.926
	20	25.46	0.775	31.25	0.875	26.71	0.885	39.56	0.901	45.29	**0.912**
	30	23.78	0.736	29.35	0.846	25.28	0.858	37.28	0.875	43.31	**0.901**
	40	21.28	0.716	27.25	0.814	23.25	0.841	35.78	0.810	37.58	**0.868**
	50	20.13	0.685	26.23	0.802	21.25	**0.825**	29.36	0.785	32.58	0.823
Avg.		25.37	0.83	**31.54**	**0.87**	27.14	0.85	**35.70**	0.86	**41.21**	**0.89**

Table 2. Test result of the Entropy values with other denoising methods

Test Images	Noise Levels (σ)	K-SVD	LPG-PCA	BM3D-SAPCA	SAIST	Proposed
Falciparum	10	0.863	0.872	0.869	0.913	**0.894**
	20	0.842	0.851	0.842	**0.887**	0.872
	30	0.812	0.830	0.810	0.858	**0.859**
	40	0.779	0.811	0.776	0.826	**0.833**
	50	0.745	0.781	0.743	0.809	**0.817**
Vivax	10	0.872	0.882	0.868	0.876	**0.924**
	20	0.857	0.865	0.841	0.853	**0.906**
	30	0.830	0.843	0.829	0.831	**0.875**
	40	0.819	0.821	0.808	0.818	**0.853**
	50	0.795	0.805	0.784	0.793	**0.832**
Malariae	10	0.874	0.887	0.871	0.902	**0.936**
	20	0.853	0.862	0.854	0.887	**0.917**
	30	0.828	0.847	0.836	0.854	**0.892**
	40	0.809	0.821	0.814	0.831	**0.863**
	50	0.784	0.804	0.782	0.817	**0.841**
Ovale	10	0.884	0.877	0.912	0.896	**0.927**
	20	0.861	0.853	0.885	0.864	**0.905**
	30	0.842	0.831	0.854	0.832	**0.874**
	40	0.821	0.817	0.831	0.819	**0.848**
	50	0.802	0.796	0.817	0.797	**0.829**
Avg.		0.828	0.837	0.831	**0.848**	**0.874**

performed superior quality on microscopic blood images with huge repeating patterns. Similarly, proposed method sufficiently does the sparse coding of the patches in these images through the developed procedure in stage 2 and stage 3. For example, *P. falciparum* image, on PSNR at $\sigma = 50$, the proposed technique is higher to K-SVD by 14.17(dB), to SAIST by 12.12(dB) respectively. The SSIM outcomes of up-to-date denoising procedures are also presented in Table 1. Clearly, observe that proposed technique has improved SSIM values than other denoising methods except for Plasmodium *vivax* image. In other words, the results shown that proposed techniques are competitive with K-SVD and SAIST.

The entropy experimental results are presented in Table 2. Clearly observe that the proposed technique has improved entropy values than other denoising methods discussed in related works. In other words, the experimentation of proposed technique is competitive with K-SVD and SAIST, and we say that our approach is superior to K-SVD. Clearly, Figure 3 demonstrate the denoising outcomes of Plasmodium falciparum image data with a noise level of $\sigma = 50$. From these results, the proposed methods are more prominently improved with high contrast than SAIST and LPG-PCA which are more useful than further methods like BM3D-SAPCA and K-SVD. In addition, visual assessments of Plasmodium vivax images shown in Figure 4 represents denoising effects of the noisy image Plasmodium vivax with various denoise methods.

Clearly, observe that the denoised images through K-SVD, LPG-PCA are similar to real visual sensitivity, in which few edges as well as textures are bit conserved and less edge artefacts are presented but the proposed phenomenon has more rate of visual perception as compared to BM3D-SAPCA and SAIST. Although BM3D-SAPCA and SAIST are superior to PSNR, SSIM and Entropy measures than our approach, denoised outcomes through K-SVD and hold more visible artefacts around edges, texture regularization and in smooth regions than our experimental outcomes.

The LPG-PCA performance the orthogonal transform to characterize related image patches and decreases noise levels through thresholding illustration coefficients in which extremely visible artifacts are originated and it processes the patches using normalization value of each patch value through image quality gets a bit improved

Figure 3. Visual test results on falciparum image computed by various algorithms. (i) Grayscale image, (ii) Noisy image (iii) K- SVD (iv) LPG –PCA (v) BM3D- SAPCA (vi) SAIST (vii) Proposed method

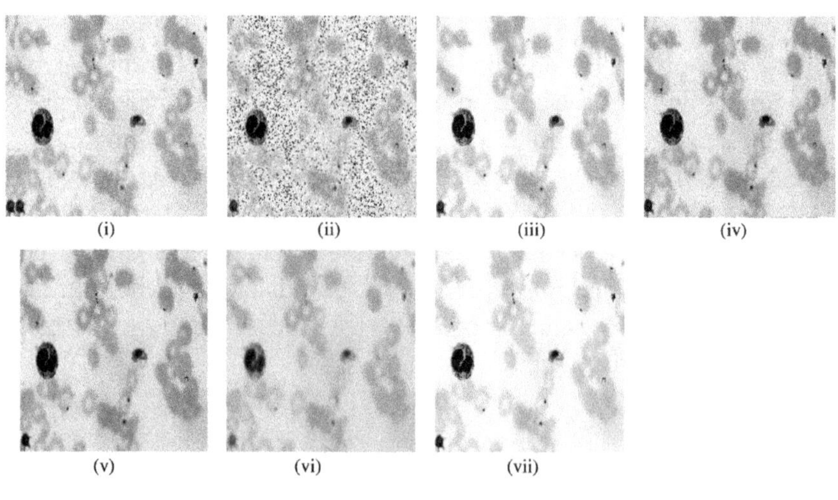

Figure 4. Visual test results on Plasmodium vivax image computed by various algorithms. (a) Grayscale image, (b) Noisy image (c) K- SVD (d) LPG –PCA (e) BM3D- SAPCA (f) SAIST (g) Proposed method

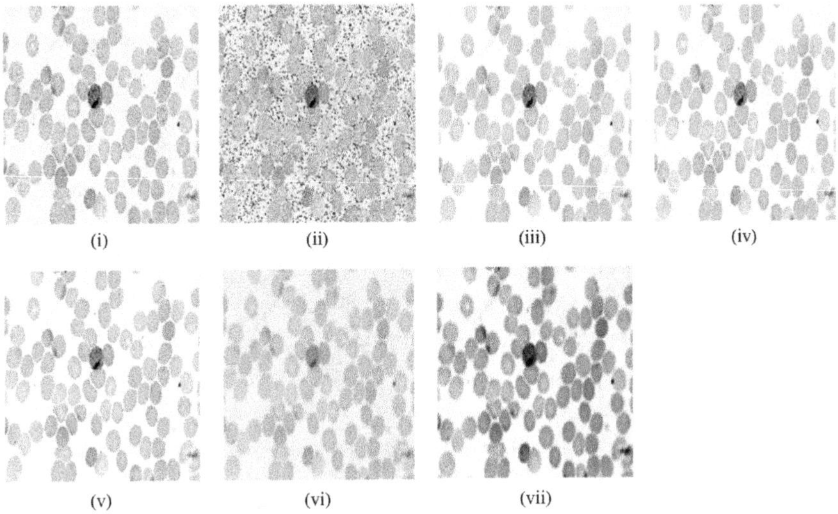

with high PSNR and Entropy values. Clearly, from the Figure 4, we clearly state that the suggested method has a more desirable performance with the other methods.

For Plasmodium malariae image, proposed method proves much superiority than compared denoising methodologies except at $\sigma = 50$, K-SVD proves as better performance in terms of PSNR than the proposed algorithms by 17.01 (dB). Whereas, in terms of SSIM at $\sigma = 40$, SAIST has shown better result the proposed methodology by the difference of 0.078 Db and Entropy values at $\sigma = 30$ K-SVD has shown better results 0.064 bits. In visual comparison from Figure 5, it is having more contrast rate than other algorithms but in texture comparison, K-SVD seems to be more efficient in texture preservation than other algorithms. Some amounts of artefacts are being noticed in the outputs of the resultant algorithms. On the basis patches regularization, the proposed methodology proves to be more efficient than other algorithms.

Figure 6 illustrates the denoising results of Plasmodium ovale image using a noise level of $\sigma = 50$. Clearly, we can observe that the results of proposed algorithms are more visually improved and high contrast than methods like K- SVD, LPG –PCA, BM3D- SAPCA and SAIST algorithm and LPG-PCA algorithm, which are improved than BM3D-SAPCA and K-SVD. In addition to which, visual comparisons of Plasmodium ovale images are shown in Figure 6, represents denoising outcomes of the noisy image of Plasmodium ovale with various denoising approaches. We examined that the denoised images through BM3D- SAPCA method and our

Figure 5. Visual test results on malariae image computed by various algorithms. (i) Grayscale image. (ii) Noisy image (iii) K- SVD (iv) LPG –PCA (v) BM3D- SAPCA (vi) SAIST (vii) Proposed method

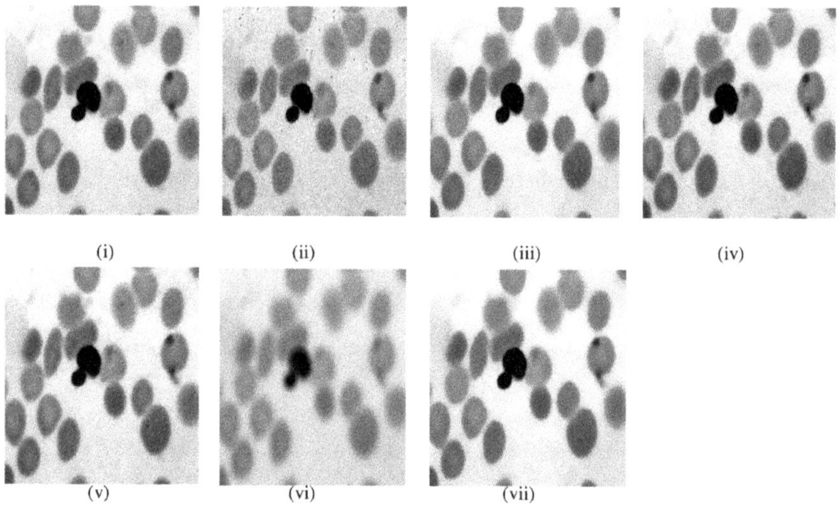

methodology are very similar. Nevertheless, the proposed phenomenon has more rate of visual perception as compared to K-SVD, method and LPG-PCA method. We noticed that the SSIM values of Plasmodium ovale image at $\sigma = 10, 20, 30$ of LPG-PCA algorithm succeeds the proposed algorithm by 0.01 (dB), 0.037 (dB), 0.055 (dB). However, we notice that the dictionary learning outperforms the reported results of aforementioned algorithms. All these noise levels lower than A = 30, although the trained global dictionary repeatedly achieves very nearby results that covers mixed-frequency based textural areas. The adaptive dictionary studies the specific training features which has a clear improvement over the globally trained dictionary with countable iterations presented with SNR = 25.

We observe that at $\sigma = 50$, the graph achieves some amount of saturation, in which non-regularized patches are removed. Thus, this result has more percentage of recovered rows through the trained dictionary. This proves the better computational efficiency in recovering with the trained dictionary generated from the test images. The PSNR, SSIM and Entropy values for the proposed technique compared with other denoising methods are shown in Figure 7 to Figure 12. The bar graphs represent the improvement in terms of dB and similarity based index performed through proposed approach with other denoising approaches such as K- SVD, LPG –PCA, BM3D- SAPCA and SAIST. From the above bar plots, it can be evidently state that proposed denoising approach have achieved the best PSNR, SSIM and Entropy values in all four benchmark datasets while compared with other denoising approaches such as BM3D- SAPCA, LPG –PCA, K- SVD, and SAIST.

Figure 6. Visual test results on Plasmodium ovale image computed by various algorithms. (i) Grayscale image. (ii) Noisy Image (iii) K- SVD (iv) LPG –PCA (v) BM3D- SAPCA (vi) SAIST (vii) Proposed method

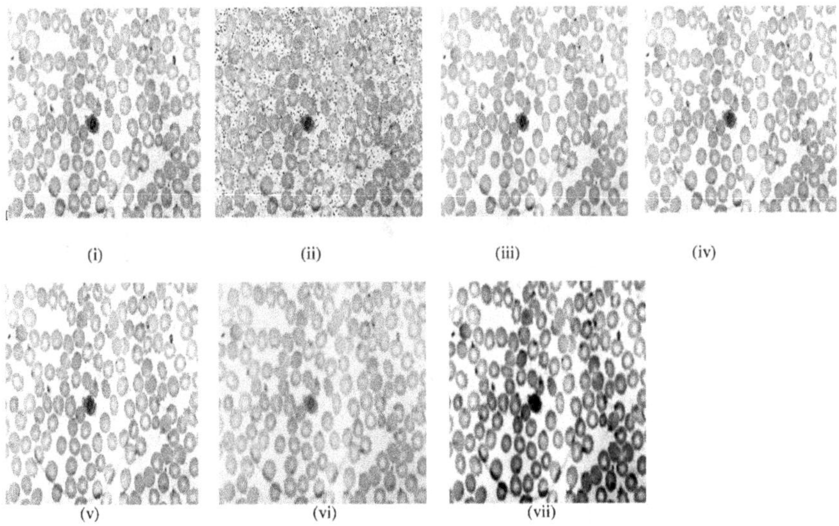

Figure 7. PSNR test results of proposed method vs other denoising methods on Plasmodium falciparum and vivax

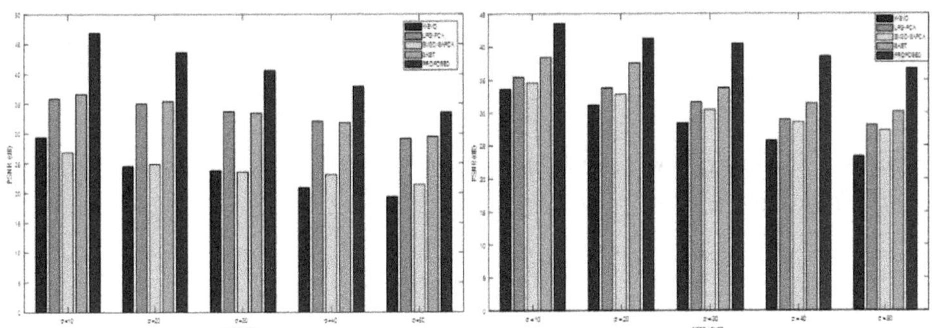

Figure 8. PSNR test results of proposed method vs other denoising methods on Plasmodium malariae and ovale

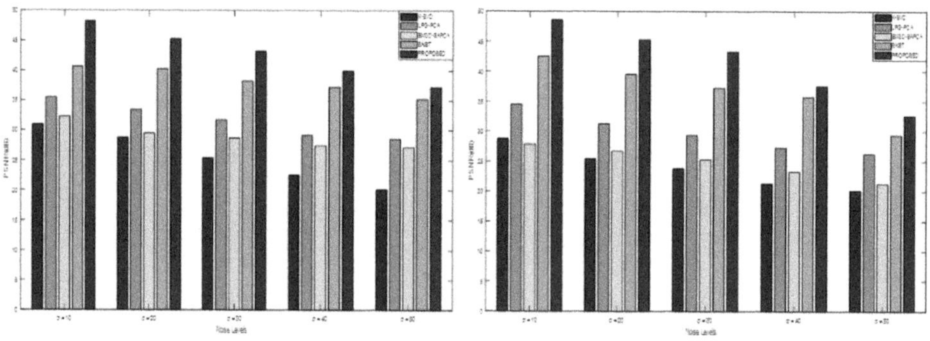

Figure 9. SSIM test results of proposed method vs other denoising methods on Plasmodium falciparum and vivax

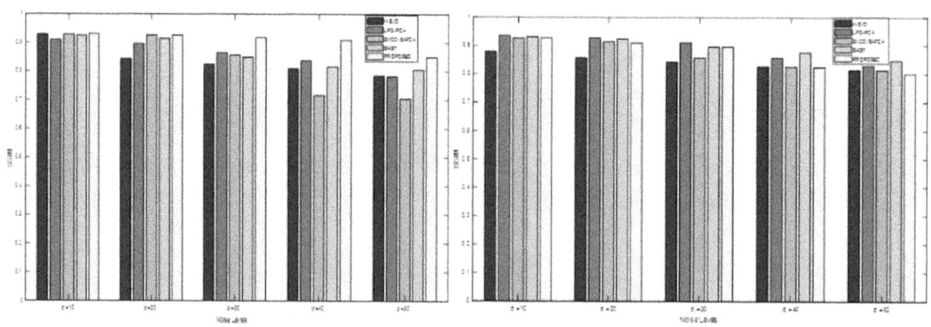

Figure 10. SSIM test results of proposed method vs other denoising methods on Plasmodium Malariae and ovale

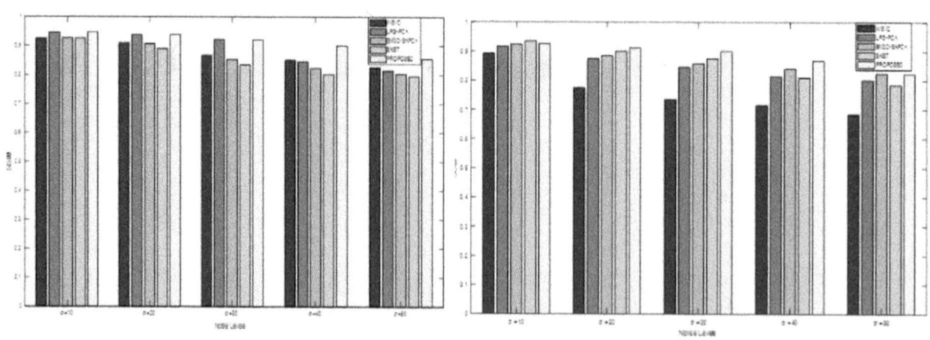

Figure11. Entropy test results of proposed method vs other denoising methods on Plasmodium falciparum and vivax

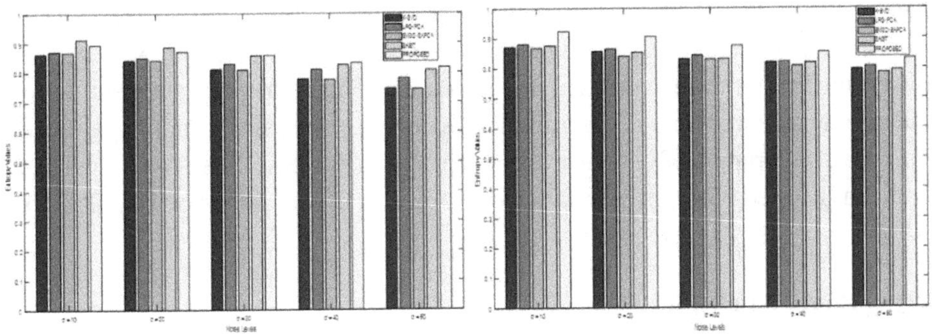

Figure 12. Entropy test results of proposed method vs other denoising methods on Plasmodium malariae and ovale

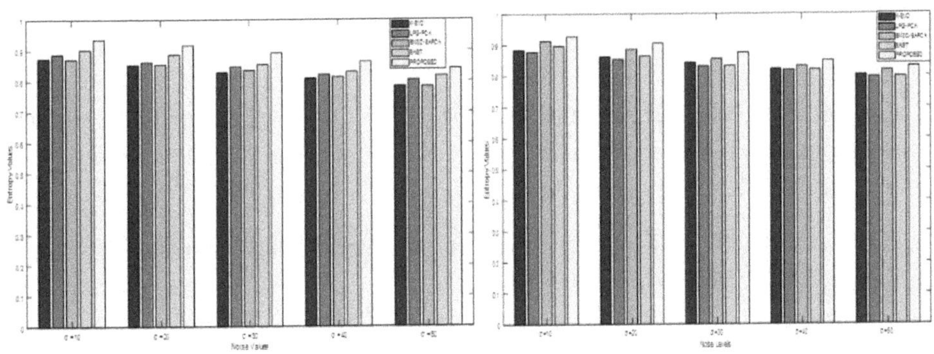

CONCLUSION

In this chapter, we have demonstrated three stage denoising technique for microscopic image analysis, which is a smooth and efficient method. We presented a patch based three-stage denoising algorithm using heap sort technique on microscopic images. This model combines the heap sort technique with an efficient dictionary learning technique such as K-SVD, to reconstruct the original images from noisy patches with improved contrast rate and homogeneity. The main contribution of this chapter was to present a better efficient algorithm for microscopic image denoising applications especially in cases of random valued and biological noises. This work concentrated on variable image patches taking into account of small sizes. The proposed method is based on local mutual coherence with heap sort for sorting out the maximum valued patches and sparse decomposition of each image block under one trained dictionary derived from the test images. The experimental results tested on various test grayscale microscopic malaria parasite images show that our proposed algorithm denoises an image effectively with comparisons shown above experimental results. Finally, it demonstrates that it is much efficient than compared algorithms with preserving local texture features in image analysis. For further improvement, we are undergoing research on using multiscale dictionaries with single tuning parameter with the development of new dictionary other than BLASS, LASSO etc. such way that it has applied on larger blocks, which is the major limitation of original K-SVD.

ACKNOWLEDGMENT

This work was supported by the DRDO-DRL, Tezpur, Assam, India (Task No. DRLT-P1- 2015/Task-64).

REFERENCES

Aharon, M., Elad, M., & Bruckstein, A. (2006). K-SVD: An Algorithm for Designing Overcomplete Dictionaries for Sparse Representation. *IEEE Transactions on Signal Processing*, *54*(11), 4311–4322. doi:10.1109/TSP.2006.881199

Buades, A., Coll, B., & Morel, J.-M. (2005). A Non-Local Algorithm for Image Denoising. *2005 IEEE Computer Society Conference on Computer Vision and Pattern Recognition (CVPR'05)*, *2*, 60-65. 10.1109/CVPR.2005.38

Carlsson, S., Chen, J., & Mattsson, C. (1996). Heaps with bits. *Theoretical Computer Science*, *164*(1-2), 1–12. doi:10.1016/0304-3975(95)00152-2

Dabov, K., Foi, A., Katkovnik, V., & Egiazarian, K. (2007). Image Denoising by Sparse 3-D Transform-Domain Collaborative Filtering. *IEEE Transactions on Image Processing*, *16*(8), 2080–2095. doi:10.1109/TIP.2007.901238 PMID:17688213

Dabov, K., Foi, A., Katkovnik, V., & Egiazarian, K. (2009). BM3D image denoising with shape-adaptive principal component analysis. SPARS'09 - Signal Processing with Adaptive Sparse Structured Representations.

Dai, T., Lu, W., Wang, W., Wang, J., & Xia, S.-T. (2017). Entropy-based bilateral filtering with a new range kernel. *Signal Processing*, *137*(C), 223–234. doi:10.1016/j.sigpro.2017.02.005

de Fontes Guillermo, F., Barroso, A., Coupé, P., & Hellier, P. (2011). Article. *Journal of Real-Time Image Processing*, *6*(15), 15–22. doi:10.100711554-010-0158-5

Dong, W., Shi, G., & Li, X. (2013). Nonlocal image restoration with bilateral variance estimation: A low-rank approach. *IEEE Transactions on Image Processing*, *22*(2), 700–711. doi:10.1109/TIP.2012.2221729 PMID:23047875

Gao, L., Wang, G., & Liu, J. (2015). Image denoising based on edge detection and prethresholding Wiener filtering of multi-wavelets fusion. International Journal of Wavelets, Multiresolution and Information Processing, 13(5).

Gu, K., Tao, D., Qiao, J.-F., & Lin, W. (2018). Learning a no-reference quality assessment model of enhanced images with big data. *IEEE Transactions on Neural Networks and Learning Systems*, *29*(4), 1301–1313. doi:10.1109/TNNLS.2017.2649101 PMID:28287984

Guo, Q., Zhang, C., Zhang, Y., & Liu, H. (2016). An efficient SVD-based method for image denoising. *IEEE Transactions on Circuits and Systems for Video Technology*, *26*(5), 868–880. doi:10.1109/TCSVT.2015.2416631

Han, Y., Xu, C., Baciu, G., & Li, M. (2015). Lightness biased cartoon-and-texture decomposition for textile image segmentation. *Neurocomputing*, *168*(C), 575–587. doi:10.1016/j.neucom.2015.05.069

He, Y., Gan, T., Chen, W., & Wang, H. (2011). Adaptive denoising by singular value decomposition. *IEEE Signal Processing Letters*, *18*(4), 215–218. doi:10.1109/LSP.2011.2109039

Hung, K.-W., & Siu, W.-C. (2012). Robust soft-decision interpolation using weighted least squares. *IEEE Transactions on Image Processing*, *21*(3), 1061–1069. doi:10.1109/TIP.2011.2168416 PMID:21937348

Hwang, H., & Haddad, R. A. (1995). Adaptive median filters: New algorithms and results. *IEEE Transactions on Image Processing*, *4*(4), 499–502. doi:10.1109/83.370679 PMID:18289998

Ko, S. J., & Lee, Y. H. (1991). Center weighted median filters and their applications to image enhancement. *IEEE Transactions on Circuits and Systems*, *38*(9), 984–993. doi:10.1109/31.83870

Larkin, K. G. (2015). Structural Similarity Index SSIMplified: Is there really a simpler concept at the heart of image quality measurement? *Occasional Texts in the Pursuit of Clarity and Simplicity in Research*, *1*(1), 1–4.

Liang, H., & Weller, D. S. (2016). Comparison-Based Image Quality Assessment for Selecting Image Restoration Parameters. *IEEE Transactions on Image Processing*, *25*(11), 5118–5130. doi:10.1109/TIP.2016.2601783 PMID:27552759

Mairal, J., Elad, M., & Sapiro, G. (2008). Sparse representation for color image restoration. *IEEE Transactions on Image Processing*, *17*(1), 53–69. doi:10.1109/TIP.2007.911828 PMID:18229804

Mairal, J., Sapiro, G., & Elad, M. (2008). Learning multiscale sparse representations for image and video restoration. *Multiscale Modeling & Simulation*, *7*(1), 214–241. doi:10.1137/070697653

Skretting, K., & Engan, K. (2010). Recursive least squares dictionary learning algorithm. *IEEE Transactions on Signal Processing*, *58*(4), 2121–2130. doi:10.1109/TSP.2010.2040671

Tomasi, C., & Manduchi, R. (1998). Bilateral Filtering for Gray and Color Images. In *6th International Conference on Computer Vision (ICCV '98)*. IEEE Computer Society. 10.1109/ICCV.1998.710815

Urban, J. (2016). *Information Entropy, Applications from Engineering with MATLAB Concepts Jan Valdman*. IntechOpen. doi:10.5772/63401

Wang, G., Wang, Z., & Liu, J. (2017). A New Image Denoising Method Based on Adaptive Multiscale Morphological Edge Detection. Journal of Mathematical Problems in Engineering.

Wang, Z., Bovik, A. C., Sheikh, H. R., & Simoncelli, E. P. (2004). Image Quality Assessment: From Error Visibility to Structural Similarity. *IEEE Transactions on Image Processing*, *13*(4), 1–13. doi:10.1109/TIP.2003.819861 PMID:15376593

Wu, H.-T., Huang, J., & Shi, Y.-Q. (2015). A reversible data hiding method with contrast enhancement for medical images. *Journal of Visual Communication and Image Representation*, *31*(C), 46–153.

Yang, J., Bouzerdoum, A., & Phung, S. L. (2009). A New Approach to Sparse Image Representation Using MMV and K-SVD. In *International Conference on Advanced Concepts for Intelligent Vision Systems*. Springer-Verlag. 10.1007/978-3-642-04697-1_19

Zhang, L., Dong, W., Zhang, D., & Shi, G. (2010). Two-stage image denoising by principal component analysis with local pixel grouping. *Pattern Recognition*, *43*(4), 1531–1549. doi:10.1016/j.patcog.2009.09.023

ADDITIONAL READING

Aharon, M., Elad, M., & Bruckstein, A. (2006). K-SVD: An Algorithm for Designing Overcomplete Dictionaries for Sparse Representation. *IEEE Transactions on Signal Processing, 54*(11), 4311–4322. doi:10.1109/TSP.2006.881199

Dabov, K., Foi, A., Katkovnik, V., & Egiazarian, K. (2007). Image Denoising by Sparse 3-D Transform-Domain Collaborative Filtering. *IEEE Transactions on Image Processing, 16*(8), 2080–2095. doi:10.1109/TIP.2007.901238 PMID:17688213

Elad, M. (2010). Image Denoising. In *Sparse and Redundant Representations*. New York, NY: Springer. doi:10.1007/978-1-4419-7011-4_14

Wang, X., Wang, H., Yang, J., & Zhang, Y. (2016). A New Method for Nonlocal Means Image Denoising Using Multiple Images. *PLoS One, 11*(7), e0158664. doi:10.1371/journal.pone.0158664 PMID:27459293

Zhang, M., & Gunturk, B. K. (2008). Multiresolution bilateral filtering for image denoising. *IEEE Transactions on Image Processing, 17*(12), 2324–2333. doi:10.1109/TIP.2008.2006658 PMID:19004705

KEY TERMS AND DEFINITIONS

Block Matching: A block-matching algorithm is a method of locating matching macroblocks in a sequence of image or video frames for the resolutions of motion estimation.

Denoising: A way of noise reduction method or it is any signal processing approach that reconstructs a signal from a noisy one.

Dictionary Learning: It is the process whose goal is to find the over-complete basis in terms of minimum approximation error and equivalent solution gave a set of vectors.

Entropy: Entropy is a measure of randomness or disorder of the system.

Grayscale Image: The value of each pixel is a single sample representation of only an amount of light that carries of only intensity information.

Image Noise: Any random variation of brightness or color related information in the image.

K-SVD: It is a dictionary learning algorithm for creating a dictionary for sparse representations based a singular value decomposition approach. K-SVD is a generality of the k-means clustering algorithm and singular value decomposition that works iteratively alternating between sparse coding the input data based on the current dictionary and updating the atoms in the dictionary that better fit the data.

Matching Pursuit: It is a sparse approximation algorithm that involves finding the "best matching" projection of multidimensional data onto the span of an over-complete dictionary.

Sparse Coding: Sparse coding is modeling data vectors into sparse linear combinations of basis elements.

Sparse Representation: SP deals with sparse solutions for systems of linear equations. It is a greedy principle that signal can be approximated by a sparse superposition of basis functions.

Chapter 8
Analysis of Medical Images Using Fractal Geometry

Soumya Ranjan Nayak
KL University, India

Jibitesh Mishra
College of Engineering and Technology, India

ABSTRACT

Fractal dimension is an emerging research area in order to characterize the complex or irritated objects found in nature. These complex objects are failed to analyze by classical Euclidian geometry. The concept of FD has extensively applied in many areas of application in image processing. The thought of the FD will work based upon the theory of self-similarity because it holds structures that are nested with one another. Over the last years, fractal geometry was applied extensively in medical image analysis in order to detect cancer cells in human body because our vascular system, nervous system, bones, and breast tissue are so complex and irregular in pattern, and also successfully applied in ECG signal, brain imaging for tumor detection, trabeculation analysis, etc. In order to analyze these complex structures, most of the researchers are adopting the concept of fractal geometry by means of box counting technique. This chapter presents an overview of box counting and its improved algorithms and how they work and their application in the field of medical image processing.

DOI: 10.4018/978-1-5225-6316-7.ch008

INTRODUCTION

The concept of fractal geometry originally initiated by (Mandelbrot, 1982) in order to characterized to complex objects. Mostly of the objects are surrounded in environment are so complicated and abnormal pattern, hence these types of abnormal structures are decline to analyzed by Euclidean geometry described by Chen et al. (2003), Asvestas et al. (1998), and Lopes and Betrouni (2009). The concept of fractal geometry will work based upon the concept of self similarity. Medical imaging system like human vascular system, nervous system, bones and breast tissue are so complex and irregular in pattern and most of the images carry self similar and statistical self similar content. In order to analysis of this complex medical images, most of the researchers are preferring the fractal concept; This is the region why fractal dimension are most popular research area now a days in the field of medical image analysis reported by Lopes and Betrouni (2009) because most of the human body organs such as tissues, brain and breast texture show complex and irritated geometric structural pattern. These types of irritated geometry structure can be characterized by means of shape properties through dissimilar scaled value. In this regard, Fractal concept shows the primary or key role when irregular surfaces comes in computation. The concept of fractal geometry was deals with self similarity objects, that means magnifying an object by means of deeper details with different scaling value and every distinct portion is look like as similar as the whole. As we discuss earlier those biomedical images generally complex and irritated in nature, that's way the fractal geometry, are widely techniques especially in medical image analysis field. In this context different researchers used different technique in medial image analysis but most of the researchers prefer box counting technique because of its simplicity and easiness. In recent literature survey of different applications of fractal geometry are progressed by means of box counting and its improved versions in both gray scale and color domain. In response to the gray scale domain many methods are presented by different researchers, but in this section we have reported some recent research topic which is related to this literature study like improved box counting at each box scale presented by Nayak et. al (2016), improved DBC by shifting box block gave by Nayak et. al (2016), Effect of error estimation by using box counting by same author (Nayak et. al (2016), Nayak et. al (2017)), comparative study was made in order to select appropriate algorithm for specific objects reported by Nayak et. al (2017), Fractal geometry the beauty of computer graphics presented by Das et. al (2017) and improved triangle box counting reported by Nayak et. al (2018). As concerned to color domain, there are very few technique are evolved like average box counting technique presented by Nayak et. al (2015), roughness subtraction technique by implementing improved differential box counting reported by Nayak et. al (2016), improved color box counting technique by Nayak et al

(2017), fundamental color processing technique by implementing CIE based human perception model reported by Nayak et. al (2017), extended differential box counting technique into color domain by implementing maximum Euclidian distance reported by Nayak et. al (2018). These box counting (BC) and their improved versions are applied in different fields of application with different domain. However, our research analysis in this charter is to revel the different application area used by means of fractal geometry in order to analysis of medical images applications. From the above literature survey we have observed that most of the box counting principle will work based upon the concept of self similarity, and almost all bio medical images are so complex and irregular in pattern at it contains self similar and statistical self similar content. Hence, from this point of view we have motivated in order carried out our further research on bio medical image processing by means of fractal geometry. In concerned to medical image analysis there are very few research work were carried out by using fractal geometry. In our next couple of passage we have presented art of the recent investigation work relevant to the box counting technique in medical image processing. Recently Ramya et. al (2016) presented cancer detection technique using fractal texture analysis by implementing box counting algorithm. Chan and Tuszynski (2016) presented tumor malignancy prediction in breast cancer by using fractal dimension. Sumitra et. al (2017) presented a review report on medical image analysis by using fractal dimension concept. Khemis et. al (2016) reported breast tissue characterization by implementing new fractal dimension algorithm based on texture measurement. Stehlik et. al (2016) presented mammary cancer detection by implementing fractal based cancer modeling. The details work flow of medical image analysis by using fractal geometry are properly discussed in section 4, and finally provides the details investigation of these techniques and describe the key ideas related to this issue. At the end this chapter may affords the guidance to fourth coming researchers in order to successful implementation of fractal concept in medical imaging applications. The main objectives in order to write this chapter to described how fractal geometry is very useful in the field of medical image analysis. The next indication of this chapter is organized as succeed: in the following passage we described fractal analysis and its corresponding importance in medical image analysis. In section 3, we have discusses the fractal methods in medical applications. In section 4 gives the different medical application area wherever fractal concept was applied. Finally our concluding remarks are presented in subsequent sections.

FRACTAL ANALYSIS AND ITS DIMENSIONS

The main intend of fractal dimension is used for guesstimate surface roughness of complicated objects. The term fractal initially presented by Mandelbrot, the Hausdorff dimensions always larger as compared to its topological dimension (TD) in fractal set. However, Euclidean geometry characterized only lines, points, cubes and planes, and these objects yields integer dimension. In general the line has the dimension of one for the region that has only able to move in single direction, similarly a two-dimensional object includes squares or a circle has to move in two directions i.e. in spatial plane. Likewise three-dimensional objects such as cubes has move in three directions. In order to characterize the fractal objects, (Mandelbrot, 1982) used this TD for characterized the shapes to describe these shapes. The concept Euclidean geometry was not permitted necessarily represent the structure and observance of these fractal entity. An essential representative of fractal entities (objects) is that the self-possessed measured characteristics like area and length are most useful measurement scale. A typical illustration to demonstrate the fractal belonging is the ‘‘length” of a coastline (Mandelbrot, 1967). In this case, author measured with a spatial scale d and the entire length of coastline $L(D)$ is estimated as a set of N number of straight line slices with length d. This indications towards the characterization of fractal (D) and associated by means of number of self similar sections. This self similar concept can be visualized when large objects can be scaling down smaller piece, and smaller piece look like as original one. More precisely, (Mandelbrot, 1983) demonstrate that the Hausdorff dimensions always larger as compared to its TD in fractal set. The Hausdorff-Besicovitch dimension D_h is represented by taking the logarithmic relationship between the numbers N of an object's with scaling factor with r.

$$D = \frac{\ln(N)}{\ln\left(\frac{1}{r}\right)} \tag{1}$$

where N are the patterns and r is the scaling factor.

Again Mandelbrot gives analytical relationship between the length (L) and measuring scale (d) and it can be represented as:

$$L(\sigma) = K \times \sigma(1 - D) \tag{2}$$

where K represents the unvarying value and D indicates FD which is a fractional number. In this regard, there are number of techniques is available in order to estimate FD and every algorithm has individual concern, although all these available follow the same fundamental concepts which are summarized in following steps:

- The heterogeneous step size will consider for measuring the object quantities.
- Perform the regression analysis between scaling factor (quantities) against step size.
- Final FD was computed from the slope of the regression line.

In line to self-similar concept, again (Mandelbrot, 1985) said fractals objects are self-affine, if and only if the fluctuation of scale in one direction inversely than the fluctuation in some else direction, However, the objects of self-similar are isotropic in nature.

FRACTAL METHODS IN MEDICAL IMAGE ANALYSIS

The conception of self-similarity is mostly used for estimation of FD. There are wide varieties of fractal methods are reported like box-counting (BC), improved BC, modified BC, deferential BC (DBC), relative DBC, fractional Brownian motion, triangular prism area methods, covering blanket method and many more. Among all these state of art techniques, the box-counting (BC) and its improvement version was well accepted and recognized among various researchers because of its easy implementation. The approach BC will work based upon the number of boxes desired to fill the complete fractal objects. The subjective grid is employed across the object and figure out the enumerate boxes that being fall in the fractal entity. In next sub sections we have presented some well-liked box counting technique and its improved version which are mostly used in medical image analysis.

Box Counting Technique

Initially, Russel et al. (1980) presented box counting technique for binary signals. In this technique they cover the binary signals with boxes of length r. According to this method the FD can be estimated by using the Eq. (3).

$$D = \lim_{r \to 0} \frac{\log\left(N\left(r\right)\right)}{\log r} \tag{3}$$

where $N\left(r\right)$ express the requisite boxes needed to cover up the whole surface and here r is called scaling factor. Mainly this technique has several restrictions, though it desire binarization of signal. Later on many drawbacks are reported by different researchers in many literatures. Based upon this drawback many improved version and modified techniques are brought forward.

Reticular Box Counting Algorithm

This is another box counting technique presented by Gangepain and Roques (1986) for evaluating fractal dimension. This algorithm look at the image in 3D space of (x,y,z), where x as well as y coordinates illustrate 2D position and third coordinate z represents image strength.

Differential Box Counting Algorithm

The extension of box-counting method is the differential box-counting method (DBC). This technique was presented by Sarkar and Chaudhuri (1984) in order to resolve some of restrictions of box count method. The main favour of BC that it will applicable for gray images. So the binarization step can be escaped. The image is divided into boxes of different scale r and $N\left(r\right)$ is calculated as the difference between the maximum and the minimum grey levels which was fall inside in i_{th} and j_{th} block respectively. This step is used again and again for entire box. FD is approximate by using in Eq. (1). This method was most popular and well like technique found in many literature survey. Based on the differential box counting techniques many modified and improved techniques are brought forward based on the some draw back found in original DBC i.e, box height, over counting, under counting and sharp gray level exist on the border of the box of block. In this regard Jin et al. (1995) explored relative DBC likely to initial DBC by considering the scale range of upper and lower part for better estimation. Similar to DBC also, Biswass et. al (1998) intended the parallel approach for prominent result. In similar way chen et. al (2003) recommended shifting DBC (SDBC) in terms of shifting operation in order to get proper experimental measure. The recent research work shows that there are some major improved techniques are recommended by various researchers for discarded some of the deficiency correlate with initial DBC. In this concern, Li et. al (2009) conferred improved technique in order to get better performance in digital domain by materialized the three alteration in original DBC. These three alterations are termed as (i) Exact grid height selection, (ii) correct box assessment, and (iii) exact surface segregation. Similarly Liu et. al (2014) recommended another three modification in addition with shifting operation in order to obtained improved DBC for better computation. These modifications are coined as (i) choosing personalized box-count, (ii) picking precise grid size, and (iii) shifting operation. The techniques are described above are the convention box-counting technique because it works only with square grid for commutation of FD. In order to precise estimation of FD in response to the convention box-counting, Kaewaramsri. et. al (2012) recommended the adaption of triangle partition of grid by means of equal size of triangle for higher precision of box-count; but this approach only meant for binary images. In order to applied this triangle box partition into gray images. kaewaramsri et. al (2015) advised some modification in partition technique. Here instead of two equal partition, they implemented four patterns by means of upper and lower right diagonal and similarly left diagonals as well. In response to the triangle partition, recently Nayak et. al (2017) given improved concerned by materializing the unsymmetrical triangle partition in addition with shifting operation in coordinate plane. This technique able to clear up all the complication linked with initial DBC and also added advantages of more exactness box–count. Nayak et. al (2018) conferred another modified DBC by adopting of correction factor in terms of mean intensity value of grid with subtraction of minimum value, and experimentally shown that this modified version is much more better than the state of the art technique. Nayak et. al (2018) extended the DBC into color domain in terms of 5D vector for assessment of FD in color domain. Recently, Nayak et al. (2018) conferred fractal study of image sets using DBC technique and reported the appropriate technique is required for specific objects. However, we have discussed regarding box counting techniques in this section are related to texture analysis but in this chapter we have confined our discussion only in medical image analysis by using different box counting and its modified techniques.

After the concept of box counting techniques being put forwarded by different researchers for describing and analysing the complex objects, it was suited one of the prominent techniques to be applied to several scientific research areas, and medical image analysis one of them the recent research area in fractal geometry by Takahashi et al. (2009). As we have discussed in our earlier section that the fractal dimension signifies the information about the geometric structures for complex objects. As we know the structure of medical images are so complex, irregular pattern and also poses some similarity pattern in different scales. This is the main region why the concept of fractal geometry was served as finest suitable technique applied in order to analysing numerous medical images. Therefore the concept of fractal geometry played important aspect in numerous fields of medical investigation analysis such as characterising the pathological tissues from healthy ones Iftekharuddin (2005) and diagnosis verity of diseases reported by Free et al. (1996). In case of brain image analysis, FD indicates a very effective outcome in assessment of structure deviation in brain images by Sarkar and Chaudhuri (1995). The key inspiration for selecting fractal concept for medical imaging analysis due to its fairly insensitiveness towards the image scaling, and its strong correlation nature with human judgment of surface roughness is also a major concern Phothisonothai and Nakagawa (2007).

Another important factor that cannot be obliterated utilization against study of noisy medicinal images. It was very much useful to identify blurred response in the edge of medical imaging. In the next section we will discuss the different medical image analysis applications where fractal geometry plays significant role.

APPLICATION AREA OF FRACTAL IN MEDICAL IMAGE ANALYSIS

Over the last years, Fractal dimension was most popular research topic in biomedical image processing in order to analysis and describe complex structure (Das et al., 2013, 2014, 2015) for diagnosis of diseases (Sahani and Das, 2018). Fractal concepts are actively applied in medical image analysis because medical images itself having a fractal character, more precisely the case where repeated sequences, for example: homologies among two separate nucleotide array of including self-similar content in mitochondrial DNA. In this section, we have broadly discussed the different fields of applications of medical image analysis where fractal geometry plays the significant role.

Mammography

Mammography is a specified tool in order to early diagnosis of breast cancer. If the breast distortion or irregularities are recognized at the early stage then this diseases can be fully cured. In order to characterise this issue, several researchers have used fractal geometry concept in order to recognize breast syndrome. Mainly there are two types of axes was followed in mammography analysis that is categorization of the contour of lesions reported by Don et al. (2009), and Abdaheer and Khan (2009) and characterization of region reported in Sankar and Thomas (2009), and Crisan et al. (2009). Nguyen and Rangayyan (2005) analysed the mammographic images by means of shape analysis of breast masses by using fractal concept. Li et al. (1996) presented the improvement on micro-calcifications of mammography image by considering the approach of fractal model. Li et al. (2007) revel additional utilization of fractal inquiry for micro classification enhancement. In his work, he explained that ductal patterns and general mammographic parenchymal can be modelled properly using fractal geometry. Guo et al. (2009) conferred fractal based model for representation of mammographic mass scratches plus architectonic alteration. In this case they took mixture of both FBM (fractional Brownian motion) FD together with lacunarity. In this counter, Mavroforakis et al. (2006) presented mammographic mass imaging classification, by the supported of fractal analysis of the texture features. Representation of architectural syndrome has now recent research problem on mind of various researches in terms of only FD and jointly with both FD techniques and texture analytic technique. Tourassi et al. (2006) reported in their article, for classification of Architectural Distortion (AD) by implementing the mammographic ROI (region of interest) in terms of FD concept. The performances were evaluated by means of circular mean power spectrum algorithm. In similar way, Banik et al. (2009) presented the combined techniques (Haralick, FD) in order to detect the architectural alteration in mammograms imaging system. For this approach author considers the statistical measures like energy, entropy, contract and homogeneity, along with the concept of FD for better characterization of breast tissue for architectural distortion.

Brain Imaging

Analysis of brain images is one of the interesting research topics where the concept of fractal geometry plays the vital role and can be applied frequently. Fractal dimension were effectively used in order to measure cells morphologies in the human brain Zook and Iftekharuddin (2005) and the brain shape magnetic resonance imaging is usually used for study. In this case the special attention was required because the fractal dimension generated from whole brain image is quite similar between healthy one and patients reported by Cook et al. (1995), and Free et al. (1996). Due to pre-processing stage and binarization step some of the important information may be lost, therefore we observed in case of brain MRI analysis by means of non-linier structures are limited in terms of abstraction of fractal atterns like identification of cortical edges as well as sub cortical edges and white matter surface. In this context, Bullmore et al. (1994) quantify the edges among the white matter including cerebral cortex for categorization of schizophrenics, manic-depressives and control, and finally mean FD were estimated by means of box-counting algorithm and it should be superior in edges counted from manic-depressive sick person as compared those counted from controls, however it was lower in schizophrenics than in controls. Finally it was recommended that the FD is a most suitable measure in clinically related differences in case of complication of MRI boundaries. Blanton et al. (2001) studied the impact of age including gender by means of asymmetry of primary cortical sulci and structural complexity. Then FD was computed of evolving children for the outline surface among the gyros and sulcus the on brain imaging (MR) system. Kedzia et al. (2002) indicates that the average FD estimated using box-counting technique was gradually increased month by month during pregnancy. This study was made from the microarchitecture of foetal brain blood vessels present during pregnancy period.

ECG Signals

The concept of FD has revealed its ability on describing the various states or to forecast the variations in phenomenon. It is usually efficiently used in ECG and EEG samples described by Jun et al. (1994). Generally fractal analysis is very much suitable for differentiating the classes of EEG pattern, which is interrelated to activities of brain. Foe ECG data compression, fractal interpolation plays vital role which was studied by Hsu et al. (2007). Kalmanti and Maris (2007) presented prominent technique known as electro encephalogram (EEG) analysing by implementing the DBC. While examine the EEG signal data, the FD also plays important appearance because it contains some fractal pattern which is random in nature. It has been seen that, fractal geometry concept will act as an emerging topic in numerous fields of applications like epilepsy, sleeping disorder and Alzheimer disease. Several FD algorithms were evolved out of which BC methods affords acceptable results. In recent research studies reveal that the concept of fractal spectra and fractal dimension are much useful as compared with Fourier transform in order to predict the brain activities in more preciously, though fractal spectra study has restrictions in experimenting multiple brain activities and stationary brain waves.

Bone Trabeculation

Over the past years, continuous researches works have been carried out on the application of fractal analysis in bone trabeculation investigation. Measuring bone strength itself a very challenging issue because structure of bone is complex in nature. Generally bone has two major part namely outer part and inner part that taken into consideration while analysis. The outer part comprising of a tube of very dense material and inner part includes the material that looks like a sea sponge that is filled with finely interlaced struts, called trabecular. In this regard most of the studies were carried out in order to authorise the use of fractal geometry in bone image analysis application because it has demonstrated that bone study (trabecular bone micro architecture on calcaneus radiographs) contains self-similarity which is one of the major characteristics of fractal geometry. Majumdar et al. (1999) presented some essential characteristics using fractal analysis and in this analysis they used three methods to evaluate the fractal dimension which are surface-area technique, semi-variance technique and Fourier transform technique. Another researcher indicates that the analysis of bone trabeculation through fractal analysis is very dynamic nature described by Messent et al. (2005). Some experimental works have proved that the bone organization is anisotropic in nature for osteoporotic patients than for healthy subjects. Jennane et al. (2006) calculated the degree of anisotropy of fractal for bone X-ray images and showed its complex nature in terms of their textured character, non-stationary and anisotropy.

FUTURE RESEARCH DIRECTIONS

In this chapter we have made case study analysis on fractal geometry in the field of medical image analysis. We have observed that most of the analysis was made based on early age box counting algorithm, but recent research in fractal domain reveals that there are many modified and improved version box counting technique were evolved in order to remove the drawback of early age box counting algorithm. The second most important point we have observed that there is no such research has been made in order to measure the cancer growth at different stages. From this point of view we will carry our further research for measurement of cancer growth by using improved differential box counting technique.

CONCLUSION

Fractal geometry has most popular and prominent research area in various applications of medical images. The core sense of adoption of fractal geometry in order to analysis of medical images is in fragmented and complex nature. It is conspicuously used for recognizing vigorous and injured area. But selecting the appropriate method for fractal dimension estimation is an important foremost issue. In the most of the medical image applications the box counting technique and its modified and improved technique were used whereas other method like differential box counting technique, triangular prisms, and Power spectrum method are also useful. One more parameter we have remark related to fractal called multi fractal, in this case the peculiar value of FD occasionally shows the properties of multi fractal activity. Hence, this point should take into consideration while analysing of medical images.

ACKNOWLEDGMENT

I owe my deep gratitude to the department of Computer Science and Engineering, KLEF, Andhra Pradesh, India to providing such good environment for successfully completing our research work. Also, I would like to extend our sincere esteems to all authors of reference.

REFERENCES

Abdaheer, S. M., & Khan, E. (2009). Shaped based classification of breast tumors using fractal analysis. In *Proceeding of IEEE conference of Multimedia, Signal Processing and Communication Technologies* (pp. 272-275). Aligarh, India: IEEE.

Asvestas, P., Matsopoulos, G. K., & Nikita, K. S. (1998). A power differentiation method of fractal dimension estimation for 2-D signals. *Journal of Visual Communication and Image Representation*, *9*(4), 392–400. doi:10.1006/jvci.1998.0394

Biswas, M. K., Ghose, T., Guha, S., & Biswas, P. K. (1998). Fractal dimension estimation for texture images: A parallel approach. *Pattern Recognition Letters*, *19*(3-4), 309–313. doi:10.1016/S0167-8655(98)00002-6

Blanton, R., Levitt, J., Thompson, P., Narr, K., Capetillo, C. L., Nobel, A., & Singerman, J. (2001). Mapping cortical asymmetry and complexity patterns in normal children. *Psychiatry Research*, *107*(1), 29–43. doi:10.1016/S0925-4927(01)00091-9 PMID:11472862

Bullmore, E., Brammer, M., Harvey, I., Persaud, R., Murray, R., & Ron, M. (1994). Fractal analysis of the boundary between white matter and cerebral cortex in magnetic resonance images: A controlled study of schizophrenic and manic-depressive patients. *Psychological Medicine*, *24*(03), 771–781. doi:10.1017/S0033291700027926 PMID:7991759

Chan, A., & Tuszynski, J. A. (2016). Automatic prediction of tumour malignancy in breast cancer with fractal dimension. *Royal Society Open Science*, *3*(12), 1–10. doi:10.1098/rsos.160558 PMID:28083100

Chaudhuri, B., & Sarkar, N. (1995). Texture segmentation using fractal dimension. *IEEE Transaction on Pattern Analysis*, *17*(1), 72–77. doi:10.1109/34.368149

Chen, W. S., Yuan, S. Y., & Hsieh, C. M. (2003). Two algorithms to estimate fractal dimension of gray-level images. *Optical Engineering (Redondo Beach, Calif.)*, *42*(8), 2452–2464. doi:10.1117/1.1585061

Cook, M., Free, S., Manford, M., Fish, D., Shorvon, S., & Stevens, J. (1995). Fractal description of cerebral cortical patterns in frontal lobe epilepsy. *European Neurology*, *35*(6), 327–335. doi:10.1159/000117155 PMID:8591799

Crisan, D. A., Coculescu, C., & Stanica, J. L. (2009). Using fractal techniques to reduce haziness in medical imaging. In Proceedings of Computer Science and Information Technology (pp. 92-95). Beijing, China: Academic Press.

Das, H., Jena, A. K., Nayak, J., Naik, B., & Behera, H. S. (2015). A novel PSO based back propagation learning-MLP (PSO-BP-MLP) for classification. In *Computational Intelligence in Data Mining* (Vol. 2, pp. 461–471). New Delhi: Springer. doi:10.1007/978-81-322-2208-8_42

Das, H., Jena, A. K., Rath, P. K., Muduli, B., & Das, S. R. (2015). Grid computing-based performance analysis of power system: a graph theoretic approach. In *Intelligent Computing, Communication and Devices* (pp. 259–266). New Delhi: Springer. doi:10.1007/978-81-322-2009-1_30

Das, H., Mishra, S. K., & Roy, D. S. (2013). The topological structure of the Odisha power grid: a complex network analysis. *IJMCA*, *1*(1), 012-016.

Das, H., Naik, B., & Behera, H. S. (2018). Classification of Diabetes Mellitus Disease (DMD): A Data Mining (DM) Approach. In *Progress in Computing, Analytics and Networking* (pp. 539–549). Singapore: Springer. doi:10.1007/978-981-10-7871-2_52

Das, H., Naik, B., Pati, B., & Panigrahi, C. R. (2014). A survey on virtual sensor networks framework. *International Journal of Grid and Distributed Computing*, *7*(5), 121–130. doi:10.14257/ijgdc.2014.7.5.11

Das, H., Panda, G. S., Muduli, B., & Rath, P. K. (2014). The complex network analysis of power grid: a case study of the West Bengal power network. In *Intelligent Computing, Networking, and Informatics* (pp. 17–29). New Delhi: Springer. doi:10.1007/978-81-322-1665-0_3

Das, H., & Roy, D. S. (2013). A grid computing service for power system monitoring. *International Journal of Computers and Applications*, *62*(20).

Das, S. K., Nayak, S. R., & Mishra, J. (2017). Fractal Geometry: The Beauty of Computer Graphics. *Journal of Advanced Research in Dynamical and Control Systems*, *9*, 76-82.

Don, S., Revathy, D., Chung, K., Choi, E., & Min, D. (2009). A Neural Network Approach to Mammogram Image Classification Using Fractal Features. In *Proceedings of IEEE International Conference of Intelligent Computing and Intelligent Systems* (pp. 444-447). Shanghai, China: IEEE. 10.1109/ICICISYS.2009.5357653

Free, S., Sisodiya, S., Cook, M., Fish, D., & Shorvon, S. (1996). Three-dimensional fractal analysis of the white matter surface from magnetic resonance images of the human brain. *Cerebral Cortex*, *6*(6), 830–836. doi:10.1093/cercor/6.6.830 PMID:8922340

Gangepain, J. J., & Carmes, C. R. (1986). Fractal approach to two dimensional and three dimensional surface roughness. *Wear*, *109*(1-4), 119–126. doi:10.1016/0043-1648(86)90257-7

Guo, Q., Shao, J., & Ruiz, V. F. (2009). Characterization and classification of tumor lesions using computerized fractal-based texture analysis and support vector machines in digital mammograms. *International Journal of Computer Assisted Radiology and Surgery*, *4*(1), 11–25. doi:10.100711548-008-0276-8 PMID:20033598

Hsu, W. Y., Lin, C. C., Ju, M. S., & Sun, Y. N. (2007). Wavelet-based fractal features with active segment selection: Application to single-trial EEG data. *Journal of Neuroscience Methods*, *163*(1), 145–160. doi:10.1016/j.jneumeth.2007.02.004 PMID:17379316

Iftekharuddin, K. (2005). Techniques in fractal analysis and their applications in brain MRI. *Journal of Medical Imaging Systems: Technology and Applications, 1*, 63-86.

Jin, X. C., Ong, S. H., & Jayasooriah. (1995). A practical method for estimating fractal dimension. *Pattern Recognition Letters*, *16*(5), 457–464. doi:10.1016/0167-8655(94)00119-N

Jun, Y., Yoon, Y., & Yoon, H. (1994). ECG data compression using fractal interpolation. In *Proceedings of IEEE Conference of Engineering in Medicine and Biology Society* (pp. 161-162). Baltimore, MD: IEEE.

Kaewaramsri, Y., & Woraratpanya, K. (2015). Improved triangle box counting method for fractal dimension estimation. In H. Unger, P. Meesad, & S. Boonkrong (Eds.), *Recent Advances in Information and Communication Technology, In Proceedings of Advances in Intelligent Systems and Computing* (Vol. 361, pp. 53–63). Cham: Springer. doi:10.1007/978-3-319-19024-2_6

Kalmanti, E., & Maris, T.G. (2007). Fractal dimension as an index of brain cortical changes throughout life. *Journal of Fractal Analysis, 21*, 641-646.

Kedzia, A., Rybaczuk, M., & Andrzejak, R. (2002). Fractal dimensions of human brain cortex vessels during the fetal period. *Medical Science Monitor*, *8*, 46–51. PMID:11887041

Khemis, K., Lazzouni, S. A., Messadi, M., Loudjedi, S., & Bessaid, A. (2016). New Algorithm for Fractal Dimension Estimation based on Texture Measurements: Application on Breast Tissue Characterization. *International Journal of Image, Graphics and Signal Processing*, *4*(4), 9–15. doi:10.5815/ijigsp.2016.04.02

Li, H., Giger, M. L., Olopade, O. I., & Lan, L. (2007). Fractal analysis of mammographic parenchymal patterns in breast cancer risk assessment. *Academic Radiology*, *14*(5), 513–521. doi:10.1016/j.acra.2007.02.003 PMID:17434064

Li, H., Liu, K., & Lo, S. (1996). Enhancement of micro-calcifications on mammograms using a fractal modelling approach. In *Proceedings of the IEEE Conference on Engineering in Medicine and Biology Society* (vol. 3, pp. 1111-1112). Amsterdam: IEEE. 10.1109/IEMBS.1996.652732

Li, J., Du, Q., & Sun, C. (2009). An improved box-counting method for image fractal dimension estimation. *Pattern Recognition*, *42*(11), 2460–2469. doi:10.1016/j.patcog.2009.03.001

Liu, Y., Chen, L., Wang, H., Jiang, L., Zhang, Y., Zhao, J., ... Song, Y. (2014). An improved differential box-counting method to estimate fractal dimensions of gray-level images. *Journal of Visual Communication and Image Representation*, *25*(5), 1102–1111. doi:10.1016/j.jvcir.2014.03.008

Lopes, R., & Betrouni, N. (2009). Fractal and multifractal analysis: A review. *Medical Image Analysis*, *13*(4), 634–649. doi:10.1016/j.media.2009.05.003 PMID:19535282

Mandelbrot, B. (1967). How long is the coast of Britain? Statistical self-similarity and fractional dimension. *Science*, *156*(3775), 636–638. doi:10.1126cience.156.3775.636 PMID:17837158

Mandelbrot, B. (1982). *The fractal geometry of nature*. W.H. Freeman and Company.

Mandelbrot, B. (1985). Self-affine fractals and the fractal dimension. *Physica Scripta*, *32*(4), 257–260. doi:10.1088/0031-8949/32/4/001

Mandelbrot, B., & Wheeler, J. A. (1983). The Fractal Geometry of Nature. *American Journal of Physics*, *51*(3), 286–196. doi:10.1119/1.13295

Mavroforakis, M. E., Georgiou, H. V., Dimitropoulos, N., Cavouras, D., & Theodoridis, S. (2006). Mammographic masses characterization based on localized texture and dataset fractal analysis using linear, neural and support vector machine classifiers. *Artificial Intelligence in Medicine*, *37*(2), 145–162. doi:10.1016/j.artmed.2006.03.002 PMID:16716579

Nayak, S. R., Khandual, A., & Mishra, J. (in press). Ground truth study of fractal dimension of color images of similar textures. *Journal of the Textile Institute*.

Nayak, S. R., & Mishra, J. (2016). An improved method to estimate the fractal dimension of colour images. *Perspectives on Science*, *8*, 412–416. doi:10.1016/j.pisc.2016.04.092

Nayak, S. R., & Mishra, J. (2017). On estimation of fractal dimension of noise images. *Indian Journal of Science and Technology*, *10*, 1–6.

Nayak, S. R., & Mishra, J. (2017). On calculation of fractal dimension of color images. *International Journal of Image, Graphics and Signal Processing*, *9*, 33-40.

Nayak, S. R., & Mishra, J. (2018). A modified triangle box-counting with precision in error fit. *Journal of Information and Optimization Sciences*, *39*(1), 113–128. doi:10.1080/02522667.2017.1372155

Nayak, S. R., Mishra, J., & Jena, P. M. (2018). Fractal analysis of image sets using differential box counting techniques. *International Journal of Information Technology*, *10*, 39-47.

Nayak, S. R., Mishra, J., Khandual, A., & Palai, G. (2018). Fractal Dimension of RGB Color Images. *International Journal for Light and Electron Optics*, *161*, 136–145. doi:10.1016/j.ijleo.2018.02.024

Nayak, S. R., Mishra, J., & Padhy, R. (2016). An improved algorithm to estimate the fractal dimension of gray scale image. In *Proceedings of IEEE International conference on signal processing, Communication, Power and Embedded System* (pp. 1109-1114). IEEE. 10.1109/SCOPES.2016.7955614

Nayak, S. R., Mishra, J., & Palai, G. (2018). An extended DBC approach by using maximum Euclidian distance for fractal dimension of color images. *International Journal for Light and Electron Optics*, *166*, 110–115. doi:10.1016/j.ijleo.2018.03.106

Nayak, S. R., Mishra, J., & Palai, G. (2018). A modified approach to estimate fractal dimension of gray scale Images. *International Journal for Light and Electron Optics*, *162*, 196–205. doi:10.1016/j.ijleo.2018.02.066

Nayak, S. R., Mishra, J., & Routray, S. (2017). Effect of noise determination on estimation of fractal dimension of digital images. *International Journal of Pure and Applied Mathematics*, *117*, 57–63.

Nayak, S. R., Mishra, J., Sethy, A., & Mohapatra, S. (2017). A comparative analysis on estimation of fractal dimension of gray scale images. *International Journal of Pure and Applied Mathematics*, *117*, 323–329.

Nayak, S. R., Padhy, R., & Mishra, J. (2016). On estimation of fractal dimension of gray scale images using modified differential box counting method. *International Journal of Computer Science and Information Security*, *14*, 764-772.

Nayak, S. R., Padhy, R., & Mishra, J. (2018). A new extended differential box counting method by adopting unequal partitioning of grid for estimation of fractal dimension of digital images. In *Proceedings of Computational Signal Processing and Analysis* (Vol. 490, pp. 45–57). LNEE Book Series. doi:10.1007/978-981-10-8354-9_5

Nayak, S. R., Ranganath, A., & Mishra, J. (2015). Analysing Fractal Dimension of color Images. In *Proceedings of IEEE International Conference on Computational Intelligence and Networks* (pp. 156-159). IEEE.

Nguyen, T., & Rangayyan, R. (2005). Shape Analysis of Breast Masses in Mammograms via the Fractal Dimension. In *Proceedings of the IEEE Engineering in Medicine and Biology* Society (vol. 3, pp. 3210-3213). Shanghai, China: IEEE.

Phothisonothai, M., & Nakagawa, M. (2007). Fractal-based EEG data analysis of body parts movement imagery tasks. *The Journal of Physiological Sciences; JPS*, *57*(4), 217–226. doi:10.2170/physiolsci.RP006307 PMID:17637165

Ramya, R., Shridhar, R., Latha, K. C., & Balasubramanian, S. (2016). Endometrial cancer detection using fractal based texture analysis: A box counting Algorithm. *International Journal of Applied Research, 2*, 243-245.

Russel, D., Hanson, J., & Ott, E. (1980). Dimension of strange attractors. *Physical Review Letters*, *45*(14), 1175–1178. doi:10.1103/PhysRevLett.45.1175

Sahani, R., Rout, C., Badajena, J. C., Jena, A. K., & Das, H. (2018). Classification of Intrusion Detection Using Data Mining Techniques. In *Progress in Computing, Analytics and Networking* (pp. 753–764). Singapore: Springer. doi:10.1007/978-981-10-7871-2_72

Sankar, D., & Thomas, T. (2009). Analysis of Mammograms using Fractal Features. In Proceedings of Nature & Biologically Inspired Computing (pp. 936-941). Coimbatore, India: Academic Press.

Sarkar, N., & Chaudhuri, B. B. (1984). An efficient differential box-counting approach to compute fractal dimension of image. *IEEE Transactions on Systems, Man, and Cybernetics*, *24*(1), 115–120. doi:10.1109/21.259692

Shantanu, B., Rangayyan, R. M., & Desautels, J. E. L. (2009). Detection of Architectural Distortion in Prior Mammograms of Interval-cancer Cases with Neural Networks. In *Proceedings of the IEEE Conference on Engineering in Medicine and Biology Society* (pp. 6667-6670). Minneapolis, MN: IEEE.

Stehlik, M., Hermann, P., & Nikolis, O. (2016). Fractal based cancer modelling. *Revstat Statistical Journal, 14*, 139–155.

Takahashi, T., Kosaka, H., Murata, T., Omori, M., Narita, K., Mitsuya, H., ... Wada, Y. (2009). Application of a multifractal analysis to study brain white matter abnormalities of schizophrenia on T2-weighted magnetic resonance imaging. *Psychiatry Res. NeuroImage*, *172*(3), 177–188. doi:10.1016/j.pscychresns.2008.03.009

Tourassi, G. D., Delong, D. M., & Floyd, C. E. Jr. (2006). A study on the computerized fractal analysis of architectural distortion in screening mammograms. *Physics in Medicine and Biology*, *51*(5), 1299–1312. doi:10.1088/0031-9155/51/5/018 PMID:16481695

Woraratpanya, K., Kakanopas, D., & Varakulsiripunth, R. (2012). Triangle-box Counting Method for Fractal Dimension Estimation, *ASEAN. Engineering Journal (New York)*, (Part D): 1, 5–16.

Zook, J., & Iftekharuddin, K. (2005). Statistical analysis of fractal-based brain tumor detection algorithms. *Magnetic Resonance Imaging*, *23*(5), 671–678. doi:10.1016/j.mri.2005.04.002 PMID:16051042

ADDITIONAL READING

Borra, S., Thanki, R., Dey, N., & Borisagar, K. (2018). *Secure transmission and integrity verification of color radiological images using fast discrete curvelet transform and compressive sensing*. Smart Health.

Das, A. K., Pradhan, M., Das, A. K., Pradhan, C., & Das, H. (2018) “A Constructive Machine Translation System for English to Odia Translation”, in *7th International Conference on Communication and Signal Processing*, IEEE India

Das, H., Jena, A. K., Badajena, J. C., Pradhan, C., & Barik, R. K. (2018). Resource Allocation in Cooperative Cloud Environments. In *Progress in Computing, Analytics and Networking* (pp. 825–841). Singapore: Springer. doi:10.1007/978-981-10-7871-2_79

Dey, N., & Ashour, A. S. (2017). *Meta-Heuristic Algorithms in Medical Image Segmentation: A Review* (p. 185). Advancements in Applied Metaheuristic Computing.

Dey, N., Ashour, A. S., & Hassanien, A. E. (2018). Feature detectors and descriptors generations with numerous images and video applications: a recap. In *Computer Vision: Concepts, Methodologies, Tools, and Applications* (pp. 571–600). IGI Global. doi:10.4018/978-1-5225-5204-8.ch022

Dey, N., Rajinikanth, V., Ashour, A., & Tavares, J. M. (2018). Dey, Nilanjan, Venkatesan Rajinikanth, Amira S. Ashour, and João Manuel RS Tavares. "Social Group Optimization Supported Segmentation and Evaluation of Skin Melanoma Images. *Symmetry*, *10*(2), 51. doi:10.3390ym10020051

(2018). Dey, Nilanjan, Amira S. Ashour, Fuqian Shi, Simon James Fong, and João Manuel RS Tavares. "Medical cyber-physical systems: A survey. *Journal of Medical Systems*, *42*(4), 74. PMID:29525900

Mishra, B. S. P., Das, H., Dehuri, S., & Jagadev, A. K. (2018). *Cloud Computing for Optimization: Foundations, Applications, and Challenges* (Vol. 39). Springer. doi:10.1007/978-3-319-73676-1

Nayak, J., Naik, B., Jena, A. K., Barik, R. K., & Das, H. (2018). Nature Inspired Optimizations in Cloud Computing: Applications and Challenges. In *Cloud Computing for Optimization: Foundations, Applications, and Challenges* (pp. 1–26). Cham: Springer. doi:10.1007/978-3-319-73676-1_1

Nayak, S. R., & Mishra, J. (2018). *Fractal Dimension of Gray Scale images. Progress in Computing, Analytics and Networking* (Vol. 710, pp. 225–234). Singapore: Springer. doi:10.1007/978-981-10-7871-2_22

Nayak, S. R., Padhy, R., & Mishra, J. (2017). Texture Analysis: A Brief Review. *Journal of Advanced Research in Dynamical and control systems,* 9(11), 46-52.

Nayak, S. R., Routray, S., & Mohapatra, S. (2017). A Comparative Study on Image Segmentation Techniques: Thresholding, K-means and Ant colony optimization. *International Journal of Pure and Applied Mathematics*, *117*(19), 65–70.

P. K. Pattnaik, S. S. Rautaray, H. Das, & J. Nayak (Eds.). (2018). Progress in Computing, Analytics and Networking: *Proceedings of ICCAN 2017* (Vol. 710). *Springer*.

Pradhan, C., Das, H., Naik, B., & Dey, N. (2018). *Handbook of Research on Information Security in Biomedical Signal Processing* (pp. 1–414). Hershey, PA: IGI Global; doi:10.4018/978-1-5225-5152-2

Rajinikanth, V. (2018). Suresh Chandra Satapathy, Nilanjan Dey, and R. Vijayarajan. "DWT-PCA Image Fusion Technique to Improve Segmentation Accuracy in Brain Tumor Analysis. In *Microelectronics, Electromagnetics and Telecommunications* (pp. 453–462). Singapore: Springer. doi:10.1007/978-981-10-7329-8_46

Rajinikanth, V., Dey, N., Satapathy, S. C., & Ashour, A. S. (2018). Nilanjan Dey, Suresh Chandra Satapathy, and Amira S. Ashour. "An approach to examine magnetic resonance angiography based on Tsallis entropy and deformable snake model. *Future Generation Computer Systems*, *85*, 160–172. doi:10.1016/j.future.2018.03.025

Reddy, K. H. K., Das, H., & Roy, D. S. (2017). *A Data Aware Scheme for Scheduling Big-Data Applications with SAVANNA Hadoop. Futures of Network*. CRC Press.

Sarkhel, P., Das, H., & Vashishtha, L. K. (2017). Task-Scheduling Algorithms in Cloud Environment. In *Computational Intelligence in Data Mining* (pp. 553–562). Singapore: Springer. doi:10.1007/978-981-10-3874-7_52

Shriranjani, D., Tebby, S. G., Satapathy, S. C., Dey, N., & Rajinikanth, V. (2018). Kapur's Entropy and Active Contour-Based Segmentation and Analysis of Retinal Optic Disc. In *Computational Signal Processing and Analysis* (pp. 287–295). Singapore: Springer. doi:10.1007/978-981-10-8354-9_26

Tuan, T. M., Fujita, H., Dey, N., Ashour, A. S., Vo, T. N. N., & Chu, D.-T. (2018). Dental diagnosis from X-Ray images: An expert system based on fuzzy computing. *Biomedical Signal Processing and Control*, *39*, 64–73. doi:10.1016/j.bspc.2017.07.005

KEY TERMS AND DEFINITIONS

AD: Architectural distortion.

BC: Box counting.

CIE L*a*b: Color space specified by the International Commission on Illumination.

DBC: Differential box counting.

ECG: Electrocardiogram.

EEG: Electroencephalogram.

FD: Fractal dimension.

FBM: Fractional Brownian motion.

IBC: Improved box counting.

IDBC: Improved differential box counting.

ITBC: Improved triangle box counting.

MDBC: Modified differential box counting.

MRI: Magnetic resonance imaging.

RDBC: Relative differential box counting.

ROI: Region of interest.

SS: Self similarity.
SDBC: Shifting differential box counting.
TBC: Triangle box counting.
TD: Topological dimension.
TBMACR: Trabecular bone micro-architecture on calcaneus radiographs.

Chapter 9
Analysis of Color Image Encryption Using Multidimensional Bogdanov Map

R. N. Ramakant Parida
Kalinga Institute of Industrial Technology, India

Swapnil Singh
Kalinga Institute of Industrial Technology, India

Chittaranjan Pradhan
Kalinga Institute of Industrial Technology, India

ABSTRACT

Image encryption is a main concern in digital transmission of data over communication network. As encryption and decryption of image has got considerable attention in the past decades, its effectiveness and compatibility need to be taken care of. The work reported in this chapter is mainly concerned with enhancement of dimension in image encryption technique. The work mainly deals with pixels shuffling of an image using Bogdanov chaotic map for both gray and color image, where encryption and decryption process are associated with the key. In color image, the image is divided into all three planes (RGB) individually. Scrambling is done with all three planes individually. All the three planes are summed up into a single plane which gives us the final result. In Bogdanov map, old pixel position is replaced with new pixel position. Further, the authors analyzed security of image encryption techniques with two parameters called NPCR and UACI. The efficacy of the encryption process can be seen in experimental results.

DOI: 10.4018/978-1-5225-6316-7.ch009

INTRODUCTION

This is a technological era where most of the work is done digitally. Computer is a revolution in itself and so as computer networks. Now one person can send and receive information with the help of computer. In modern era, travelling of data or information is more convenient than ever. Information can be audio, video and images etc. Where computer network offers many advantages but also it sets up illegal use of information. To secure information, it needs to be hidden from unauthorized people. Nowadays, not only textual but also multimedia data is transferred over networks. To prevent unauthorized user, lots of methods can be used such as Image encryption technique, Cryptographic system, Watermarking techniques etc. The image encryption methods can prevent from illegal access. To deal with illegal access of digital data there are diversity of techniques used such as Arnold's cat map, baker map, henon map, cross chaotic map, logistic map, duffing map, bogdanov map, tent map etc.

IMAGE ENCRYPTION

Image encryption is the process to convert a message in such way that only authorized person can access it. In an encryption process, the intended information or message, referred to as plaintext, is encrypted using an encryption algorithm and generating cipher text that can be read only if decrypted with authorized person. An encryption process generally uses a pseudo- random encryption key generated by an algorithm. An authorized receiver can easily decrypt the message with the key provided by the sender to receiver but not to unauthorized users.

Image encryption usually consist two parts:-

1. Encryption
2. Decryption

In encryption process, image can be encrypted through keys such as pseudo random number from original image into encrypted image. In Decryption process, encrypted image can be decrypted into original image through keys and only authorized person can decrypt the image. Figure 1 and Figure 2 shows block diagram of image encryption and decryption process.

Figure 1. Process of image encryption

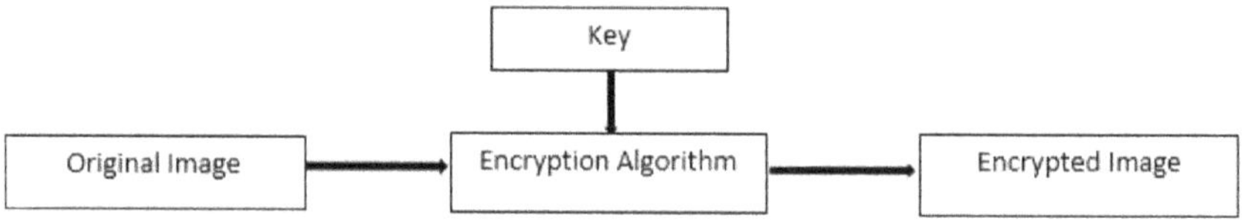

Figure 2. Process of image decryption

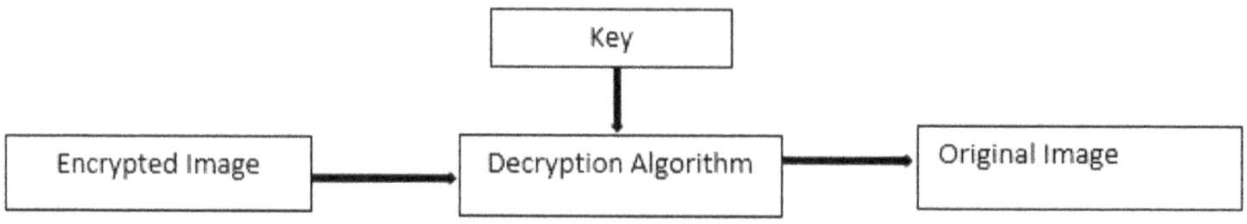

BASIC CONCEPT

Image Encryption Techniques

Image encryption techniques classified into two groups named as spatial domain in which pseudo random numbers or watermark (watermarking is the process to embed information into host image or cover image) inserted into intensity value of images and transform domain in which pseudo random numbers or watermark inserted in form of transform coefficients (Goel et al., 2010).

Spatial Domain

Spatial Domain is the easiest way of methodologies of encrypting image. It creates a sequence of random number and reforms the Least Significant Bits (LSB) of gray values or intensity values and finally extracts the original bits through spatial cross-correlation. Simply in spatial domain pseudo random numbers can embed into original or host image by changing intensity values or gray values of pixels in original image.

The main drawback of these methods is that in case of geometric deformation it is less robust and for JPEG compression it has less resistance. LSB is simple and basic method to encrypt image through using 2D matrix of pixels to hold hidden data. As we know casting algorithm of image encryption can only be used to embed few bits in order to respect the unobstructed requirement, they seem to offer a low bit capacity.

Transform Domain

This method can work on a complete digital image of a block or for minor blocks gradually of 8×8 or 16×16. Transform domain method basically works on wavelet, the image is decomposed in the bands consisting of the space of embed. Transform domain is of three types as follows (Kumar et al., 2015):

- Discrete Fourier Transform (DFT)
- Discrete Cosine Transform (DCT)
- Discrete Wavelet Transform (DWT)

Discrete Fourier Transform (DFT)

French mathematician Joseph Fourier introduced fourier series to represent continuous-time periodic signal. The signal can be decomposed into a linear weighted sum called "spectrum" of harmonically related complex exponential. When the signal becomes non-periodic, its spectrum became continuous and period became infinite. A spatial image function is decay into a set of orthogonal functions by fourier transform and the spatial intensity image is transformed into its frequency domain (Cox et al., 2007). If f(a, b) denotes a digital image in spatial domain and F(x, y) denotes a transform image information in a frequency domain, the 2D DFT equation is:

$$F(x,y) = \frac{1}{MN}\sum_{x=0}^{M-1}\sum_{y=0}^{N-1} f(a,b)\exp\left[-2j2\pi\left(\frac{xa}{M}+\frac{yb}{N}\right)\right] \quad (1)$$

For x = 0, 1, 2 . . . M-1 and y = 0, 1, 2 . . . N-1.

The inverse DFT can be represented as:

$$f(a,b) = \sum_{x=0}^{M-1}\sum_{y=0}^{N-1} F(x,y)\exp\left[j2\pi\left(\frac{xa}{M}+\frac{yb}{N}\right)\right] \quad (2)$$

For a = 0, 1, 2 . . . M-1 and b = 0, 1, 2 . . . N-1.

DFT can be used in phase modulation in between watermark image and its carrier and for dividing image into perceptual bands to record watermark. Phase modulation has less visual effect so that DFT uses phase modulation rather than magnitude components to encrypt message.

Discrete Cosine Transform (DCT)

For compressing data to frequency domain from spatial domain, DCT is used, for example JPEG compression. DCT uses existing parts of DFT which carries cosine terms. This method usually transforms space domain and time domain of existing input into elementary frequency components. The DCT grants an image to decay into various frequency bands like low, high, middle frequency bands. Low frequency bands having higher strength if any alteration is done over host image its effect reduces the quality of host image. High frequency bands having less strength, in this case if any alteration is done over host image, it can be removed by watermarking algorithm and it will not affect the quality of host image. Mid frequency is appropriate enough to insert watermark into host image. This is because mid frequencies sidestep many essential visual parts of image (low frequencies) without over disclosing themselves to removal through compression and noise attack (high frequencies) (Cox et al., 2007).

Two-dimensional discrete cosine transformation and its inverse transform for a square image are defined as follows:

$$C(g,h) = \alpha(g)\alpha(h)\sum_{a=0}^{N-1}\sum_{b=0}^{N-1}\cos\left[\frac{\pi(2a+1)g}{2N}\right]\cos\left[\frac{\pi(2b+1)h}{2N}\right] \tag{3}$$

$$f(x,y) = \sum_{g=0}^{N-1}\sum_{h=0}^{N-1}\alpha(g)\alpha(h)C(g,h)\cos\left[\frac{\pi(2a+1)g}{2N}\right]\cos\left[\frac{\pi(2b+1)h}{2N}\right] \tag{4}$$

where, g, h = 0, 1, 2 . . . N-1 and a, b = 0, 1, 2 . . . N-1, and where, C(g, h) is the new matrix value obtained after applying DCT on blocks of f(a, b) and further IDCT is applied on C(g, h) to perform inverse DCT to transform to spatial domain again. Alpha is the embedding strength factor. DCT puts most of an image's energy at low frequencies.

Discrete Wavelet Transform (DWT)

Discrete Wavelet Transform (DWT) converts the image from spatial domain to frequency domain, it able to provide representation for both spatial and frequency as one. Wavelet analysis can be used to split the information of an image into approximation and detailed sub signal. The approximation sub signal display the general trend of pixel value, and three detailed sub signal show vertical, horizontal and diagonal details or changes in image. If all these details are very small than these detail can be set to zero without much changing the image. If the number of zeroes is greater than the compression ratio is also greater. Two types of wavelet is used in DWT. First is Continuous wavelet transform and second is discrete wavelet transform. Filter bank is used to compute wavelet analysis. Two types of filters can be used as (Cox et al., 2007):

- **High Pass Filter:** High frequency information is kept, low frequency information is lost.
- **Low Pass Filter:** Low frequency information is kept, high frequency information is lost.

Therefore, signal gradually splits into two halves, at first high frequency (detailed part) and secondly low frequency (approximation part). Details of level 1 is horizontal, details of level 2 is vertical, and details of level 3 is diagonal in case of image signal. Generally high frequency has mostly edge components of signals. The next lower frequency is again subdivided into two parts low and high frequencies. The above procedure is repeated a random number of time that is generally predicted by application.

In the 2D case, the 1D analysis filter bank is first applied to the columns of the image and then applied to the rows. If the image has R1 rows and R2 columns, then after applying the 1D analysis filter bank to each column we have two sub band images, each having R1/2 rows and R2 columns; after applying the 1D analysis filter bank to each row of both of the two sub band images, we have four sub band images, each having R1/2 rows and R2/2 columns. The 2D synthesis filter bank merge the four sub band images to obtain the original image of size R1 by R2.The three level wavelet decomposition is shown in Figure 3.

Evaluation of Performance

The performance of the decrypted image can be calculated on the basis of peak signal to noise ratio and NPCR & UACI values. We have also evaluated on the basis of encryption and decryption time (Ahmad et al., 2009).

Peak Signal to Noise Ratio (PSNR)

Efficiency and effectiveness of decrypted image can be evaluated by PSNR (peak signal to noise ration). If PSNR value is more than 30 db then it is considered to be acceptable image. Higher PSNR value means quality of the decrypted image is better. PSNR value calculated as:

Figure 3. Three-level decomposition in DWT

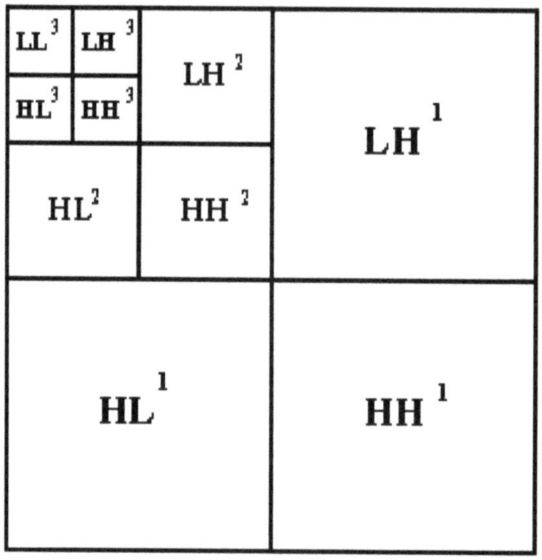

$$MSE = \frac{1}{mn}\sum_{m-1}^{i=0}\sum_{n-1}^{j=0}\left[I(i,j) - K(i,j)^2\right] \tag{5}$$

$$PSNR = 10\log_{10}\left(\frac{R}{MSE}\right) \tag{6}$$

where, MSE is the mean square error of the decrypted image and the original image and m is the number of rows and n is the number of columns. I and K are the original and decrypted images. When PSNR is higher than 30db, it is tough to differentiate between original image and the reconstructed image.

Number of Pixel Change Rate (NPCR) and Unified Averaged Changed Intensity (UACI)

To check the strength of image, we evaluate two terms NPCR and UACI in between cipher text or decrypted image and plain text or original image. A high NPCR score or low UACI score is usually interpreted as a high resistance to differential attacks. Although these two tests are defined and easy to calculate, test scores are difficult to interpret in the sense of whether the performance is good enough. Even the difference of a single pixel can bring about a significant change in the encrypted images. NPCR is used to calculate this difference in pixels where UACI is used to calculate the degree of security provided. It is used to calculate what percentages of pixels are different in two images. NPCR and UACI calculated as (Ahmad et al., 2009 and Kabi et al., 2014):

$$NPCR = \frac{\sum_{i,j} K(i,j)}{a \times b} \times 100\% \tag{7}$$

Let P and Q be two differential images, varying with 1 pixel only. Another matrix K is calculated which is shown below:

$$K(i,j) = \begin{cases} 0, & if \;\; P(i,j) = Q(i,j) \\ 1, & if \;\; P(i,j) \neq Q(i,j) \end{cases} \tag{8}$$

$$UACI = \frac{\sum_{i,j} \frac{|\, p(i,j) - Q(i,j) \,|}{255} \times 100\%}{a \times b} \tag{9}$$

where,

a = height of image P & Q and
b = width of image P & Q.

CHAOTIC MAPS

Chaotic maps are used for image encryption which shows various chaos features like randomness, periodicity, non-deterministic, dependent on initial conditions, long-term unpredictability, certainty etc. In physics and mathematics, chaos theory deals with the behaviour of certain nonlinear dynamics system that exhibits a phenomenon under certain circumstances known as chaos. Some of chaotic map are Arnold's cat map, Bogdanov map, Henon map etc. (Wu et at., 2011 and Kumar et al., 2015).

1D Chaotic Maps

Logistic Map

It shows various chaotic properties like randomness, periodicity, non-deterministic etc. which is derived from non-dynamical discrete systems and generates a sequences of random number. It is described in (Kabi et al., 2014):

$$X_{n+1} = g \times X_n \times (1 - X_n) \tag{10}$$

X_n is the initial parameter; g is a control parameter which lies between 3 and 4. X_n lies between 0 and 1. X_{n+1} is the new parameter value. The result is shown in Figure 4.

Tent Map

The tent map is described in (Hassani et al., 2013 and Borujeni et al., 2009):

$$f(X_n) = X_{n+1} = \begin{cases} \dfrac{X_n}{a}, & if \ \ 0 \le X_n \le a \\ \dfrac{(1-X_n)}{(1-a)}, & if \ \ a \le X_n \le 1 \end{cases} \tag{11}$$

where a is control parameter and lies between [0, 1] but not equal to 0.5 when a = 0.5, the system enters a chaotic state and initial values is $X_n = [0,1]$. The name of tent map being due to the tent-like figure of the graph. For the values of the parameter

Figure 4. Image encryption using 1D logistic map

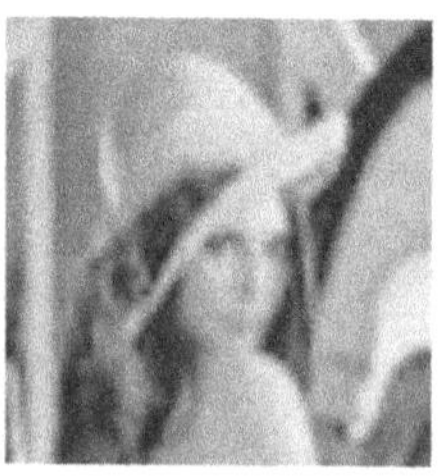

a. Original Image

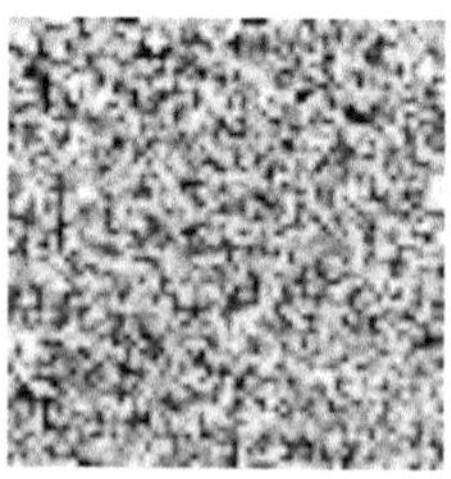

b. Encrypted Image

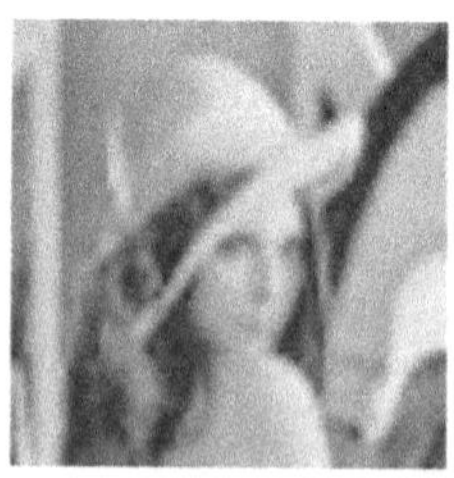

c. Decrypted Image

a within 0 and 1, f (X_n) maps the unit interval [0, 1] into itself, thus defining a discrete-time dynamical system on it. In specific, iterating a point X_n in [0, 1] gives increasing sequence. The result is shown in Figure 5.

2D Chaotic Maps

Arnold's Cat Map

It is based on pixel shuffling where old pixels position of image is changed into new pixels position after several iterations of pixels matrix from old pixels this time called Arnold period. Its 2D map is described in (Ahmad et al., 2009):

$$\begin{aligned} i' &= (i + x \times j) \bmod N \\ j' &= (y \times i + ((x \times y) + 1) \times y) \bmod N \end{aligned} \tag{12}$$

The result is shown in Figure 6.

Duffing Map

A system which is dynamic that is in discrete-time which shows the chaotic behaviour is referred as Duffing map (It is also called as "Holmes map"). 2D Duffing map maps a new point after taking a point (X_i, Y_i) in the plane. It is described in (Liu et al., 2015 and Stoyanov et al., 2014):

$$\begin{aligned} X_{i+1} &= Y_i \\ Y_{i+1} &= -b \times X_i + a \times Y_i - a \times Y^3 \end{aligned} \tag{13}$$

Figure 5. Image encryption using tent map

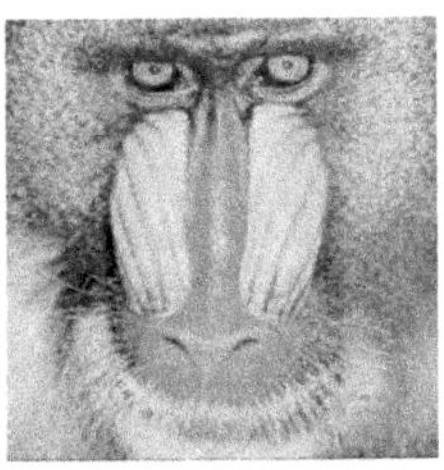

a. Original Image

b. Encrypted Image

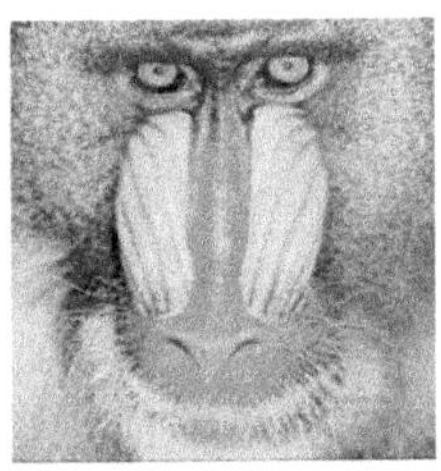

c. Decrypted Image

Figure 6. Image encryption using Arnold's map

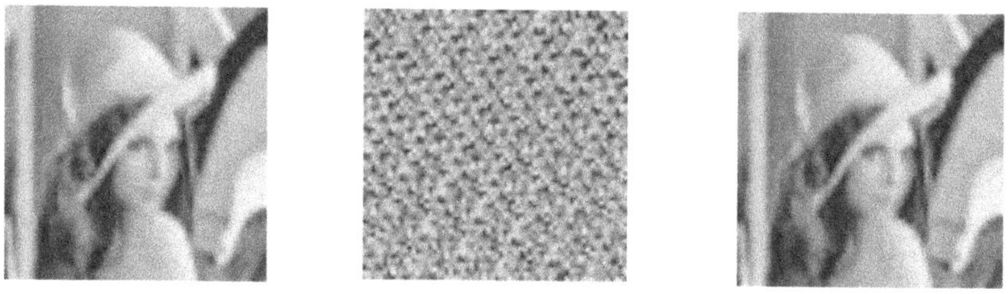

a. Original Image b. Encrypted Image c. Decrypted Image

where *a* and *b* are control parameters; initial values are X_i and Y_i; X_{i+1} and Y_{i+1} are new pixel positions. The quantization equation converts the random number to binary format. For image encryption, firstly we create pseudo random numbers and they are quantized into binary format and this quantization equation is Xored bit by bit with size of m×m input gray image which generates encrypted image and vice versa. The result is shown in Figure 7.

Baker Map

The extension of Tent map in chaotic map is known as 2D Baker Map. Baker map also shows various chaos features like randomness, periodicity, non-deterministic etc. Baker map described as follows (Kabi et al., 2014):

Figure 7. Image encryption using Duffing map

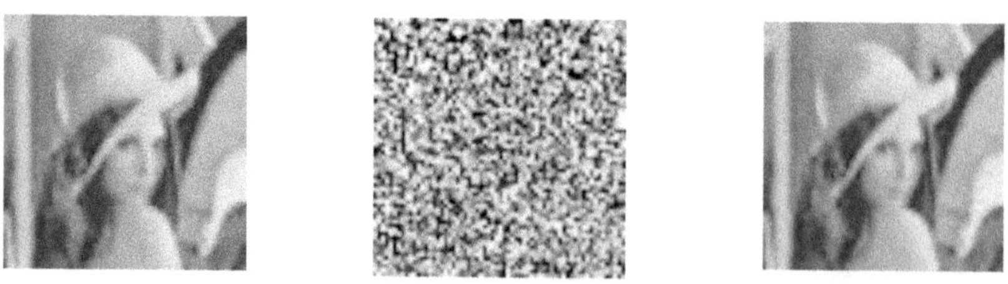

a. Original Image b. Encrypted Image c. Decrypted Image

$$M(a) = \begin{cases} \left((2 \times a), \frac{b}{2}\right), & for \quad 0 \leq a \leq 0.5 \\ \left((2 - 2 \times a), 1 - \frac{b}{2}\right), & for \quad 0.5 \leq a \leq 1 \end{cases} \tag{14}$$

where a and b are initial parameter. The result is shown in Figure 8.

Henon Map

Michel Henon introduced the henon map. It generates pseudo random key which is used to encrypt the image. Henon map described as follows (Kabi et al., 2014):

$$\begin{aligned} N_{i+1} &= b \times M_i \\ M_{i+1} &= N_i + 1 - a \times M_i^2 \end{aligned} \tag{15}$$

where a and b are control parameter and M_i and N_i are initial parameters. The result is shown in Figure 9.

Chaotic neural networks can be used in Image encryption and decryption technique, where neural network is made up of chaotic neuron layer and to construct block cipher a linear neuron layer is used to transforms the plain text data into unintelligible form with the help of a key. Chaotic neural networks (CNN) are categorized into two groups stream cipher and block cipher. Stream cipher generates the sequences of pseudo random numbers through neural networks. Block cipher uses the property of chaotic neural network to encrypt the plain text block by block. Stream cipher's security depends on the random sequences. Encryption process consist of two parts

Figure 8. Image encryption using Baker map

a. Original Image b. Encrypted Image c. Decrypted Image

Figure 9. Image encryption using Henon map

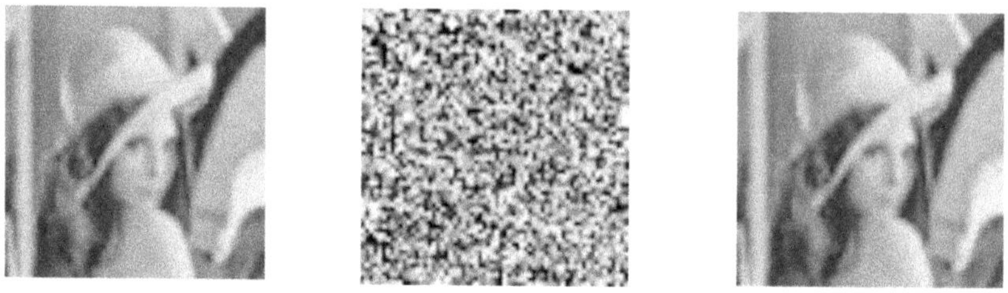

a. Original Image b. Encrypted Image c. Decrypted Image

i.e. data diffusion and data confusion. Data diffusion realizes the chaotic neuron layer and data confusion realizes the linear neuron layer. Chaotic neural networks consist only diffusion layer where image pixels xored with the binary sequence number which is generated by chaotic maps which is not secure to differential attack. To resist attack confusion layer is used to make CNN a product cipher where triple key is used for chaotic image encryption techniques (Lian, S. (2009), Bigdeli et al., (2012) and Jain et al., (2012)).

2D BOGDANOV MAP

V. J. Subashini and S. Poornachandra proposed image encryption technique in 2017 by taking the image of matrix size of m×m and then applying chaos on the image. The pixel position value of image can be converted or shifted to undistinguished cipher image and apply reverse procedure on it to get plain text. Bogdanov map is named after Rifkat Ibragimovich Bogdanov, a Soviet Russian mathematician. It is a chaotic 2D map related to Bogdanov-Takens bifurcation. It is given by Ref. (Subashini et al., (2017) and Arrowsmith et al., (1993))

$$\begin{aligned} i' &= i + j' \\ j' &= j + \varepsilon \times j + k \times i \times (i-1) + \mu \times i \times j \end{aligned} \tag{16}$$

where ε and μ are correlated to u_1 and u_2 in Bogdanov vector field correspondingly. Bogdanov vector field [11] is describe as follows

$$
\begin{aligned}
&i' = j \\
&j' = u_1 \times j + i(i-1) + u_2 \times i \times j \times \\
&Q(i, u_1, u_2) + u_2^2 \times j^2 \times \varphi(i, j, u_1, u_2)
\end{aligned}
\tag{17}
$$

Bogdanov vector field is discretized by applying the backward and forward Euler discretization methods to the equations with step length h. Then the outcome of Euler map is given as

$$
\begin{aligned}
&i' = i + h \times j \\
&j' = j + h \times u_1 \times j + h \times i(i-1) + h \times u_2 \times \\
&i \times j \times Q(i, u_1, u_2) + h \times u_2^2 \times j^2 \times \varphi(i, j, u_2, u_2)
\end{aligned}
\tag{18}
$$

The Bogdanov map is defined by assigning $Q(i, u_1, u_2) = 1$, $\varphi(i, j, u_1, u_2) = 0$, $h \times j = j'$, $h \times u_1 = \varepsilon$, $h \times u_2 = \mu$, and $h = k$ where $\varepsilon, \mu, k \in R$.

To scramble the pixels of image and to makes use of bogdanov map, discretization is applied in equation (16) and maintain the Hamiltonian nature by assigning ε and μ as zero. Then the resultant map's equation is describe as:

$$
\begin{aligned}
&i' = i + j' \\
&j' = j + k \times i \times (i-1)
\end{aligned}
\tag{19}
$$

i and j is the old pixel position in an image whereas i' and j' is the new pixel position in an image k is the any positive integer.

2D Bogdanov Map in Gray Image

This algorithm is depended on the scrambling of pixels in an image where the old pixel position replaced by new pixel position in original image. The key k uses at the scrambling time same uses at the unscrambling time to get original image. Bogdanov map scramble images of any dimension without dividing them into blocks. So, there is no limitation in the size of images. In Bogdanov, original image is restored after a certain number of iterations. For restoring the initial position pixels the no of repetition required is known as the period of Bogdanov map.

Scrambling Algorithm

```
Input: Original image, O, and any positive integer k
Output: Scrambled image, S
Step 1: [r, c] ←size (O), r represent the rows and c represent the columns.
Step 2: For every pixel position (i, j) in O, perform Step 3 to Step 5.
Step 3: j' ← mod (j+ k×i×(i-1), c) +1
Step 4: i' ← mod (i+ j', r) +1
Step 5: S (i', j') ←O (i, j)
```

Unscrambling Algorithm

```
Input: Scrambled image, S, and the positive integer k
Output: Plain image, O
Step 1: [r, c] ←size (S), r represent the rows and c represent the columns.
Step 2: For every pixel position (i', j') in S perform Step 3 to Step 7
Step 3: i ←mod (i'-j', r) -1
Step 4: If (i <0) then i ← i+ r; else if (i = 0) then i ←r
Step 5: j ←mod (j'-k×i'× (i' -1), c) -1
Step 6: If (j < 0) then j ←j+ c; else if (j = 0) then j ←c
Step 7: O (i, j) ←S (i', j')
```

Taking standard image "Baboon.bmp" and values k = 5, the result has been shown in Figure 10.

2D Bogdanov Map in Color Image

For image scrambling in RGB plane, image divided into all three planes (RGB) individually (Kumar et al., 2015). All the individual planes are again reverted into a 2D plane; thus making the scrambling more versatile. All the three planes are summed up into a single plane which gives us the final scramble image. For the unscramble process, first unscramble image divided into three plane then unscrambling process is applied on all three plane individually. Then after all the three planes are summed up into a single plane which gives us the final unscramble image.

For experimental result, taking standard image "Barbara.png" and values k = 5, the result has been shown in Figure 11 and Figure 12.

Figure 10. Scrambling and Unscrambling through 2D Bogdanov Map in Gray Image

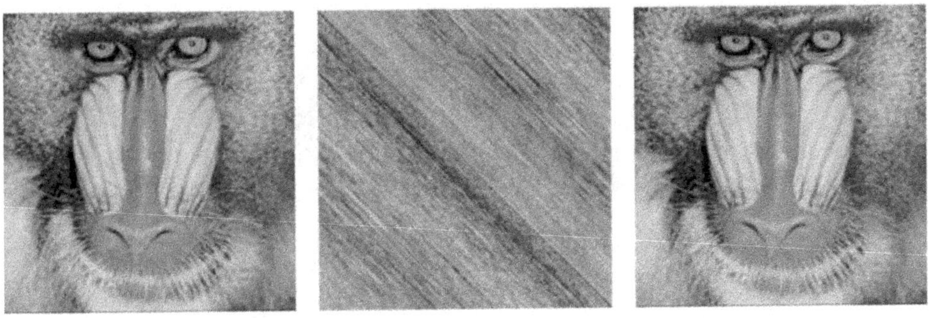

a. Original Image b. Scramble Image c. Unscramble Image

Figure 11. Scramble through 2D Bogdanov Map in Color Image

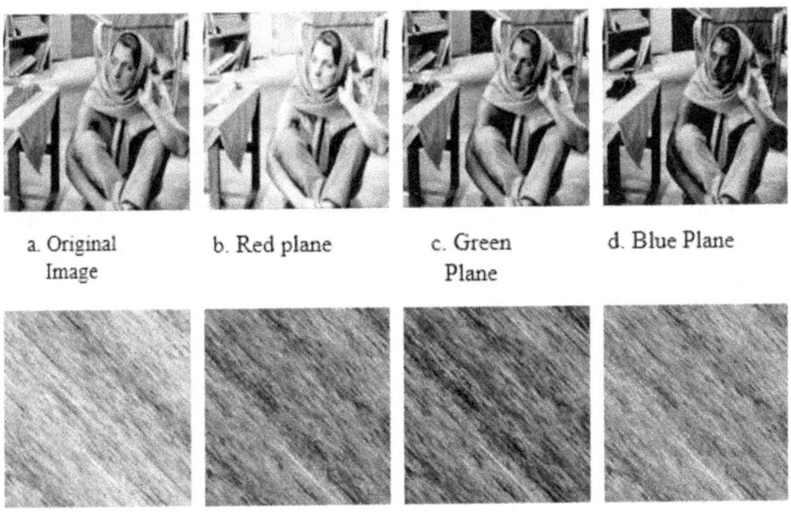

a. Original Image b. Red plane c. Green Plane d. Blue Plane

e. Scramble in red plane f. Scramble in Green Plane g. Scramble in Blue Plane h. Final scramble Image

**For a more accurate representation see the electronic version.*

PROPOSED ALGORITHM

Here, we have proposed 3D Bogdanov map which is the extension of 2D Bogdanov map through increasing dimension, number of keys and parameters to improve security, robustness and efficiency of image. 2D Bogdanov map have one key k (positive integer) whereas 3D Bogdanov map include three more keys z, d, e (positive

Figure 12. Unscramble through 2D Bogdanov Map in Color Image

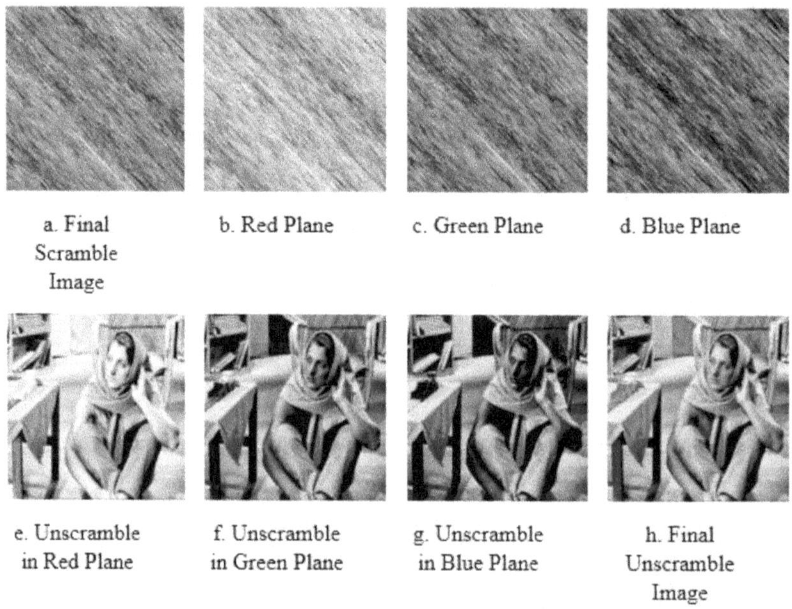

**For a more accurate representation see the electronic version.*

integer) so that it increases the effectiveness and robustness of chaotic map. 3D Bogdanov map can also enhance dimensions to increase efficiency and secrecy. 3D Bogdanov map is described below:

$$i' = i + j'$$

$$j' = j + k \times i \times (1 - 1) \quad (20)$$

$$z = d \times e$$

$$i'' = i' \bmod z$$

$$j'' = j' \bmod z$$

Scrambling Algorithm

```
Input: Original image, O, and any positive integer k, z, d, e
Output: Scrambled image, S
Step 1: [r, c] ←size (O), r represent the rows and c represent
the columns.
Step 2: For every pixel position (i, j) in I perform Step 3 to
Step 8.
Step 3: j' ← mod (j + k×i× (i-1), c) +1
Step 4: i'← mod (i+ j', r) +1
Step 5: z ←mod (d X i X j, c)+1
Step 6: j'' ←mod ((j'+ z), c) +1
Step 7: i''←mod ((i'+z), r) +1
Step 8: s (i'', j'') ←O (i, j)
```

Unscrambling Algorithm

The unscrambling process is the reverse process by taking the scramble image, S and the positive integers k, z, d, e to produce the final image. This process also involves in generating the chaotic sequence which is used in the decryption method.

```
Input: Scrambled image, S, and the positive integer k, z, d, e
Output: Plain image
Step 1: [r, c]←size (S), r represent the rows and c represent
the columns.
Step 2: For every pixel position (i'', j'') in S perform Step 3
to Step 24
Step 3:  z ←d×e
Step 4:  i'←mod ((i'' - z), r)-1
Step 5:  if (i' <0) then  i'←i'+r; else if (i'=0) then  i'←r
Step 6:  j' ←mod (j'' - z), c)-1
Step 7:  if (j'<0) then  j' ←j' +c; else if (j'=0) then  j' ←c
Step 8:  i ←mod ((i' - j'), r)-1
Step 9:  if (i<0) then  i ←i + r; else if (i=0) then   i ←r
Step 10: j ←mod (j' - (ki (i-1)), c)-1
Step 11: if (j<0) then  j ←i + c; else if (j=0) then  j ←c
Step 12:   O (i, j) ←S(i'',j'')
```

3D Bogdanov Map in Gray Scale

This algorithm is depended on the scrambling of pixels in an image where the old pixels (i, j) position replace by new pixel (i'', j'') position in original image. The key k, d, e (positive integer) uses at the scrambling time same uses at the unscrambling time to get original image. Bogdanov map scramble images of any dimension without dividing them into blocks. So, there is no limitation in the size of images. In Bogdanov, original image is restored after a certain number of iterations. For experimental result, taking standard image "Baboon.bmp" and values k = 5, d = 6, e = 7, the result is shown in Figure 13.

3D Bogdanov Map in Color Image

For image scrambling in RGB plane, image divided into all three planes (RGB) individually. All the individual planes are again reverted into a 2D plane; thus making the scrambling more versatile. All the three planes are summed up into a single plane which gives us the final scramble image. For the unscramble process, first unscramble image is divided into three planes individually and then unscrambling process is applied on all three planes individually. Then after all the three planes are summed up into a single plane which gives us the final unscramble image.

For experimental result, taking standard image "Barbara.png" and values k = 5, d = 6, e = 7, we get the result as shown in Figure 14 and Figure 15.

Figure 13. Scrambling and Unscrambling through 3D Bogdanov Map in Gray Image

a. Original Image b. Scramble Image c. Unscramble Image

Figure 14. Scramble through 3D Bogdanov Map in Color Image

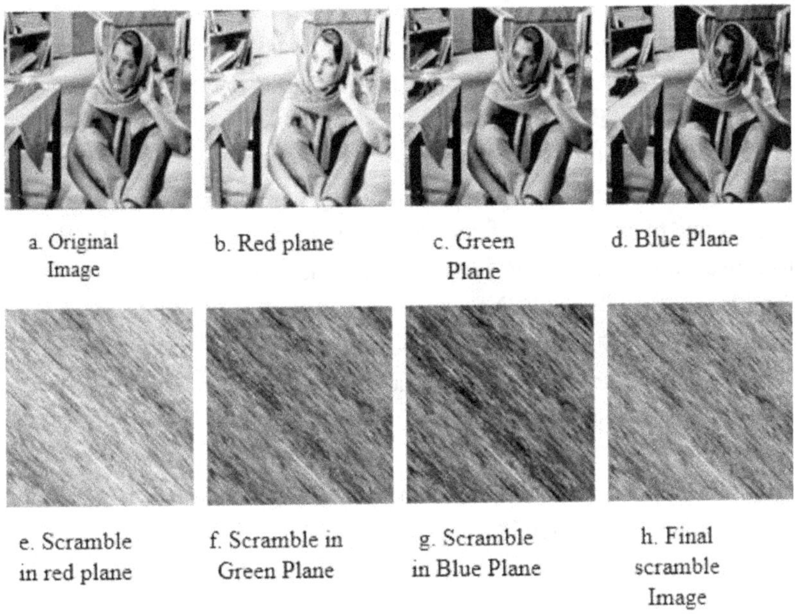

**For a more accurate representation see the electronic version.*

Figure 15. Unscramble through 3D Bogdanov Map in Color Image

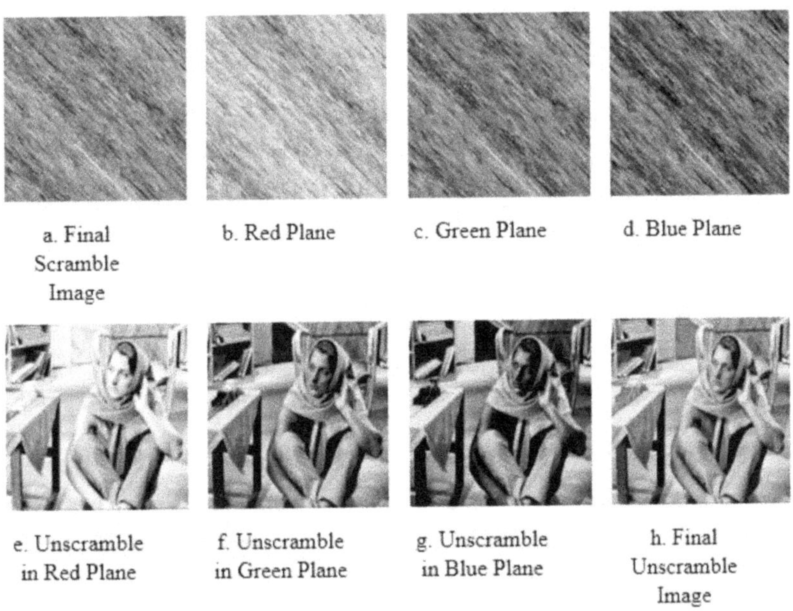

**For a more accurate representation see the electronic version.*

RESULT ANALYSIS

We have implemented a new 3D chaotic map named 3D Bogdanov map. There are three terms which is used to evaluate the performance of decrypted image such as NPCR, UACI and PSNR. Now, we check the degree of security. NPCR and UACI are two parameters through which we can analyse the difference of pixels in terms of percentage between encrypted image and original image.

Efficiency and effectiveness of decrypted image can be evaluated by PSNR (peak signal to noise ration). If PSNR value is more than 30 db then it is considered to be acceptable image. Higher PSNR value means quality of the decrypted image is better (Ahmad et al., 2009).

Table 1 describes the NPCR, UACI and PSNR values of Bogdanov map for the image size of 512×512 pixels.

We have also calculated the encryption time and decryption time for image size of 512×512 pixels which is shown in Table 2. From the result, we can say that the 3D Bogdanov map is more efficient and robust in comparison to 2D Bogdanov map.

Table 3 shows the encryption and decryption of various chaotic maps with various image sizes which may used in medical field to secure the customer report or files or data from unauthorized users. Table 4 shows the efficiency and effectiveness of various chaotic maps in form of these parameter such as NPCR, UACI and PSNR value and encryption and decryption time.

Table 1. NPCR, UACI and PSNR values

Image Size	Chaotic Map	NPCR Value	UACI Value	PSNR Value(db)
512×512	2D Gray Bogdanov Map	98.46	33.85	34.56
	2D Color Bogdanov Map	98.46	33.85	35.55
	3D Gray Bogdanov Map	98.80	33.39	34.221
	3D Color Bogdanov Map	99.80	33.39	35.24

Table 2. CPU Encryption & decryption time

Image Size	Chaotic Map	Encryption Time (sec)	Decryption Time (sec)
512×512	2D Gray Bogdanov Map	0.9375	0.6406
	2D Color Bogdanov Map	2.7813	2.7969
	3D Gray Bogdanov Map	0.6875	0.8125
	3D Color Bogdanov Map	3.0000	5.3437

Table 3. Encryption and decryption of various images

Image Size	Chaotic Map	Original Image	Encrypted Image	Decrypted Image
512×512	2D Gray Bogdanov Map	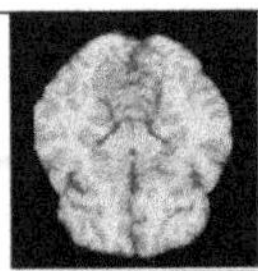	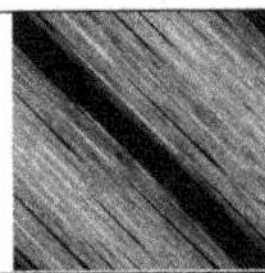	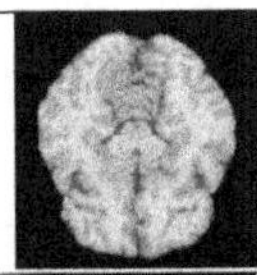
128×128	2D color Bogdanov Map	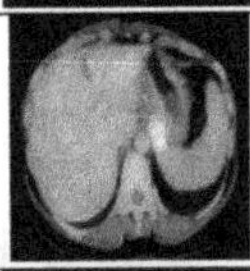	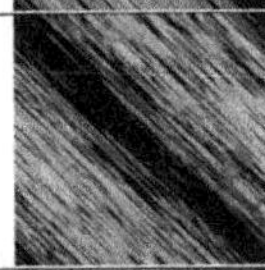	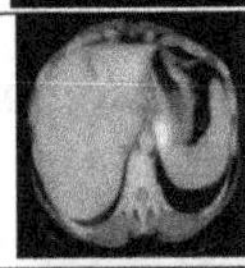
128×128	3D Gray Bogdanov Map	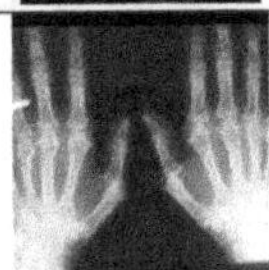	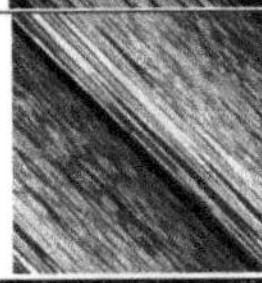	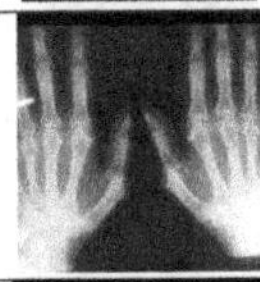
256×256	3D color Bogdanov Map	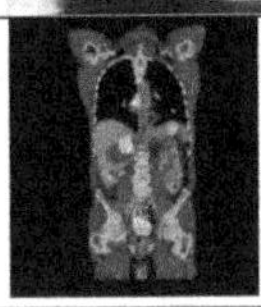	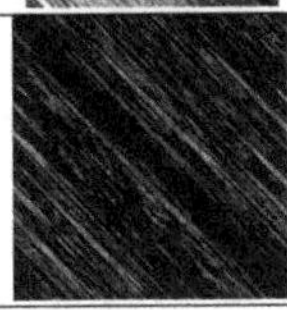	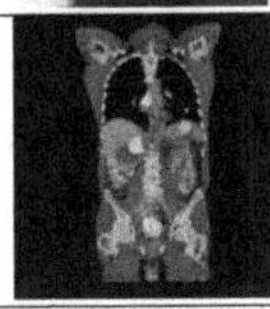

Table 4. NPCR, UACI, PSNR values and encryption and decryption TIME

Image Size	Chaotic Map	NPCR Value	UACI Value	PSNR Value(db)	Encryption Time(sec)	Decryption Time(sec)
512×512	2D Gray Bogdanov Map	99.80	33.39	34.55	0.85937	0.60937
128×128	2D color Bogdanov Map	99.22	33.59	34.65	2.1250	2.00
128×128	3D Gray Bogdanov Map	99.22	33.59	35.33	1.1563	0.7813
256×256	3D color Bogdanov Map	99.61	33.46	35.44	2.82812	3.45312

CONCLUSION AND FUTURE WORK

In this chapter, we implemented a new image encryption technique using 3D Bogdanov map. This map is more robust, effective and secure as compared to 2D Bogdanov map. This has been proven by the evaluation parameters like NPCR and UACI as well as encryption and decryption times. NPCR values assure the decrypted image is good enough and get pixel difference between original image and decrypted image and UACI values assure the average difference between original image and decrypted image.

In this, further development is possible for proposed algorithm in terms of robustness and embedding technique. This method can be more versatile so that it will takes more time to recover the original image than this.

REFERENCES

Ahmad, M., & Alam, M. S. (2009). A New Algorithm of Encryption and Decryption of Images using Chaotic Mapping. *International Journal on Computer Science and Engineering*, *02*(01), 46–50.

Arrowsmith, D. K., Cartwright, J. H. E., Lansbury, A. N., & Place, C. M. (1993). The Bogdanov Map: Bifurcations, Mode Locking, and Chaos in a Dissipative System. *International Journal of Bifurcation and Chaos in Applied Sciences and Engineering*, *3*(04), 803–842. doi:10.1142/S021812749300074X

Bigdeli, N., Farid, Y., & Afshar, K. (2012). A novel image encryption/decryption scheme based on chaotic neural networks. *Engineering Applications of Artificial Intelligence, Elsevier*, *25*(4), 753–765. doi:10.1016/j.engappai.2012.01.007

Borujeni, S. E., & Eshghi, M. (2009). *Chaotic Image Encryption Design using Tompkins-Paige Algorithm. Mathematical Problems in Engineering*.

Cox, I. J., Miller, M. L., Bloom, J. A., Fridrich, J., & Kalker, T. (2007). *Digital watermarking and steganography*. Morgan Kaufmann publisher.

Goel, A., Sahu, O. P., Gupta, R., & Gupta, S. (2010). Improved digital watermarking techniques and data embedding in multimedia. *International Journal on Computer Science and Engineering*, *02*(02), 164–168.

Hassani, E., & Eshghi, M. (2013). Image encryption based on chaotic tent map in time and frequency domains. *The ISC International Journal of Information Security*, *5*(1), 97–110.

Jain, A., & Rajpal, N. (2012). A two layer chaotic network based image encryption technique. *National Conference on Computing and Communication Systems*, 1-5. 10.1109/NCCCS.2012.6413005

Kabi, K. K., Pradhan, C., Saha, B. J., & Bisoi, A. K. (2014). Comparative Study of Image Encryption using 2D Chaotic Map. *International Conference on Information Systems and Computer Networks*, 105-108. 10.1109/ICISCON.2014.6965227

Kalra, G. S., Talwar, R., & Sadawarti, H. (2011). Robust blind digital image watermarking using DWT and dual encryption technique. *International Conference on Computational Intelligence, Communication Systems and Networks*, 225-230. 10.1109/CICSyN.2011.56

Kumar, S., Sinha, B., & Pradhan, C. (2015). Comparative Analysis of Color Image Encryption using 2D Chaotic Maps. *Information Systems Design and Intelligent Applications, Springer*, *2*, 379–387. doi:10.1007/978-81-322-2247-7_39

Lian, S. (2009). A block cipher based on chaotic neural networks. *Neurocomputing, Elsevier*, *72*(4), 1296–1301. doi:10.1016/j.neucom.2008.11.005

Liu, H., & Kadir, A. (2015). Asymmetric Color Image Encryption Scheme using 2D Discrete-Time Map. *Signal Processing, Elsevier*, *113*, 104–112. doi:10.1016/j.sigpro.2015.01.016

Mahdi, A., Jawad, A. K., & Hreshree, S. S. (2016). Digital Chaotic Scrambling of Voice Based on Duffing Map. *Communications Engineering Journal*, *1*(2), 16–21.

Pradhan, C., Rath, S., & Bisoi, A. K. (2012). Non blind digital watermarking technique using DWT and cross chaos. *Procedia Technology, Elsevier*, *6*, 897–904. doi:10.1016/j.protcy.2012.10.109

Stoyanov, B., & Kordov, K. (2014). *Novel Image Encryption Scheme Based on Chebyshev Polynomial and Duffing Map. The Scientific World Journal*, 1–11.

Subashini, V. J., & Poornachandra, S. (2017). Chaos Based Image Encryption Using Bogdanov Map. *Journal of Computational and Theoretical Nanoscience*, *14*(9), 4508–4514. doi:10.1166/jctn.2017.6768

Wu, Y., Noonan, J. P. & Agaian, S. (2011). NPCR and UACI Randomness Tests for Image Encryption. *Cyber Journals: Multidisciplinary Journals in Science and Technology, Journal of Selected Areas in Telecommunications*, 31-38.

ADDITIONAL READING

Dey, Nilanjan, Ashour, Amira S., Shi, Fuqian, & Fong, Simon James, and João Manuel RS Tavares. (2018). Medical cyber-physical systems: A survey. [PubMed]. *Journal of Medical Systems*, *42*(4), 74.

Pradhan, C., Das, H., Naik, B., & Dey, N. (2018). *Handbook of Research on Information Security in Biomedical Signal Processing* (pp. 1–414). Hershey, PA: IGI Global; doi:10.4018/978-1-5225-5152-2

Chapter 10
Automatic Computerized Diagnostic Tool for Down Syndrome Detection in Fetus

Michael Dinesh Simon
Anna University, India

Kavitha A. R.
Anna University, India

ABSTRACT

Down syndrome is a genetic disorder and the chromosome abnormality observed in humans that can cause physical and mental abnormalities. It can never be cured or rectified. Instead it has to be identified in the fetus and prevented from being born. Many ultrasonographic markers like nuchal fold, nasal bone hypoplasia, femur length, and EIF are considered to be the symptoms of Down syndrome in the fetus. This chapter deals with the creation of automatic and computerized diagnostic tool for Down syndrome detection based on EIF. The proposed system consists of two phases: 1) training phase and 2) testing phase. In training phase, the fetal images with EIF and Down syndrome is analyzed and characteristics of EIF are collected. In testing phase, detection of Down syndrome is performed on the fetal image with EIF based on the knowledge cluster obtained using ESOM. The performance of the proposed system is analyzed in terms of sensitivity, accuracy, and specificity.

DOI: 10.4018/978-1-5225-6316-7.ch010

INTRODUCTION

Down syndrome is the chromosomal abnormality caused in humans when extra genes from chromosome 21 are transferred to a newly produced embryo. It causes a change in the fetal development leading to physical and mental abnormalities. The babies with Down syndrome have a distinguished appearance than normal babies. The child suffering from Down syndrome are likely to have retardation in growth and the mental problems. Down syndrome in general cannot be cured; it can be prevented by discontinuing the pregnancy based on the symptoms observed in the fetus.

There exist multiple ultrasonographic markers like nuchal fold, nasal bone hypoplasia, femur length that can lead to Down syndrome child. Recently, Echogenic Intracardiac Foci (EIF) had been added as a new observation in this line. Many clinical researches prove that presence of EIF acts as a possible symptom of Down syndrome. An EIF is defined as a bright white shape that is spotted in the heart of the fetus and it can be clearly visualised in an ultrasound image. An article "Ultrasound findings" reports that EIF is seen in about 1 out of every 20 or 30 pregnancies (~3-5%). If an EIF is observed in an ultrasound image, the mothers carrying the fetus with EIF undergo terrible mental pressure fearing that they would deliver Down syndrome child. This mental pressure created in the pregnant women can have undesirable impact on the fetus. To bring the down the mental pressure of the pregnant women and to ensure the fetus is unaffected with Down syndrome, women with EIF fetuses are suggested to undergo Chorionic villus sampling and amniocentesis.

Amniocentesis and Chorionic villus sampling methods are well known non-ultrasonic method for detecting Down syndrome. Amniocentesis is a process of collecting small quantity of the amniotic fluid that encircle the fetus and analyzing it for trisomy 21.It is performed with the help of ultrasonic guidance. It has disadvantage such as leaking amniotic fluid, miscarriage, needle injury to fetus and infection transmission. Chorionic villus sampling is a process of performing chromosomal analysis of cells taken from the placenta. It suffers from miscarriage and uterine infection problems.

Down syndrome is no more a rare phenomena; the affected rate is gradually improving throughout the world. A statistical report show that i) the risk of Down syndrome in the overall birth rate is 0.00125% ii) women in the age group of 30 and below have 0.001% risk of Down syndrome iii) women in the age group of 45 have 0.022% risk of Down syndrome. Inspite of Down syndrome affected rate is being high, there doesn't exist an easy diagnostic method for its detection. This acts as the driving force for this research.

The major contributions of the chapter are i) a new medical parameter EIF is used for the detection of Down syndrome ii) extended region growing (ERG) is utilised to detect EIF in the fetus iii) cross correlation technique (CCT) is used to confirm Down syndrome by analysing the nasal bone in training phase iv) enhanced self organising map (ESOM) is used to distinguish the benign EIF from the EIF related to Down syndrome.

Introduction of the problem statement, need for this research and challenges involved in this research had already been well discussed in section 1. The rest of the chapter is organized as follows. A brief review of related researches related to the proposed techniques is presented in section 2. The proposed technique is presented in section 3.The systematic experimental results and discussions are presented in section 4.The conclusion and future works are presented in section 5.

Background

This section presents a report of the recent researches carried out in the detection of Down syndrome using ultrasound. Rebecca et.al (2001) performed experiments to determine the accuracy of second-trimester ultrasound in detecting Down syndrome in fetuses. The structural malformation and ultrasonographic markers are the lying essences behind this research. The results proved that the ultrasonographic markers without associated structural malformations did not distinguish well between the normal fetus and the fetus with Down syndrome. Considering the markers as a deciding factor to offer amniocentesis may lead to more number of fetal losses.

Lauren Lynch et.al (1989) discovered the ultrasonic parameter nuchal fold was very informative than the other parameters such as biparietal diameter and femur length for detection of Down syndrome. Patrick Rozenberg et.al (2006) suggested the inclusion of first trimester ultrasound scan also for the diagnosis of Down syndrome in addition to the second trimester ultrasound. The accurate detection of the ultrasonographic marker, nuchal fold, biparietal diameter and femur length is highly complex task as they can be easily confused with the speckle noise. Detection of these markers demands highly skilled sonologists, obstetricians and fetal medicine professionals. This provided shift in paradigm for the automated diagnosis of Down syndrome from the ultrasound images.

Yenhui Deng et al (2010) have projected an ordered structural model for the automated detection of nuchal translucency region. Anzalone et al (2013) wholly automated the system for nuchal translucency measurement which operates on the images obtained from the ultrasound. Nirmala. S and Palanisamy. V (2009) segmented the region of nuchal translucency using the imaging techniques mean shift analysis and canny operators. The thickness of nuchal translucency was calculated using blob analysis. Sonia. R and Shanthi. V (2016) later used morphological operations and otsu thresholding for the segmentation of nuchal translucency region.

Lai K Wee et.al (2010) proposed the usage of neural network to locate the region of nuchal translucency. The boundary region of nuchal translucency layer is detected using instinctive computerized algorithm. After the detection of the boundary region, the optimum thickness of the region is calculated based on intensity continuity and edge strength.

Yan Du et.al (2017) performed fetal karyotype examination among Chinese women and discovered that absence of nasal bone in the second trimester has a high risk of abnormal. Iliescu Dominic-Gabriel and Drăgușin Roxana-Cristina (2018) reviewed various schemes in early genetic screening and ultrasound evaluation and came to a conclusion that first-trimester ultrasound examination has the potential to diagnose the majority of fetal abnormalities.

Shafia Shakoor, Humera Ismail and Shama Munim (2012) studied the outcome in fetuses with echogenic intracardiac focus. The experiment was performed in Pakistan and the results showed that 95.77% of the fetuses were normal, 4.2% had cardiac defects and 0% had Down syndrome. Aaron B. Caughey, Deirdre J. Lyell et.al (2001) studied the impact of isolated EIF for screening Down syndrome. The experiment clearly demonstrated the usage of EIF as a screening parameter may lead to huge number of amniocenteses and miscarriages to discover a rare Down syndrome fetus.

The following noteworthy observation can be made from the previous researches carried on this field i) The most commonly used parameters for the detection of Down syndrome are nuchal translucency, femur length and nasal bone hypoplasia ii) Association of Dosun syndrome and EIF is relatively low iii) There is a need of automatic computerised tool for detecting Down syndrome, as the manual intervention requires some artifacts.

Issues, Controversies, Problems

Histopathology is the study of tissues in the diseased area. The drastic increase in the computational of the image analysis had given rise to a new perspective called computer assisted diagnosis. Analogous to the role of computer-assisted diagnosis (CAD) algorithms in medical imaging to complement the opinion of a radiologist, CAD algorithms have begun to be developed for disease detection, diagnosis, and prognosis prediction to complement to the opinion of the pathologist. Detection of Down syndrome based on EIF is one of the challenging issues that could be solved by CAD algorithms. The power of image analysis and CAD algorithm can be collectively employed to replace the conventional Down syndrome detection methods like Amniocentesis and chronic sampling.

Proposed Solution and Recommendations

The proposed system utilizes a new medical parameter EIF for the detection of Down syndrome. It is designed with the aim of discriminating the benign EIF from Down syndrome related EIF. It involves two phases i) training phase ii) testing phase. Not all fetuses with EIF can be associated with the Down syndrome. Hence training is performed with the fetal image with EIF and Down syndrome positive. In training phase, the feature of the fetal image like intensity, size and location of EIF is obtained. The presence of Down syndrome in the fetus is diagnosed by confirming the presence of nasal bone using CCT. In testing phase, ESOF had been employed to diagnose the positivity of Down syndrome using the features of EIF. An architecture diagram of the proposed system is given below in the Figure 1.

Training Phase

Not all the EIF fetus are malignant that can cause Down syndrome. Only certain patterns of EIF can cause Down syndrome. The motto of this phase is to obtain the characteristics of the malignant EIF related to Down syndrome. The training phase includes five phases i) image pre-processing using neuro fuzzy filter ii) detection of EIF using ERG iii) detection of nasal bone using CCT iv) Learning of features of EIF. The flowchart representation of training phases is shown in Figure 2.

Image Pre-Processing

The ultrasound devices attain high quality, real-time images but it is often degraded with speckle noise. Speckle noise spoils the quality of the images thus making

Figure 1. Architecture of the proposed system

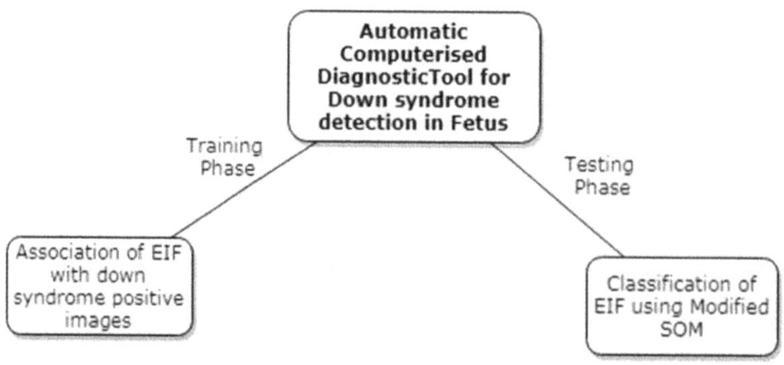

Figure 2. A flowchart representation of training phase

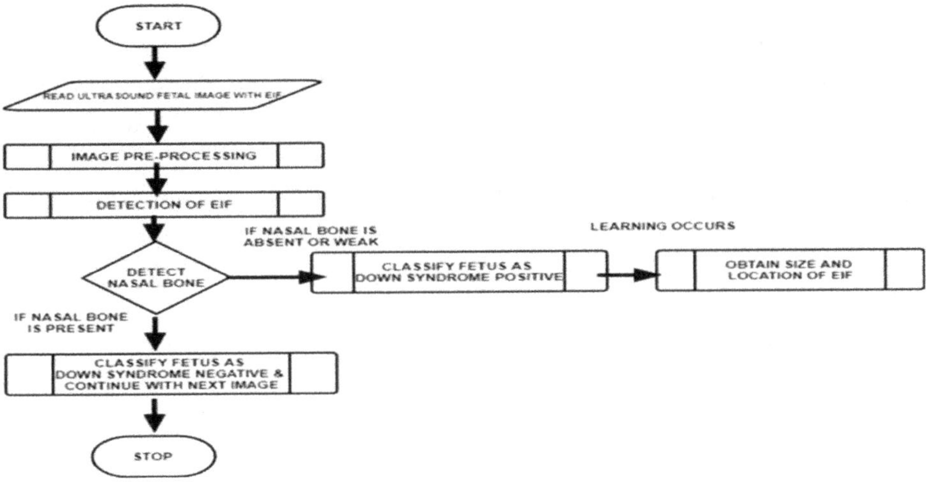

the identification of the edges, patterns a complex task. It is capable of producing artificial edges, echoes the patterns in the images thus hinders the diagnosis process.

The image pre-processing is the first and foremost step of the training phase. In pre-processing; a neuro fuzzy filter that works based on neuro-fuzzy and evolutionary learning. The neural network possesses the ability to train and the knowledge for the training is fed into the system in fuzzy format. Speckle noise is deducted on based on the local statistical characters using the fuzzy knowledge. A memetic algorithm is used to optimize neuro fuzzy filter. Algorithm of neuro fuzzy filter mechanism is shown as follows

Procedure: Neuro fuzzy filter
Input: Noisy image
Output: Pre-processed image

Algorithm

1. For a single noisy image A_1, there exists 25 membership function (M)
2. Membership function outputs 25 intermediate $Y_1, Y_2....Y_{25}$
3. Obtain weighting factor for each individual membership
4. Calculate the weighted average of the individual rule outputs and form Yo output.

Detection of EIF

Detection of EIF is the next step in the training phase following the image pre-processing. ERG technique is used to detect the EIF in the ultrasound images. Extended Region growing is a three stage process which involves gridding, seed point selection, employing region growing to the point (A.R.Kavitha, 2012). The conventional Region Growing considers only the intensity constraint whereas the extended region growing takes the orientation as an additional constraint. Algorithm of extended region growing is presented below

Procedure: Extended Region Growing
Input: Pre-processed image
Output: Detection of EIF

1. Start
2. Find image gradient in x and y direction
3. Obtain gradient vector with the help of equation 1

$$g = \left(1 / \left(1 + \left(Ix + Iy\right)^2\right)\right) \tag{1}$$

4. Convert gradient vector into orientation of the pixel
5. Set intensity (T_I) and orientation (T_O) threshold
6. Fragment the image into the grids
7. For each grid, select a seed point based on histogram
8. If neighbouring pixel satisfies the intensity and orientation threshold, the region grows using equations 2 and 3.

$$|| I_P - I_N || <= T_I \tag{2}$$

Ip is the intensity at the seed point

I_N is the intensity at the neighbouring pixel

$$|| O_P - O_N || <= T_O \tag{3}$$

Op is the orientation at the seed point

O_N is the orientation at the neighbouring pixel

9. Stop

Detection of Nasal Bone

The presence of Down syndrome is confirmed by the absence of nasal bone using CCT.CCT is a template matching algorithm that works based on correlation. The algorithmic description of CCT is displayed below (Thomas C. Winter, 2000).

Procedure: Cross correlation technique
Input: Pre-processed image
Output: 3D surface plotted graph

1. Start
2. Let S be target image, T be template image.
3. Take the ultra sound image S for which nasal bone has to be detected

$$S'i,j = \frac{1}{mxn}\sum_{i=0,j=0}^{n-1,m-1} S\left(i+x, j+y\right) \quad (4)$$

where $S_i \rightarrow$ subset of target *im* age, *i* and *j* are co-ordinates of template *im* age, and *x* and *y* are co-ordinates of target image...

4. Take the ultra sound image T with nasal bone detected

$$T' = \frac{i}{mxn}\sum_{i=0,j=0}^{n-1,m-1} Ti,j \quad (5)$$

where $T' \rightarrow$ subset of template *im* age

5. Select subset image(I) in T image that include nasal bone area
6. Search for I in S image
7. If I is present in S, obtain the location of I
8. Obtain cross correlation matrix for the template image and target image

$$\partial = \frac{J\left(Si+x, j+y-S'i,j\right)\left(Tx,y-T'\right)}{\sqrt{J\left(Si+x-S'i,j\right)2 * J\left(Tx,y-T'\right)2}} \quad (6)$$

Where $J = \sum_{x=0,y=0}^{n-1,m-1}$ -> summation of co-ordinates in the template image

9. Correlation matrix is converted into surface plotting graph
10. Based on the graph, the maximum value of image correlation will be used for detection of nasal bone
11. If peak of graph was less than 0.35, it can be decided that nasal bone is absent
12. stop

Learning the Features of EIF

This phase occurs only, when the nasal bone is absent or nasal hypoplasia occurs. The size and location of EIF is collected and clustered based on the similarity. The similarity parameter used for clustering are i) size of EIF and ii) position of EIF namely left ventricle and right ventricle. These clusters act as the knowledge base for ESOM involved in the testing phase.

Testing Phase

Testing phase involves discriminating the malignant EIF from the benign EIF. The knowledge acquired in the training phase plays the crucial role in the determination of Down syndrome related EIF. Enhanced Self Organising Map (ESOF) maps the testing image with the cluster map formed in the training phase, thus detecting the malignant EIF. The flowchart representation of the testing phase is shown in Figure 3.

Enhanced Self Organising Map

ESOM unsupervised learning plays the crucial role mapping the test image into Down syndrome positive or negative clusters. For a single learning two iteration of ESOM has to be performed. In the first step, the size of EIF acts as the weight vector and in the second the position of EIF is treated as the weight vector. This method breaks the input neuron groups into two types i) normal group ii) far group.

Figure 3. Flowchart representation of testing phase

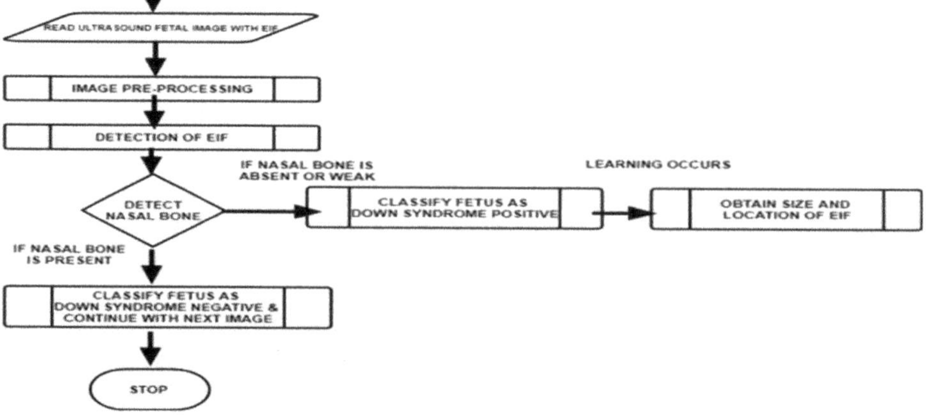

Neurons that are far away from the input are known as far group. Self organising map does not handle far group neurons and it is treated as dead units. On the contrary, ESOM treats far group neurons and thereby improves the learning rate and achieving the better results. Algorithm of ESOM learning algorithm is explained as follows:

```
1.          Weight vectors wi of m × n neurons, where i= 1,
2,...., mn, are initialized.
2.          Randomly select an input vector x(t) and x(t)
becomes the input for all neurons simultaneously.
3.          The winner neuron c, i.e., BMU is found with the
help of equation 7
         C = arg (min 1<= i <= mn { || wi(t) - x(t) })       (7)
4.          Euclidean formula computes the distance of all
neurons from the input x(t) and identify the distant neuron for
this input.
5.          Update the weight vectors of winner and its
neighbours except the distant neurons with the help of equation
8
        Wi(t+1) = Wi(t) + hc,i(t)[x(t) - wi(t)]                (8)
        Where t is learning step
        hc,i(t) is neighbourhood function
6.          Update the weight vectors of distant neurons using
the equation 9:
        Wk (t+1) = Wk(t) +αd(t) hc,k(t)[x(t) - wk(t)]          (9)
        Where αd(t)  is the learning rate
        hc,k(t) is neighbourhood function
7.          Iterate the steps 2 to 6 for all the input data.
```

Results and Discussion

This section describes the experimental results of the proposed techniques. Automatic Computerised Diagnostic Tool for Down syndrome Detection in Fetus is implemented using software Scilab. Scilab was utilized for image and mathematical processing needs. Scilab is open source and free software that can perform extensive numerical computation for engineering and scientific applications.

Dataset Description

The experiment was performed with 35 ultrasound fetal images that was collected from various online and offline sources. The fetal images belong to the age group of 24 – 26 weeks. There were 20 ultrasound fetal images with EIF and Down syndrome confirmed. The ultrasound fetal image with EIF and Down syndrome negative was 5 in numbers. There were also 10 ultrasound fetal images with EIF and no clue for Down syndrome was used. Some of the fetal image with EIF that was used for the experiment was shown in the Figure 4.

Experimental Results

Training was performed with 25 Down syndrome diagnosed images. It was performed in five iterations and the learning rate was continuously improving. The result of the training phase was shown in Table 1. The average learning rate of the training phase was 80%, while the rejection rate was only 20%.

Experimental results of the training phase is given as follows i) detectionof EIF using ERG is shown in Figure 5 ii) detection of nasal bone using CCT in Figure 6 iii) the rejected fetal image (A. Normal) and the learned fetal image (B. Down syndrome) in the training phase in Figure 7.

The knowledge obtained from training phase about the location and size of EIF is show in Table 2.

The testing phase was performed to diagnose Down syndrome in 5 fetal images with EIF is shown in Table 3.

Figure 4. Dataset of the fetal images with EIF

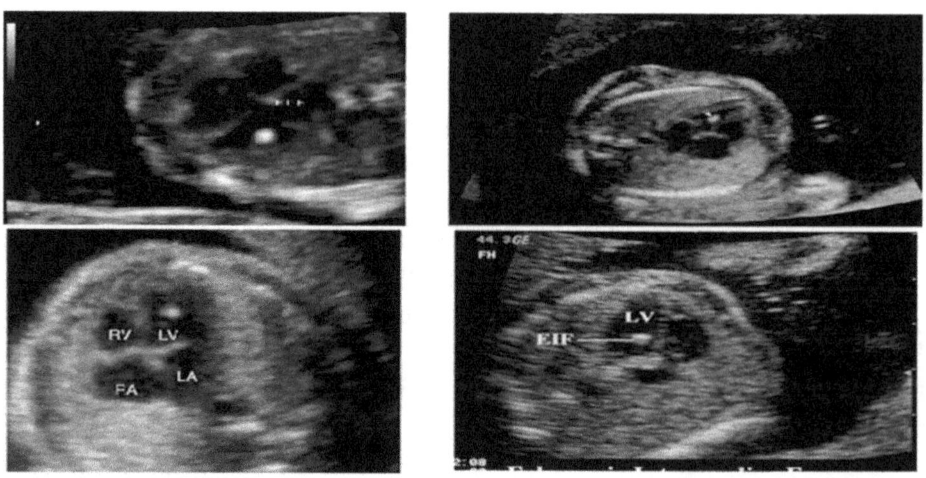

Table 1. Results of training phase

Iteration No#	No. Of Input Images	Learning Rate	Rejection Rate
1	1	1	0
2	2	2	0
3	4	3	1
4	8	6	2
5	10	8	2

Figure 5. Detection of EIF

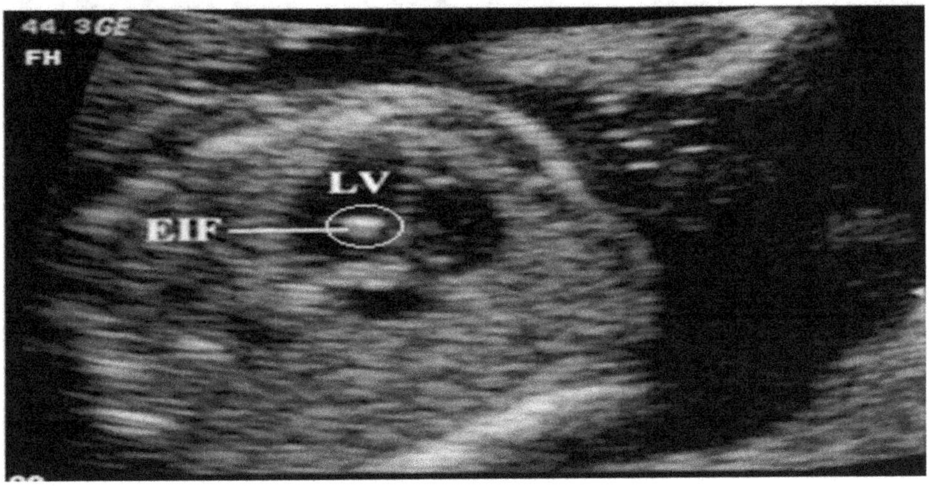

Figure 6. Detection of nasal bone

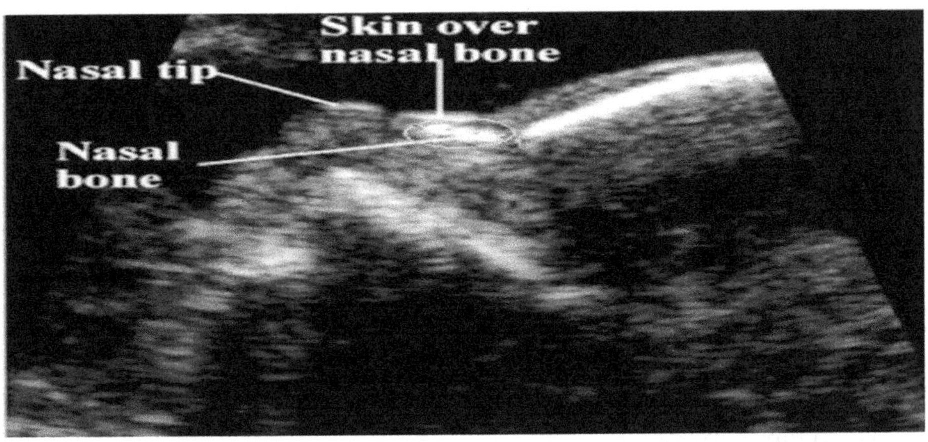

Figure 7. Results of training phase

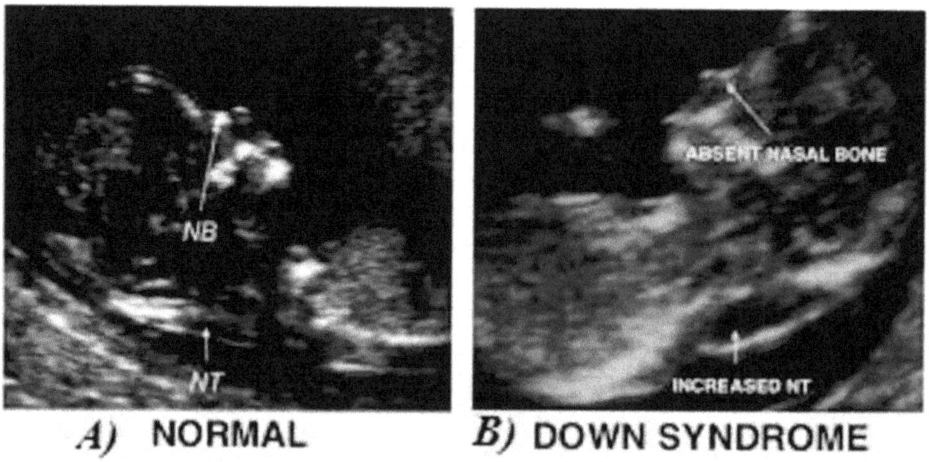

Table 2. Clustered knowledge from training phase

S.No	Size of EIF	Location of EIF	Other Ultrasound finding
1	>= 6mm	Left Ventricle	Nasal Bone Absence

Table 3. Results of testing phase

Experiment No #	Tested images	Down Syndrome Positive	Down Syndrome Negative
1	5	2	3

The fetal image with EIF that was diagnosed for Down syndrome in the testing phase and found to be Down syndrome negative is shown in Figure 8.

Performance Analysis Using Evaluation Metrics

The evaluation of Down syndrome detection is performed using parameters such as sensitivity, specificity and accuracy. Sensitivity is the quantity of true positives that are rightly acknowledged by a diagnostic test. It tells how good the diagnostic test is detecting a disease.

Figure 8. Fetus termed as Down syndrome negative in testing phase

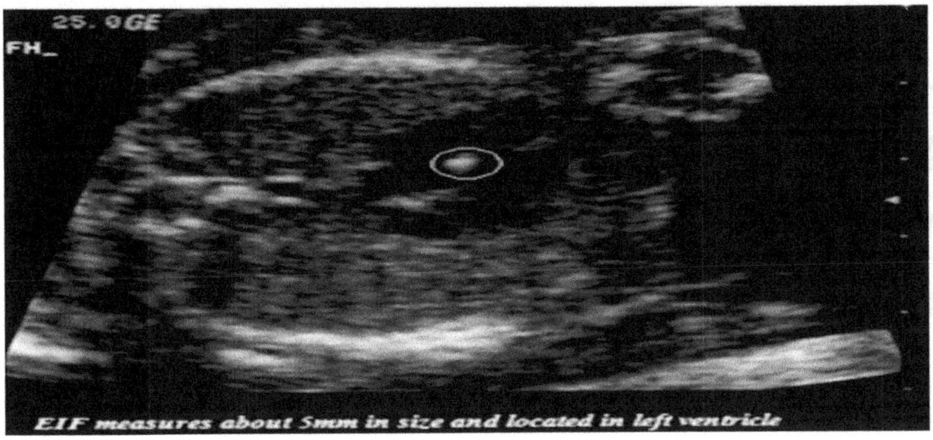

Sensitivity = True Positive/(True Positive + False Negative) (10)

Specificity is the quantity of the true negatives rightly acknowledged by a diagnostic test. It suggests how good the test is identifying normal (negative) condition.

Specificity = True Negative/(True Negative + False Positive) (11)

Accuracy is the quantity of true results, either true positive or true negative, in a population. It measures the degree of veracity of a diagnostic test on a condition.

Accuracy = (True Negative + True Positive)/(True Negative + True Positive + False Negative + False Postive) (12)

The performance metrics of the proposed system is shown in Figure 9.

Future Research Directions

The proposed system was able to clearly differentiate Down syndrome related fetus from the benign fetus. It was producing very accurate results when operated on the fetal ultrasound images with a single EIF. In future works, the fetal images with multiple EIF can be used for detection of Down syndrome. The soft markers like nuchal fold, femur length can be used instead of nasal bone hypoplasia in the training phase.

Figure 9. Performance Metrics Graph

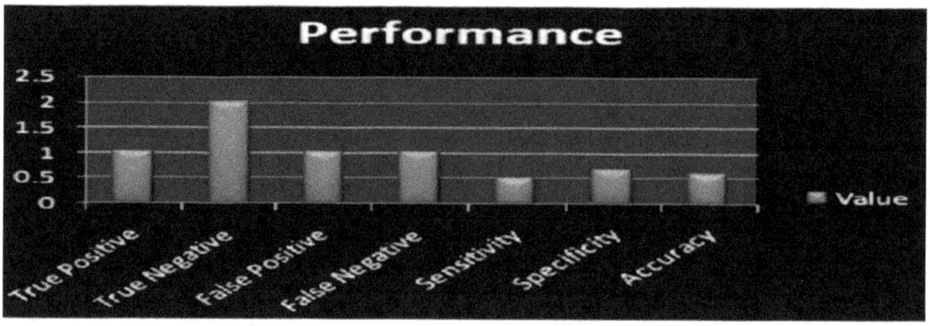

CONCLUSION

This chapter presented a new idea to detect Down syndrome based on EIF in computerised way. The proposed system was able to clearly differentiate Down syndrome causing EIF from the benign EIF. It achieved better results in terms of the parameters like accuracy, sensitivity and specificity. Moving forward from the research phase to the implementation phase, this system can be added as a feature in the ultrasound fetal scan. It can also replace the conventional Down syndrome diagnostics like Amniocentesis and Chorionic villus sampling.

ACKNOWLEDGMENT

This research received no specific grant from any funding agency in the public, commercial, or not-for-profit sectors. I feel an immense pleasure to thank my guide Dr. A. R. Kavitha, for her precious suggestions and kind co-operation to the completion of this work. I wish to express a sense of gratitude and love to my niece Natalie Nashley, as I would have never come across this problem statement without her. Last but not least I express gratitude to my family and friends for their moral support and consistent motivation.

REFERENCES

Anzalone, A., Fusco, G., Isgro, F., Orlandi, E., Prevete, R., Sciortino, G., ... Valenti, C. (2013). A System for the Automatic Measurement of the Nuchal Translucency Thickness from Ultrasound Video Stream of the Foetus. *Proceedings of the 26th IEEE International Symposium on Computer-Based Medical Systems*, 239-44. 10.1109/CBMS.2013.6627795

Caughey, A. B., Lyell, D. J., Filly, R. A., Washington, E. A., & Norton, M. E. (2001). The Impact of the Use of the Isolated Echogenic Intracardiac Focus as a Screen for Down Syndrome in Women under the Age of 35 Years. *American Journal of Obstetrics and Gynecology, 185*(5), 1021–1027. doi:10.1067/mob.2001.117674 PMID:11717625

Cristina, D. R. (2011). Prenatal Diagnosis of Down Syndrome. In *Advances in Research on Down Syndrome* (pp. 75-92). INTECH. doi:10.5772/intechopen.71064

Deng, Y., Wang, Y., & Chen, P. (2010). Automated Detection of Fetal Nuchal Translucency Based on Hierarchical Structural Model. *2010 IEEE 23rd International Symposium on Computer-Based Medical Systems (CBMS),* 78-84. 10.1109/CBMS.2010.6042618

Du, Y., Ren, Y., Yan, Y., & Cao, L. (2017). Absent Fetal Nasal Bone in the Second Trimester and Risk of Abnormal Karyotype in a Prescreened Population of Chinese Women. *Acta Obstetricia et Gynecologica Scandinavica, 97*(2), 180–186. doi:10.1111/aogs.13263 PMID:29164604

Echogenic Intracardiac Focus. (2017, January) *Kaiser Permanente.* Retrieved from https://mydoctor.kaiserpermanente.org/ncal/Images/GEN_US EIF handout_tcm63-9941.pdf

Kavitha, Chellamuthu, & Rupa. (2012). An Efficient Approach for Brain Tumour Detection Based on Modified Region Growing and Neural Network in MRI Images. *2012 International Conference on Computing, Electronics and Electrical Technologies (ICCEET*). doi:.10.1109/icceet.2012.6203809

Lynch, L., Berkowitz, G. S., Chitkara, U., & Wilkins, I. A. (1989). Ultrasound Detection of Down Syndrome: Is It Really Possible? *Journal of Diagnostic Medical Sonography: JDMS, 5*(4), 217. doi:10.1177/875647938900500445 PMID:2521379

Nirmala, S., & Palanisamy, V. (2009, June 4). Measurement of Nuchal Translucency Thickness in First Trimester Ultrasound Fetal Images for Detection of Chromosomal Abnormalities. *International Conference on Control, Automation, Communication and Energy Conservation*. Retrieved from https://ieeexplore.ieee.org/document/5204467/media

Rozenberg, P., Bussières, L., Chevret, S., Bernard, J. P., Malagrida, L., Cuckle, H., ... Ville, Y. (2006). Screening for Down Syndrome Using First-trimester Combined Screening Followed by Second-trimester Ultrasound Examination in an Unselected Population. *American Journal of Obstetrics and Gynecology*, *195*(5), 1379–1387. doi:10.1016/j.ajog.2006.02.046 PMID:16723105

Shakoor, S., Ismail, H., & Munim, S. (2012). Intracardiac Echogenic Focus and Fetal Outcome – Review of Cases from a Tertiary Care Centre in Karachi, Pakistan. *The Journal of Maternal-Fetal & Neonatal Medicine*, *26*(1), 2–4. doi:10.3109/14767058.2012.703724 PMID:22708618

Smith-Bindman, R., Hosmer, W., Feldstein, V. A., Deeks, J. J., & Goldberg, J. D. (2001). Second-Trimester Ultrasound to Detect Fetuses With Down Syndrome. *Journal of the American Medical Association*, *285*(8), 1044–1055. doi:10.1001/jama.285.8.1044 PMID:11209176

Sonia, R., & Shanthi, V. (2016). Early Detection of Down Syndrome Marker by Measuring Fetal Nuchal Translucency Thickness from Ultrasound Images during First Trimester. *Indian Journal of Science and Technology*, *9*(21), 1–6. doi:10.17485/ijst/2016/v9i21/95174

Wee, L. K., Min, T. Y., Arooj, A., & Supriyanto, E. (2010, August). Nuchal Translucency Marker Detection Based on Artificial Neural Network and Measurement via Bidirectional Iteration Forward Propagation. *WSEAS Transactions on Information Science and Application*, *7*(8), 1025–1036.

What Is Down Syndrome? (n.d.). *Right Diagnosis*. Retrieved from http://www.rightdiagnosis.com/d/down_syndrome/basics.htm

Winter, T. C., Anderson, A. M., Cheng, E. Y., Komarniski, C. A., Souter, V. L., Uhrich, S. B., & Nyberg, D. A. (2000). Echogenic Intracardiac Focus in 2nd-Trimester Fetuses with Trisomy 21: Usefulness as a US Marker. *Radiology*, *216*(2), 450–456. doi:10.1148/radiology.216.2.r00au32450 PMID:10924569

KEY TERMS AND DEFINITIONS

Down Syndrome: An inherited disorder caused due to chromosomal defect, resulting in brain impairment and physical abnormalities.

Echogenic Intracardiac Focus: A bright spot near the heart of the fetus that can observed in ultrasound examination.

Femur Length: It refers to the length of thigh bone.

Nasal Bone Hypoplasia: A sonographic observation where the fetal has weak nasal bone or no nasal bone.

Nuchal Fold: A normal fold of skin seen at the back of the fetal neck during the second trimester of pregnancy.

Chapter 11
Adaptive Prediction Methods for Medical Image/Video compression for Telemedicine Application

Ketki C. Pathak
Sarvajanik College of Engineering and Technology, India

Jignesh N. Sarvaiya
Sardar Vallabhbhai National Institute of Technology Suart, India

Anand D. Darji
Sardar Vallabhbhai National Institute of Technology Suart, India

ABSTRACT

Due to rapid development of multimedia communication and advancement of image acquisition process, there is a crucial requirement of high storage and compression techniques to mitigate high data rate with limited bandwidth scenario for telemedicine application. Lossless compression is one of the challenging tasks in applications like medical, space, and aerial imaging field. Apart from achieving high compression ratio, in these mentioned applications there is a need to maintain the original imaging quality along with fast and adequate processing. Predictive coding was introduced to remove spatial redundancy. The accuracy of predictive coding is based on the choice of effective and adaptive predictor which is responsible for removing spatial redundancy. Medical images like computed tomography (CT) and magnetic resonance imaging (MRI) consume huge storage and utilize maximum available bandwidth. To overcome these inherent challenges, the authors have reviewed various adaptive predictors and it has been compared with existing JPEG and JPEG LS-based linear prediction technique for medical images.

DOI: 10.4018/978-1-5225-6316-7.ch011

INTRODUCTION

Due to advancement of wireless communication, remote diagnosis of emergency medical events is possible in real time. The medical records are required to transmit for remote assessment with effective compression techniques, so that optimum bandwidth utilization is achieved without loss of visual quality of images. For every medical images diagnostically affected part are considered to be more important than other part of the image, which is known as Region of Interest (ROI). Telemedicine system involves many health care centers which are equipped with highly efficient software platform and devices. For any telemedicine system, it is essential to use compression algorithms to improve channel utilization and to reduce storage requirement. It is also equally important to preserve diagnosis area with high resolution so that, it can be further decoded to reproduce the processed image at various resolutions for different end terminal devices. High resolution with high compression ratio is the major challenge to design efficient ROI based medical image compression for health care centers for telemedicine system.

Efficient medical image compression involves three basic processing steps.

- Suitable transform techniques for de-correlation based higher compression rate.
- Suitable prediction based entropy coding scheme for error control.
- Reproducible compressed image with compatible resolution level for end terminal.

Image compression techniques are widely classified as lossless and lossy compression techniques. Each of these techniques removes trivial and unnecessary data to decrease image size. Lossy techniques gains higher compression ratio compared to lossless techniques but degrades the image quality as there is permanent loss of information whereas lossless compression protects all details of original image. In case of medical images non-degraded images are essential for radiologists to interpret disease and to extract related diagnostic information. Also degraded images affect the efficiency of Computer Aided Diagnosis (CAD) system. Also legal reasons also require the non-degraded images that have suffered no loss of information. As a result lossless compression methods are mainly used for medical image storage. The medical and information technology community has acknowledged that the lossless compression is a really pertinent way to minimize the transmission and archive resources related to medical imaging while ensuring its ideal reconstruction. Compared to its precursor H.264/AVC, High Efficiency Video Coding has shown a remarkable enhancement in the encoding efficiency of video sequences, acquiring a decrease in bit-rate of 50% while ensuring the same perceived quality.

The transform algorithm or de-correlation algorithm decomposes the medical image, than analyze the data redundancies and determine higher correlation co-efficient, which is optimum for prediction based entropy system. Prediction based entropy system predicts and selects most suitable coefficient and ignore lower resolution coefficient. Finally, the image is reconstructed as per resolution requirement of the end terminal. Thus, compression techniques of medical images are having many algorithms to fulfill the healthcare and Telemedicine requirements.

For remove spatial redundancy we need process which is called prediction. Prediction function is the core part for improving coding efficiency of any lossless, near-lossless or lossy compression methods. It is s used for efficient compression by removing spatial redundancy. The prediction function predicts the next value with prior knowledge of previous data in such a manner that the differences between the original value and the predicted value should be as minimum as possible for perfect reconstruction (Chen, Y.T,2007). We can improve compression ratio by making proper choice of Predictor. Predictive coding approach minimizes the relevance pixels in time and space domain. Linear prediction based method improves the compression performance at the cost of higher computation complexity. There are various compression standard who have propose various predictor for compression. Joint Picture Expert Group –Lossless standard(JPEG-LS) uses simple predictor namely Median Edge Detection (MED) predictor (Shirsat, T.G. & V.K. Bairagi,2013). It predicts optimal predictor among three sub predictor namely vertical edge, horizontal edge and smooth region. For context based predictor, one of the popular predictor is Context based Adaptive Lossless Image CODEC (CALIC) which utilizes Gradient Adjusted Predictor(GAP). This predictor selects and adjust co-efficient of predictor based on estimation of local gradients. Gradient Edge Detection (GED) predictor combines best features like simplicity and accuracy of MED predictor and GAP predictor respectively (Shirsat, T.G. & V.K. Bairagi,2013).

Irrespective of noise, the performance of lossless compression method is based on exact reconstruction of image. Degree of Compression is the quantitative measure for any Predictor's accuracy. The purpose of any adaptive predictor is to remove spatial redundancy in such a way that after prediction stage, entropy coding stage provides highest compression. Thus, prediction stage never performs the compression, it only improves compression. For precise diagnosis and loss of important clinical information is eliminated. Perfect reconstruction is the essential requirement for medical imaging. Due to limited bandwidth, delay in transmission of progressive image sequences leads problem to patient and retaining patient records demand huge storage at health care centers. These are some of crucial issues of Telemedicine application. So, advancement in lossless compression algorithms is one of critical research field for researcher. Linear predictor is one the basic predictor which can predict current pixel by its two neighbouring pixels. But it is not proper predictor in many application due to its inability to remove spatial redundancy for non-stationary features like textures and edges. So, Adaptive predictor is the optimal choice for non-stationary features. Some basic predictors such as MED, Differential Adaptive Run Coding (DARC) and Graham work on principle of tracking the edges in horizontal and vertical directions. Other than these, Gradient based selective predictor first analyzes the edges and then tracks the edges in four directions. GAP is one of the special predictor which first tracks edges in horizontal and vertical directions. Apart from tracking, it also classifies edges like weak edges, normal edges and sharp edges. It also tracks edges in more directions precisely. Main prospective of this algorithm is to design highly adaptive and an efficient predictor that can be incorporated in the modeling step of image compression system. By examining surrounding pixels of an unknown pixel we try to find the maximum intensity change level to find edges value. Intra frame coding with linear predicator are also used to improve compression performance. For medical image sequence or Ultrasound medical video we have to consider Differential Pulse Code Modulation (DPCM) based fast gradient edge based prediction techniques as a part of Intra coding. Because DPCM based intra prediction will provide highest compression ratio and it works accurately in non-stationary situation like edges and texture based local features. Advance prediction algorithm along with video coding standard is one of the challenging task as it require complex mode operation, but medical video compression standard provides high compression rate and allowing high frame rate compared to JPEG-LS based low complexity predictor.

Main goal of this chapter is to review and identify the suitable combination of adaptive predictor to minimize the prediction error followed by efficient entropy coding techniques to boost compression rate for lossless medical image/video compression.

BACKGROUND

Prediction function is used to de-correlate the image pixel from its available neighbouring pixels. Prediction based lossless compression algorithms are adopted in JPEG LS compression standard JPEG-LS (Weinberger, M. J., Seroussi, G., & Sapiro, G., 2000). There are varieties of prediction algorithm which exploits spatial correlation property among neighbouring pixels (Bairagi, V. K., & Sapkal, A. M. 2013). The different between original pixel and predicted pixel is known as prediction error or residue error. Residue error does not guarantee about compression but its minimum value surely performs lossless compression This error residue is further encoded by entropy coders like Huffman coding, Arithmetic and Run length coding, bit plane coding to improve coding gain.

Prediction algorithm can be designed along with some stastical modelling or markov modelling. It can also design with advanced image and video compression standard. The detail algorithm categories are shown in Figure 1.

The combination of LS based predictor and CALIC shows significant improvement in compression ratio (Tiwari, A. K., & Kumar, R. R., 2009). In some advance prediction algorithms uses edge detection and logal gradient estimation (Avramović, A., & Savić, S. 2011). In Hierarchical prediction scheme (Babu, P. S., & Sathappan, S., 2015) the vertical, horizontal, diagonal (left up, left down and right up, right down pixels) pixels are predicted to progress with the compression process which preserve the sharpness of original image and to reduce the bit rates.

Need of Compression in Medical Images

In Telemedicine application, there are few important requirements like adequate bandwidth, Huge storage and Retention of Medical reports. Progressive healthcare records of patient require huge storage and to download previous records we need adequate bandwidth. Perfect reconstruction compression is an essential requirement in many recent technologies. Region of Interest based Lossless image compression algorithm provide solution of huge storage and it also ensures proper visual quality of diagnostic part of medical imaging. This concept is demonstrated in Figure 2.

In any prediction based compression algorithm two stages are important. First stage is prediction which estimate current pixel from its available neighbouring pixels to minimize residue error and reduces spatial redundancy. Second stage is entropy coder which encodes the residue error to improve coding gain Entropy coders are capable enough to remove further redundancy from prediction error and improve coding efficiency. Overall compression will be improved based on the accuracy of prediction stage to minimize prediction error and coding efficiency of entropy

Figure 1. Overall classification of Medical image compression algorithms

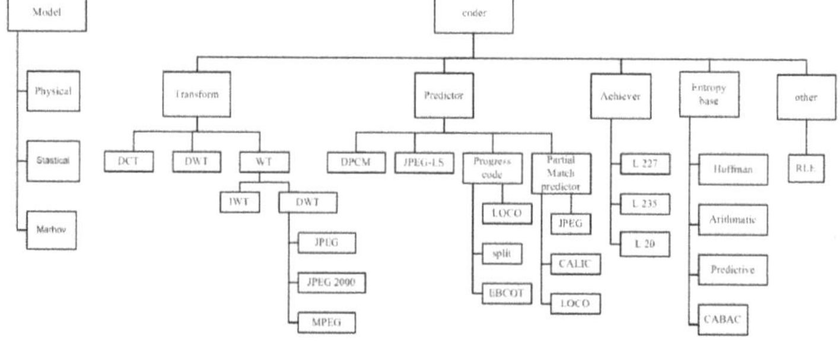

Figure 2. Basic diagram of Image Compression (Redrawn from Sophia, P. E., & Anitha, J., 2015)

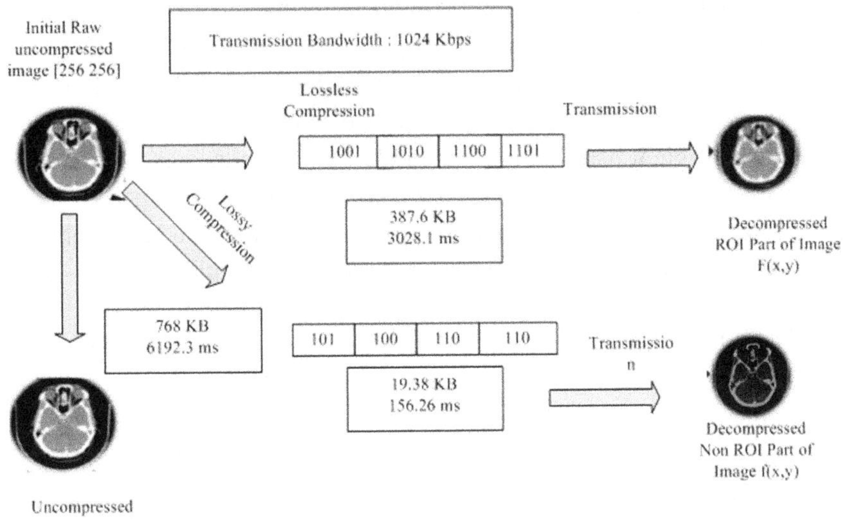

coder to reduce bit rate and ultimately improves compression factor. Overall block diagram is shown in Figure 3

ISSUES, CONTROVERSIES, PROBLEMS

Motivation

Telemedicine is one the important part for health care centers situated at rural part. It provides benefits to rural patients for better health care treatment. Limited or poor

Figure 3. Overall block diagram of Prediction based Compression (Rad, R. M., Attar, A., & Shahbahrami, A. (2013)

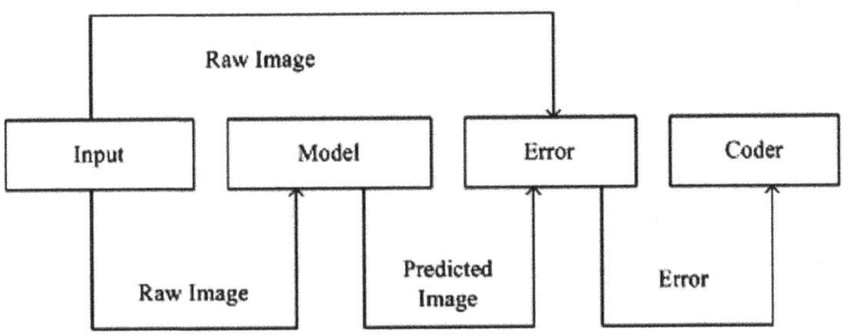

transmission bandwidth and insufficient infrastructure facility at rural health care center may results in delay of patient information transmission or may transmit poor visual quality of diagnostically important image, which may lead wrong information and patient may not get initial treatment at proper instant of time. At initial arrival of patient for the treatment, low quality of image can be tolerated because original image can be available for subsequent download as or when required. But lack of storage and insufficient bandwidth may lead loss of diagnostically important data. Due to this there is no provision of previous medical records and not adequate bandwidth for subsequent download. This kind of situation creates problems for rural health care Centre's doctors and also troublesome to patient health. (Banu, N. M., & Sujatha, S., 2015)

Progressive transmission provides the benefit to improve visual quality gradually by the use of latest wavelet based compression method. DWT or Integer based DWT (IWT) based compression are the optimal choice for progressive transmission of medical image sequences. IWT based facility to improve gradually image visual quality. Progressive transmission is suitable for telemedicine application as it gradually improve low quality image to high resolution image by proper entropy encoder. It also reduces bitrate and lossless information recovery is also possible.

In this chapter we have reviewed and proposed an adaptive predictor along with IWT based transformed method which improves visual quality gradually with progressive transmission. This also suggests Huffman, Arithmetic and predictive entropy combination to improve coding gain and maintain moderate compression ratio. It justifies improvement in visual quality along with marginal trade off in compression ratio.

Issues and Challenges With Telemedicine

There are various issues and challenges for development of Telemedicine system, which are listed below.

1. With m-health, telemedicine application provide clinical health care at a distance rural area
   where no facility of hospital.
2. So reduce health-care cost, improve patient health.
3. More patient data and related information can store in limited space.
4. Sending good quality medical image/data to expert in minimum time.
5. Medical image compression is higher challenges and complicatedness which the increasing demands of the medical science.
6. It is very difficult for the hospital management to the same storage device.

In addition, such data requires a high-end network, especially for image transmission through the network, such as telemedicine

Objective

In order to meet the challenge of medical image compression for Telemedicine application, we have to analyses optimal predictor followed by entropy coder for maximal removal of spatial redundancy and obtain higher compression rate. Introduce new compression schemes which not only address the issues of higher compression performance, but also ensure that a reconstructed image has lossless diagnostically relevant information.

ORGANIZATION OF THE CHAPTER

Initially, basics of predictive coding for medical image compression are explained first. Then overview of different linear predictors is described. In later part of the chapter adaptive prediction method along with Integer wavelet transformed based proposed methods and result analysis are discussed. Finally challenges and future scope is described.

BASICS OF PREDICTIVE CODING FOR MEDICAL IMAGE COMPRESSION

In today's electronic media, total annual records of the patients' can be more than tens of Terabytes. These rapid growth leads to huge storage, efficient online transmission bandwidth and maintenance of perceptual quality of diagnostic imaging data for rural healthcare Centre for further treatment investigation. In medical field also recently they have adopted new approaches like 3D and 4D imaging, which demands even higher storage requirement, so lossless compression is inescapable.

Role of Predictive Coding in Lossless Compression

In recent development of multimedia communication, most of the compression standards have been developed for general image and videos, so there is a wide scope of development of compression algorithm for medical images. For accurate diagnosis of disease perfect reconstruction is the essential requirement for medical imaging. Due to rapid development of telemedicine, there is a vital demand for bulk storage of progressive diagnostic value.In contrast with natural images, medical images have higher homogeneity at background part and Region of Interest part. So they have very high spatial correlation. Lossless compression utilizes this spatial redundancy to achieve high compression. There is a proportional relationship between compression and amount of redundancies. The role of prediction stage is to reduce the residue error between original content and predicted content by proper estimation of predicted pixel.

In Prediction base lossless compression algorithm, it exploits the degree of correlation among neighboring pixels. Prediction method models the spatial correlation properties among the neighboring pixels, other data is decorrelated and residue error i.e difference between original pixel and predicted pixel in then encoded by entropy coder to achieve higher coding gain.

Overall image data are non-stationary, i.e. each and every region of image may have different statistical properties. So we have to develop the prediction model in such a way that it adapts dominant local region property in such way that it achieves high decorrelation among neighbouring pixels. Prediction state is preformed prior to entropy coding for effective lossless compression. It is demonstrated in Figure 4

The effectiveness of prediction based image compression algorithms involves following steps

1. Design simple, adaptive and fast efficient prediction to remove spatial redundancy
2. Analyze repeating patterns in non stationary region
3. Develop efficient Entropy coder to reduce bitrate and improve coding gain

Medical Image Compression Approaches

For diagnostically important part of any medical image is very important for any patient. So those part or sometime whole medical image needs special attention for further treatment. So there are basically two methodologies for lossless compression. First approach is stastical based prediction approach which is pixel based prediction method. And second approach is transformed domain in which frequency domain analysis is preferred.

Figure 4. Prediction based model of lossless image compression (Redrawm,Banu, N. M., & Sujatha, S. (2015))

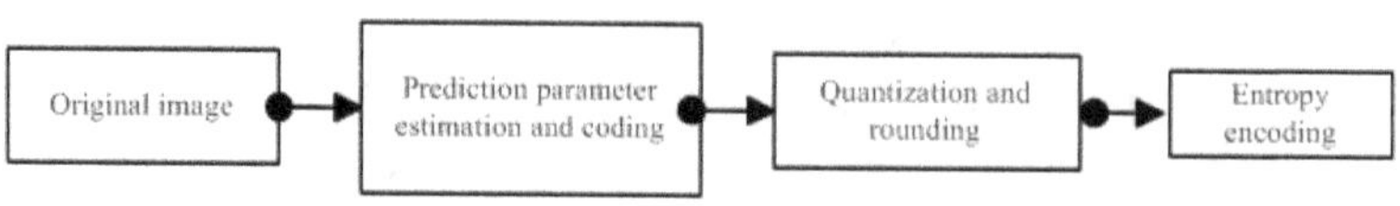

There is always trade between visual quality and compression ratio. For natural images or other than medical data visual quality is compromised while maintaining high compression ratio. But in medical field we have to improve visual quality of clinically important region at the cost of higher compression parameter.

Role of Predictor for Removing Spatial Redundancy

Predictive algorithm can be performed by two ways. One is with single class and other with two class predictor. In single class prediction, it estimates all the required parameters for compression during initial first scanning of the image. These parameters are called optimal parameters. In this class of prediction, coding is done simultaneously with optimum prediction or it can be performed as a separate task after optimal prediction. In other two class prediction algorithms, the first pass, it performs the estimation of optimal parameters for both prediction stage and coding stage by analysing image and in second pass it performs prediction and coding based on selection of optimal parameters of first pass.

Prediction stage is one of the important stage for efficient lossless compression algorithms. It removes spatial redundancy, so optimal predictor can be design based on its efficiency to remove spatial redundancy. Predictor can also be classified as linear or nonlinear predictor. In linear prediction algorithm, it selection or combined one or more suboptimal predictor on the basis of context of sub-region of images. So this class of predictor are simple to implement and fast in processing as they combine one or more sub predictor for the finite set of pixels based on smooth, texture or edge sub regions of the image. Optimization in this type of predictor is one of the challenging task. Optimization is done on the basis of adaptation of finite group of pixel characteristic which is computationally intensive. Non-linear predictor are more adaptive for different sub regions of the images.

Prediction and Contextual Based Medical Image Compression

Prediction based compression is basically lossless compression method. The efficiency measure of the prediction method is depends on stastical modelling and entropy coding. Basically in stastical analysis the correlation among neighbouring pixels is considered because in gray images neighboring pixels are highly correlated to each other. This correlation factor is useful for prediction value calculation. Prediction parameter is useful for calculating current pixel. Then in this prediction based modelling the residue error (Prediction error) is calculated between original pixel and predicted pixel. This prediction error is then stastically encoded by entropy coder to improve coding gain and hence compression is performed (Banu, N. M., & Sujatha, S. (2015). The prediction based compression techniques is shown in Figure 5

Figure 5. Prediction model for lossless Encoding/Decoding

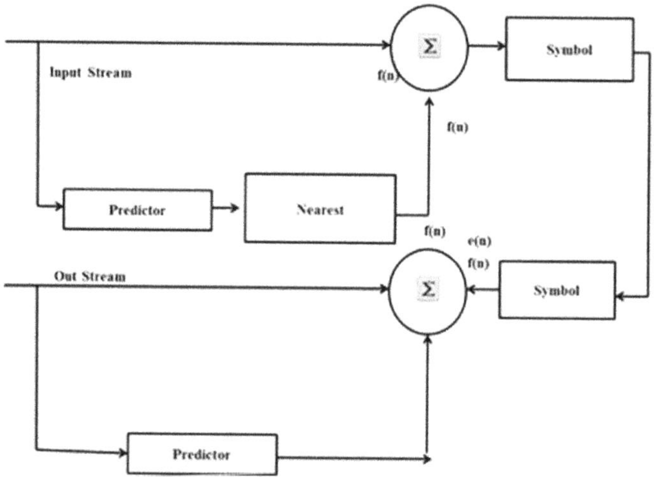

Most of the predictors are linear predictors. In linear predictors, prediction error is calculated on the stastical behaviors of neighbouring pixel by taking the averaging over the block. This type of computation is not producing exact value of prediction hence compression is not performed optimally because of dependency of neighbouring pixel over the small block. This type of problem can be overcome by considering some adaptive algorithm for predictor designing or it can be overcome by context based predictors. In context type modelling or adaptive predictor design, we have to first calculate the probability of current pixel P(xc) on the basis of previously encoded set of pixels S(x1.........xk) . The group of this pixel is known as context. So each and every time the calculation of prediction error is changes with respect to the context formed. These contexts may be smooth region, edge region, or texture region (Knezovic, J., Kovac, M., Zagar, M., Mlinarić, H., & Hofman, D., 2011). As shown in Figure 6. The basic algorithm is demonstrated as Figure 5. So in adaptive predictor switching of context should be efficient so that it can be adaptive to those region Adaptive predictors are sometime also known as non-linear predictor because of change in local information in the form of sub regions like smooth, texture or edges. Adaptive predictor reduces entropy distribution (Banu, N. M., & Sujatha, S., 2015). Performance of Lossless compression based adaptive predictor depends of efficient stastical modelling, and entropy coder.

Figure 7 shows neighbouring pixels arrangement which is used for adaptive switching of predictor to predict one of the unknown pixel X. This X pixel can be predicted with the knowledge of neighbourhood pixel s shown. Efficiency and adaptivity of predictor is based on total number of neighbour pixel used to predict corrected pixel as well as it switching activity.

Figure 6. General scheme of Prediction based lossless compression (Knezović, J., Kovač, M., Žagar, M., Mlinarić, H., & Hofman, D. (2011)

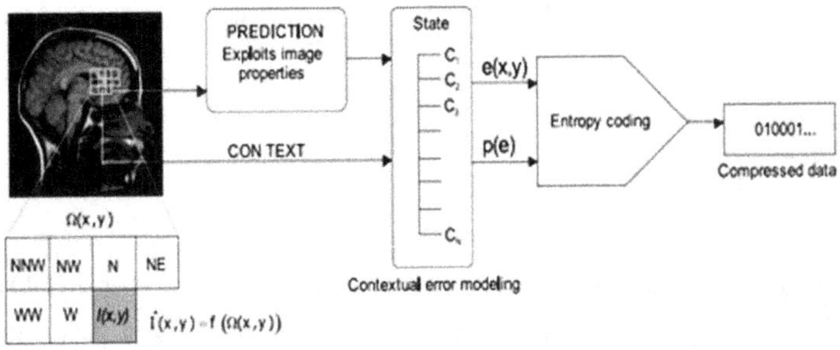

Figure 7. Neighbourhood pixel arrangement for prediction

NNWW	NNW	NN	NNE
NWW	NW	N	NE
WW	W	X (Pixel to be Predicted)	

The actual current pixel is estimated by taking the difference between the new information pixel value and predicted pixel values. When the same concept is applied for whole image, we have to select neighbouring pixels by considering its above or left position with respect to current pixel (Pathak, K. C., & Sarvaiya, J. N., 2017). Nonlinear model assigns an arbitrarily complex function to the models. Non linear model of adaptive predictor must accurately work in non-stationary situation and can able to switch between linear predictor and non-linear predictor. The accuracy of linear predictor for final decision of estimating current pixel is based on switching activity and adaptivity for non- stationary regions

Predictive Coding Based Image Compression

There are different types of lossless compression coding which are listed below:

1. Dictionary coding
2. Entropy Coding
3. Predictive coding

The three types of predictive coding are – Median Edge Detector (MED), Gradient Adjusted Predictor (GAP) and Gradient Edge Detector (GED). Dictionary based coding is not efficient for short file which consist of more bits during transmission. The limitation of Entropy coding is that it cannot differentiate same belonging codes which have same starting and ending bits. Among all these type of coding, Predictive coding is much more efficient and less complex coding techniqucs Table 1 shows the comparative analysis of different type of coding techniques.

Following Table 2 shows the comparison of basic predictive based coding techniques.

Table 1. Comparative analyses of Different types of Coding Techniques

Parameters	Entropy Coding	Dictionary	Predictive Coding	Transform Coding
Principle	In this, symbols are represented by the average number of bits. Entropy is lower bound on this average number.	In this, the values in the data structure I.e. dictionary represents the actual values of the image while transmission.	In this only the error between predicted value and actual value is transmitted.	In this, the input is transformed into another domain such as frequency to achieve compression.
Type	Lossless	Lossless	Lossless	Lossy
Complexity	Moderate	Moderate	Less	More
Example	Huffman, shanonfano coding	RLE	MED,GAP,GED etc.	JPEG

Table 2. Comparative Table for Basic Predictive based coding techniques

Predictive Method	Method	Advantages	Limitation
Median Edge Detector (MED)	It selects optimal prediction based on the image subrigion whether it is vertical edge, horizontal edge or smooth part	Optimal Combination of Simplicity and efficiency.	It found predictor in smooth region not in threshold.
Gradient adjusted predictor (GAP)	This algorithm estimates the edges around the current pixel and edges are categorized as strong edge	Combination of Edge estimation and simplicity of median predictor are used as an advantageous feature	Work also in threshold region.
Gradient Estimation Detector (GED)	In this algorithm decision of optimal predictor among three sub-predicator is done by estimation of local gradient and a threshold	The proposed predictor is based on one threshold	Complex
Blending Prediction	Non-linear predictors that are based on contextual switching	High efficiency Time efficient	Increase Complexity
Hierarchical Prediction	Divide Image Chrominance Pixel component In odd and even Pixel. Then prediction do on that Component	Prediction Done in Edge region also and decomposition of prediction is easy. Efficient in High Frequency requirement.	Mostly useful for RGB images.
Intra prediction HEVC	It exploits the spatial redundancy of reference row and previously coded neighborhood pixel and prediction angle .Best mode has been decided by sum of Absolute difference	It gives better prediction for more angular direction	Mostly useful for Video compression Increase complexity as modes are increases

LOSSSLESS JPEG BASED LINEAR PREDICTORS

Median Edge Detector(MED)

The MED is a switching type of non-linear predictor.It selects one predictor among three adjacent pixels at vertical edge, horizontal edge and smooth region to calculate unknown pixel. The value of predicted pixel is calculated by the equation as shown:

$$p = \begin{cases} Min\left(W,N\right), if\ NW \geq \max\left(W,N\right) \\ Max\left(W,N\right), if\ NW \leq \min\left(W,N\right) \\ N + W - NW, \qquad else \end{cases} \tag{1}$$

where functions min(N, W) and max(N, W) return the minimum and maximum values of W and N, respectively. It's worth noting that the output value of the MED algorithm is always limited to the range of [min(N,W),max(N,W)], and it cannot predict beyond this range.

Grahm

The Graham is a directional estimator kind of non-linear predictor that makes use of three adjacent pixels to measure the unknown pixels. The Graham algorithm evaluates the direction of gradient by calculating direction of horizontal and vertical gradients named dhand dv, respectively.

$$\begin{cases} d_h = N - NW \\ d_v = W - NW \end{cases} \tag{2}$$

In the Graham algorithm, predictor does not generate any new values, so it assigns existing values to unknown pixels. For horizontal and vertical edges, W and N, respectively, are chosen.

DARC

The DARC is a non-linear adaptive predictor that uses W, N and NW pixels to calculate the unknown pixels. Parameters dh and dv which present the direction of gradient in horizontal and vertical, respectively, are calculated as following equations:

Then final predictor predicts the unknown pixel by the following equation

$$x = \left(\frac{dv}{dh} + dh\right)W + \left(\frac{dv}{dh} + dh\right)N \tag{3}$$

The above equation shows that the weights of the pixels corresponds to dv and dh so they try to keep gradient direction. DARC's level of complexity reaches the level of MED.

GAP

Gradient adjusted prediction (GAP) is a non-linear adaptive predictor that uses seven adjacent pixels to calculate unknown pixel value. The GAP algorithm does this by calculating gv and gh using the following equation

$$gv = \left|W - WW\right| + \left|N - NW\right| + \left|N - NE\right| \tag{4}$$

$$gh = \left|W - NW\right| + \left|N - NN\right| + \left|NE - NNE\right| \tag{5}$$

The prediction coefficients and thresholds specified in the algorithm are chosen empirically. The GAP algorithm is described in Figure 8.

The complexity of GAP is not much higher than that of MED, but its output is not limited to a range similar to MED.

Gradient Based Selected Weighted (GBSW) Predictor

It estimates the average gradients in four directions and tries to select the best predictor for predicting unknown pixels. GBSW algorithm first computes four parameters to earn the gradient orientation. Parameters are computed using ten closest pixels as follows:

$$d1 = 2|WW - NW| + 2|N - NNE| + |W - N| + |NW - NN| \tag{6}$$

Figure 8. Gradient Adjusted Prediction Algorithm

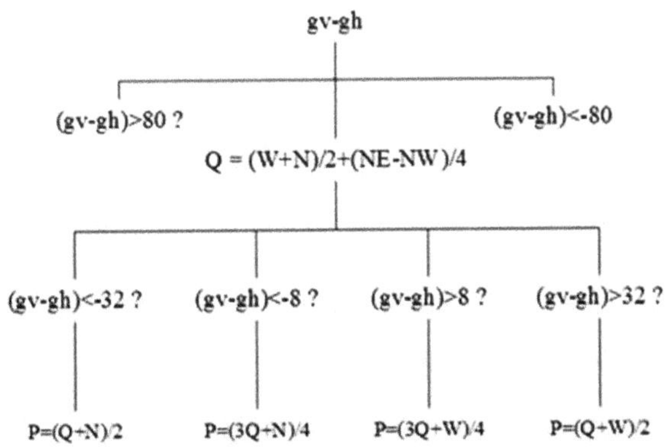

$$d2 = 2|N - NN| + 2|W - NW| + 2|NW - NNW| + 2|NE - NNE| + |WW - WWN| + |WWN - NNWW| \quad (7)$$

$$d3 = 2|W - WWN| + 2|N - NNW| + |NW - NNWW| + |NE - NN| \quad (8)$$

$$d4 = 2|W - WW| + 2|N - NW| + 2|NW - WWN| + 2|N - NE| + |NN - NNW| + |NN - NNE| \quad (9)$$

Then average gradients are estimated by considering above parameters in mentioned four directions: 45°, 90°, 135°, and 180°.

$$dNE = \left\lfloor \frac{d1}{6} + 0.5 \right\rfloor \quad (10)$$

$$dN = \left\lfloor \frac{d2}{10} + 0.5 \right\rfloor \quad (11)$$

$$dNW = \left\lfloor \frac{d3}{6} + 0.5 \right\rfloor \quad (12)$$

$$dNE = \left\lfloor \frac{d4}{10} + 0.5 \right\rfloor \quad (13)$$

After gradient estimation, This Predictor produces the prediction in a way that the neighbouring pixel in the direction with the minimal estimated gradient has the biggest contribution to the formation of final prediction. GBSW uses just two of four neighbouring pixels (N, W, NW, and NE) for final predictor. For example, if dW and dN (dW\dN) are two minimum estimated gradients around the current pixel X, then the prediction for that pixel is computed as:

$$\hat{X} = (dW \times N| + | dN \times W|) / |dw+dN| \tag{14}$$

GBSW's complexity is a bit higher than MED.

DPCM Based Predictor

In many lossy compression algorithms, 2D DCT is one of the important blocks to be implemented to improve the performance. But 2D DCT is not applicable for lossless compression algorithm quantization error. DCT co-efficient are quantized and then it is applied to encoder part which does not guarantee the prefect reconstruction which is the prime feature of Lossless coding [1]. Wavelet based approach overcome this problem by converting prediction residue in to integer transforms. These transforms co-efficient are then directly given to entropy encoder. So it eliminates quantization block and lossy coding turns into lossless coding. (Cai, X., & Lim, J. S., 2015). In PCM based approach which is highly adopted in latest video compression standard H.264 and HEVC, prediction residuals are directly applied to context based arithmetic entropy encoder for lossless coding. (Cai, X., & Lim, J. S., 2015). DPCM based approach, is highly adopted in latest H.264 and H.265 video compression standard (Cai, X., & Lim, J. S., 2015) In this approach 9 and 35 intra prediction modes can be optimize with sample wise DPCM based on image intensities along with the same direction for H.264 and H.265 respectively. This approach minimize the Mean Square Error (see Figure 9).

Consider residual pixel which is currently being coded as X. We can predict this X by considering its neighboring pixel which is denoted as U means above pixel, L means Left pixel and LU mens one immediately above left L. So predicted pixel is given by following formula by considering their respective weights w_L, w_U and w_{LU} as shown in following figure

$$X = round\left(w_L XL + w_U XU + w_{LU} X\, LU\right) \tag{15}$$

Figure 9. DPCM based prediction model

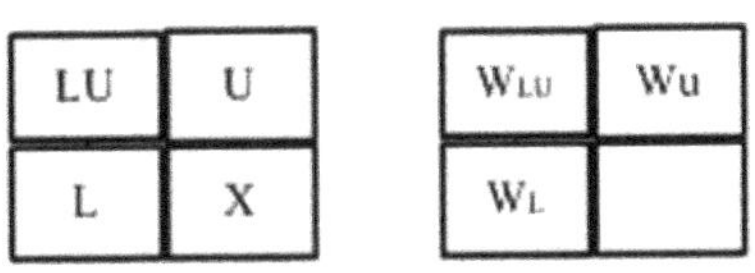

Neural Network Predictor

The advantageous feature for Neural network predictor are ability of learning stage by example and improved capacity of mapping hidden and nonlinear input output dependency in training data set.

Design Aspect of Proposed Adaptive Predictor for Lossless Medical Image Compression

Performance of any lossless compression depends on accuracy of prediction stage and efficiency of entropy coder for prediction based algorithms. Prediction function always considers neighbourhood pixels to predict current pixel and remove spatial redundancy using local non-stationary information. Again the performance of prediction algorithm is based on its switching speed from main direction to sub-direction for estimating current predicted pixel. There are two criteria to decide performance accuracy of predictor . First criteria is optimum choice of neighbouring pixel to reduce prediction error for first decision to reduce spatial redundancy of non-stationary regions. This decision is based on Total Number of Neighbouring Pixel(TNNP), which should be as minimum as possible. In Second criteria we have to choose Total Number of Neighbouring Pixel for Final Prediction of Pixel (TNNPF). This stage further ensures reduction in neighbouring pixel requirement to reduce prediction error and ensures bit rate reduction for proceeding stage of entropy coder .

On basis of above mentioned criteria, our proposed predictor is more adaptive for its switching operation from main direction to sub-direction for estimation of current predicted pixel and it is also optimum as it reduces the requirement of total number of neighbouring pixel for final accurate prediction of current pixels according

Table 3. Comparative Analysis of different Prediction Techniques

Parameters for optimum predictor selection	***LS-JPEG***	***MED***	***GAP***	***Proposed Predictor***
Total Number of Neighbouring Pixel	-	3	7	19
Total Number of Neighbouring Pixel for Final Prediction of Pixel (TNNPF)	-	3	4	2
Behavior operation (Linear /Non Linear)	Linear Predictor	Non Linear Predictor	Non Linear Predictor	Non Linear Predictor
Switching Criteria	NO	YES	YES	NO
Adaptivity Performance	None	Low	Adequate	High

to non-stationary regions like texture, smooth or edges as per local information of image .It ensures reduction in prediction error and improves the performance of entropy coder to reduce bit rate and improves coding gain for lossless compression. Table 3 shows comparative analysis of Adaptivity and switching speed of proposed adaptive predictor with reference to previous linear predictors.

Preceding edge tracking based predictors like DARC, MED and GAP are not suitable for minimizing number of final neighbouring pixel for efficient prediction decision. While our proposed predictor is more adaptive for switching for intensity variation i.e edges and texture variations by examining surrounding pixel properly for any unknown pixel. The maximum change direction can be determined by basic three steps as described below.

Step 1: The main direction $P^o$of intensity variation is decided by only considering four basic neighbourhood pixel like N,W, NW and NE

Step 2: To determine the abrupt intensity variation(edges), we have to select sub-direction which is produced by any one of the P^0, P^0+45^0 or P^0-45^0 sub-direction.

Step 3: Final optimum prediction value is obtain by following equation (16)

$$Final\ optimum\ direction = \left(2 * MD\right) + \left(\frac{1}{3} * SD\right) \tag{16}$$

where,

Figure 10. Nonlinear switching of prediction in sub-direction

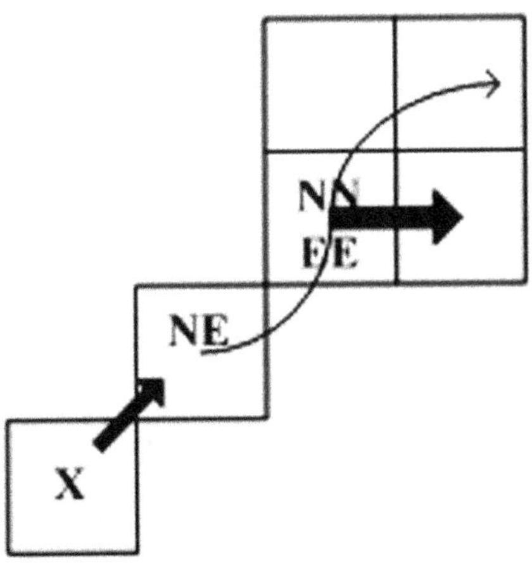

MD = Main Direction (According to Step 1)
SD = Sub Direction (According to Step 2)

As per the equation optimum final direction or each pixel prediction involves one or two neighborhood pixels. The decision is based on orientation of edges. If orientation of edges is same as main direction than just one neighborhood pixel is used for decision otherwise at least two neighborhood pixel may participate to take the decision of final prediction. First pixel resembles to main direction is multiplied by weighted factor 2 which indicates maximum changes occurrence and second pixel is multiplied with weighted factor of 1 and overall value is divided by the factor or 3 which is formulated as following equation (17).

Final predicted pixel is formulated as:

$$\tilde{x} = \frac{1}{3} * \left(2 * MD + SD\right) \tag{17}$$

Overall block diagram is shown as below Figure 11.

To check the accuracy of proposed adaptive predictor we have used several medical data base test images, which are shown collected from hospitals, which is shown in Figure 12. Efficiency of adaptive predictor based compression system is analyzed with some quantitative parameter like Compression Ratio(CR) and subjective visual quality of reconstructed image is measured using PSNR and Structural Similarity

Figure 11. Overall proposed adaptive predictor based system block diagram

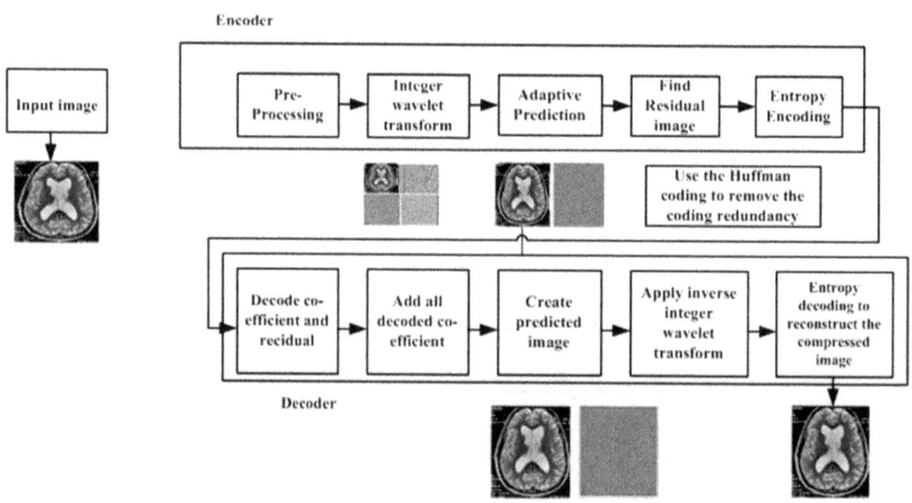

Measurement Index(SSIM). The efficacy of predictor is evaluated on the basis of Mean of Absolute Error (MAE) calculation.

Performance Parameters for Comparisons of the Compressed Images

Some of the most desirable properties of compression method for medical images include:

1. High lossless compression ratios, along with high PSNR.
2. High correlation between original and reconstructed image.
3. Resolution scalability, which is defined as decoder accuracy to retrieve the image at different resolution.

Mean Square Error (MSE)

To evaluate the performance of the reconstructed images, the peak signal-to-noise ratio (PSNR) is employed. Suppose x_{mn} is the gray value of the pixel (m, n) of the original image, and $\hat{x}_{mn}$ is the gray value of the pixel (m, n) of the reconstructed

Figure 12. Medical Image database collected from hospital

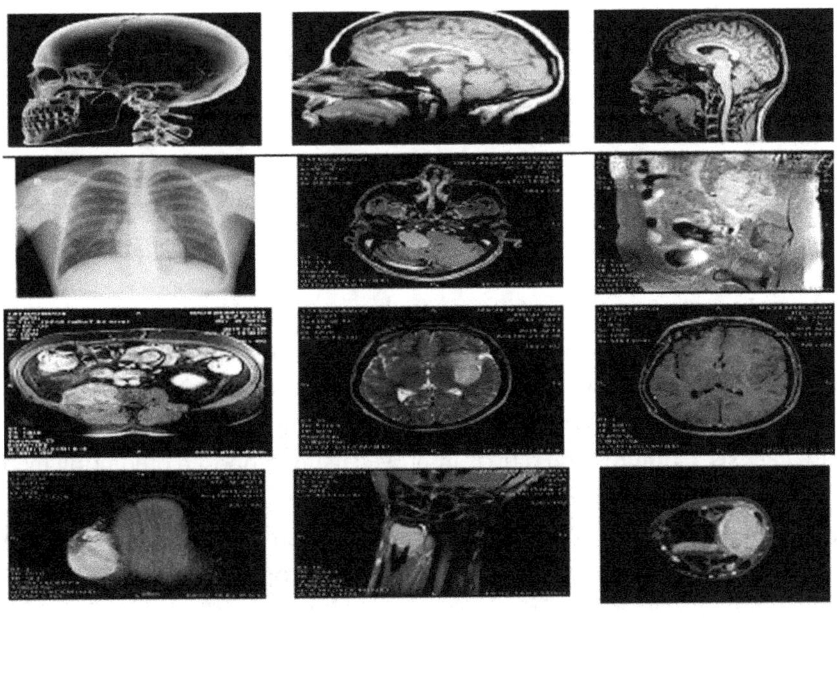

image. M and N are the numbers of the horizontal and vertical pixels, respectively. The mean square error is defined as:

$$MSE = \frac{1}{MN}\sum_{m=0}^{M-1}\sum_{n=0}^{N-1}\left(x_{mn} - \hat{x}_{mn}\right)^2 \tag{18}$$

Peak Signal to Noise Ratio (PSNR)

The PSNR is defined as,

$$PSNR = 10\log_{10}\left(255^2 / MSE\right) \tag{19}$$

Compression Ratio

Compression ratio is defined as,

CR = Size of Original Image / Size of compressed image (20)

Mean Absolute Error(MAE)

Mean Absolute Error (MAE) is calculated for performance analysis of predictor. For optimal predictor, MAE should be as minimum as possible.

$$MAE = \frac{\sum_{i=1}^{N}\sum_{j=1}^{M}\left|e_{i,j}\right|}{NxM} \tag{21}$$

The implementation results of proposed method of Gradient based adaptive method is applied on ROI part and results are shown in Figure 12.

Following Table 4 shows the comparative analysis of Compression ratio of full image of propped predictive method with other existing method. Figure 5.12 shows its chart analysis. Compression ratio is improved using proposed prediction method.

Following Table 5 compares PSNR and CR value of proposed method. Figure 15 shows comparison chart of Compression ratio of Linear prediction method with proposed method. Compression ratio is better for proposed method compared to

Figure 13. Output images of implementation of proposed system

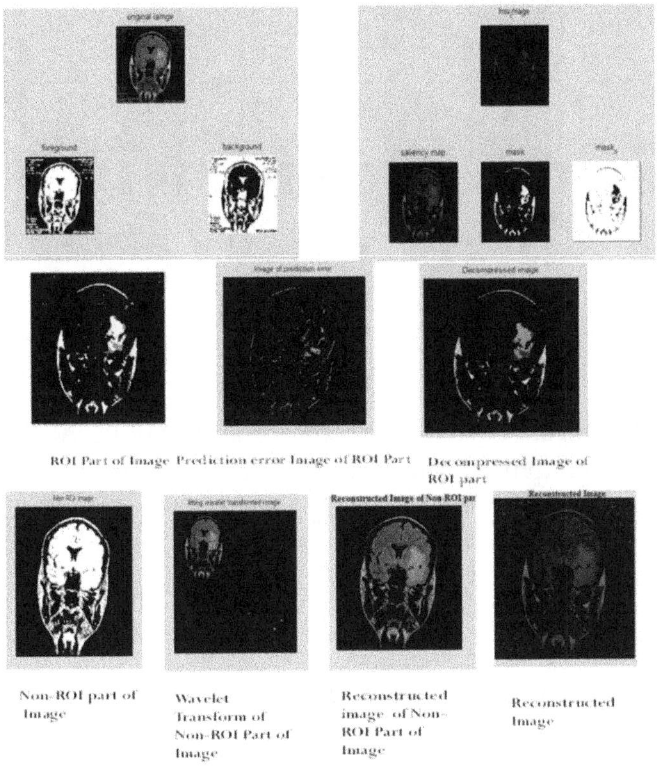

Table 4. Comparison of Compression Ratio of Full image with proposed prediction method

IMAGE NAME	LINEAR	MED	GAP	DARC	Graham	Proposed
ANDOMEN0001	1.04	1.71	2.14	1.05	1.43	4.04
BRAIN	1.03	2.02	4.70	1.06	1.37	3.73
BRAIN0001	1.38	2.32	3.18	1.39	1.69	4.58
BRAIN0002	1.20	2.01	2.69	1.21	1.88	4.06
BRAIN20001	1.31	2.10	2.81	1.32	1.74	4.49
BRAIN20002	1.35	2.07	2.92	1.36	1.70	4.79
SHOULDER0001	1.27	2.21	3.88	1.23	1.86	4.32
WRIST JOINT0001	1.32	2.40	2.18	1.33	1.98	4.43
WRIST JOINT0002	1.43	2.65	3.27	1.43	2.21	4.75
WRIST JOINT00031	1.63	3.11	3.41	1.65	2.48	4.79

Figure 14. Comparison chart for Compression ratio of proposed system with other prediction methods

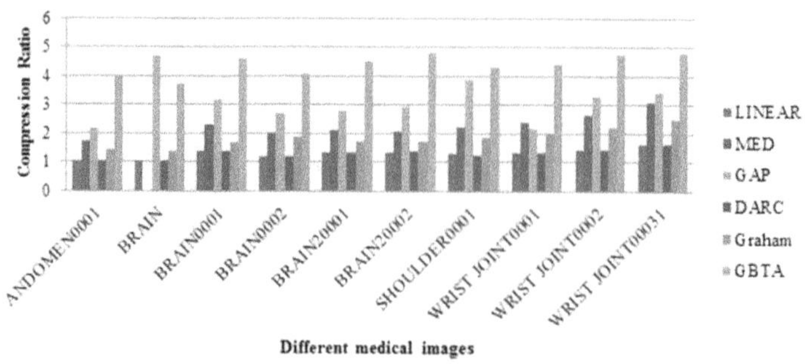

Linear prediction. Figure 16 shows the comparison chart of PSNR in dB of Linear prediction method with proposed method. PSNR values are slightly degraded in some medical images otherwise it is also visually better in most of the medical images.

SUMMARY

Inferences of the Obtained Result

1. We have implemented different predictive coding methods of ROI part of different medical images like GAP, MED, GRAHM, DARC, LINEAR and

Table 5. PSNR and CR Valuse of Proposed Adaptive Prediction method

Image Name	Linear		Proposed	
	CR	PSNR(dB)	CR	PSNR(dB)
ABDOMEN001	1.57	19.30	4.57	13.38
BRAIN10001	1.34	24.21	4.50	36.72
BRAIN10002	1.33	23.14	4.29	33.83
BRAIN10003	1.23	20.81	4.05	27.40
BRAIN20001	1.34	23.63	4.34	34.58
BRAIN20002	1.33	23.60	4.34	34.80
BRAINC1	1.40	22.36	2.73	20.37
CTSCAN CHEST1	1.26	22.42	1.58	21.39
MRI11	1.15	20.32	2.25	18.60
Brain	0.80	11.89	1.44	14.37

Figure 15. Comparison chart of Compression Ration of Linear Prediction Vs Proposed adaptive prediction

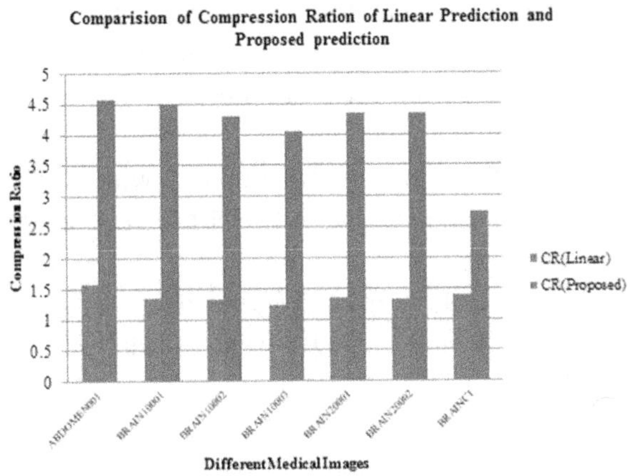

Figure 16. Comparison of values for Linear PSNR prediction Vs Proposed adaptive prediction

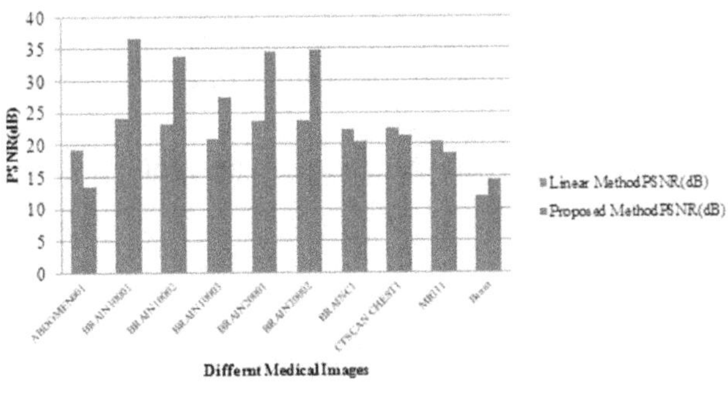

Figure 17. MAE of Proposed method vs Other prediction method

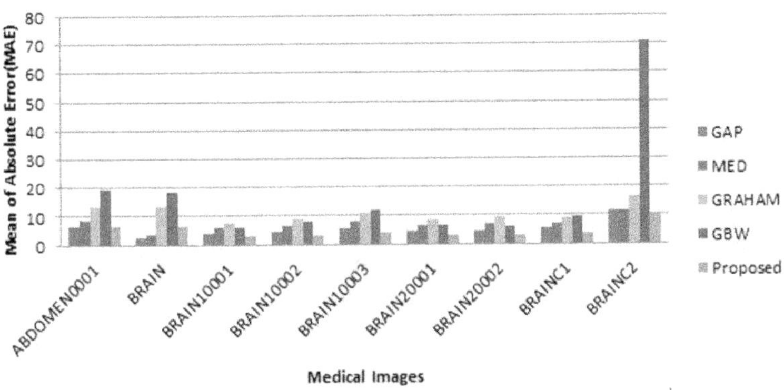

Proposed Gradient based adaptive tracking by considering minimum number of neighborhood pixel to predict the errorous or lost pixel.

2. Compared to all Predictive method proposed Gradient based Adaptive Tracking based Prediction method (GBATP) gives minimum Mean Absolute Error(MAE) which suggest less prediction error and absolute reconstruction of original image.
3. The combination of Proposed predictive coding with Huffman coding gives heighest Compression ration with good PSNR to get good perceptual quality of most of medical images.
4. Using Integer Wavelet Transform(IWT) non –ROI part is processed and finally fused image of ROI part and Non-ROI part gives better PSNR along with good compression Ratio
5. Throughout the analysis we have applied our proposed prediction method and intra prediction we have applied to ROI part as we as whole image, compared to full image compression ratio of only ROI part is better compared to full image .

The accuracy of prediction based lossless compression techniques is measured on the basis of amount of spatial redundancy removal and switching among available sub optimal predictor. As switching operation is faster among suboptimal predictor, more sub region of image can be predicted with minimum prediction error. Entropy coder also plays very important role for achieving highest compression rate. Predictive method is a lossless compression method.

DISCUSSION AND SUGGESTIONS

A loss of clinical data has the potential to compromise the value of an imaging examination to a patient as it does not contain disease information which is to be diagnosed. Also semi-automated analysis like MRI and CT includes data set which has lossless compression as it includes both clinical as well as equipment modalities and hence currently lossless compression is used by wider community. Critical issues related to lossy compression approaches for medical imaging have been studies all over the world. Various research studies have given numerous example to set acceptable limit for compression ratio for different modalities like CT, MRI, PET, Ultrasound and ECG, EEG. Among various compressions standard latest High Efficiency Video Coding has shown its performance improvement on compression of medical image sequences at minimum bitrate and optimum visual quality of diagnostically important region.

Lossy compression is marginal acceptable at some extent for certain information which is clinically not important. General conclusion is that some levels of lossy compression are suitable for some diagnoses like fracture, PET, etc.; however there remains considerable uncertainty to decide the threshold level and type of compression factors, for any particular examination or modality as if threshold is fixed than quality of image examination may get deteriorate and it leads to false or poor diagnosis of diseases. For example, while compression of digital mammograms is not permitted in the USA by the Food and Drug Administration (Banu, N. M., & Sujatha, S., 2015). If lossy compression has been implemented in the case where life of patient is not in danger than use of such compression would not increase the legal responsibility of physicians, if used and implemented appropriately as per the survey conducted by Canadian Association of Radiologists (CAR). However, this conclusion leaves wider scope for researcher because of compromise between visual quality and compression factor and improper choice may lead to inconsistent application of compression.

FUTURE SCOPE

For medical images most of the background is processed with lossy compression we apply transformation method, Wavelet transform and Discrete cosine transform and conclude that WT transform gives better result. These all Predictive Method is working on linear and Nonlinear switching. If there is more Curvature in Image then it is not working well on that new image. So, we move to the new standard of image compression which give better result when more curvature in the image and also give more visual quality. The new immerging compression standard is HEVC. Compressive sensing based prediction algorithm are also emerging algorithms for giving perfect image reconstruction and also provide lossless compression with DARC predictor along with dictionary based LZW encoding scheme. Neural network based prediction is also very useful for diagnostic purpose.

REFERENCES

Abo-Zahhad, M., Gharieb, R. R., Ahmed, S. M., & Abd-Ellah, M. K. (2015). Huffman image compression incorporating DPCM and DWT. *Journal of Signal and Information Processing*, *6*(02), 123–135. doi:10.4236/jsip.2015.62012

Agrawal, M., & Choudhary, R. R. (2016, August). Median Edge Detector for Lossless Video Coding: An efficient prediction scheme for lossless video coding. In *Proceedings of the International Conference on Advances in Information Communication Technology & Computing* (p. 40). ACM. 10.1145/2979779.2979819

Avramović, A., & Savić, S. (2011). Lossless predictive compression of medical images. *Serbian Journal of Electrical Engineering*, *8*(1), 27–36. doi:10.2298/SJEE1101027A

Ayoobkhan, M. U. A., Chikkannan, E., & Ramakrishnan, K. (2017). Feed-Forward Neural Network-Based Predictive Image Coding for Medical Image Compression. *Arabian Journal for Science and Engineering*, 1–9.

Babu, P. S., & Sathappan, S. (2015). Efficient lossless image compression using modified hierarchical prediction and context adaptive coding. *Indian Journal of Science and Technology*, *8*(34), 1–6.

Bairagi, V. K., & Sapkal, A. M. (2013). ROI-based DICOM image compression for telemedicine. *Sadhana*, *38*(1), 123–131. doi:10.100712046-013-0126-4

Banu, N. M., & Sujatha, S. (2015). 3D medical image compression: A review. *Indian Journal of Science and Technology*, *8*(12).

Cai, X., & Lim, J. S. (2015, March). Adaptive residual DPCM for lossless intra coding. In *Visual Information Processing and Communication VI* (Vol. 9410). International Society for Optics and Photonics.

Chen, Y. T., & Tseng, D. C. (2007). Wavelet-based medical image compression with adaptive prediction. *Computerized Medical Imaging and Graphics*, *31*(1), 1–8. doi:10.1016/j.compmedimag.2006.08.003 PMID:17046200

Dragoi, I. C., Coltuc, D., & Caciula, I. (2014, June). Gradient based prediction for reversible watermarking by difference expansion. In *Proceedings of the 2nd ACM workshop on Information hiding and multimedia security* (pp. 35-40). ACM. 10.1145/2600918.2600924

Karimi, N., Samavi, S., Soroushmehr, S. R., Shirani, S., & Najarian, K. (2016). Toward practical guideline for design of image compression algorithms for biomedical applications. *Expert Systems with Applications*, *56*, 360–367. doi:10.1016/j.eswa.2016.02.047

Knezović, J., Kovač, M., Žagar, M., Mlinarić, H., & Hofman, D. (2011). Novel prediction based technique for efficient compression of medical imaging data. In *Telemedicine Techniques and Applications*. InTech. doi:10.5772/18126

Li, X., & Bi, G. (2015, July). Image reconstruction based on the improved compressive sensing algorithm. In *Digital Signal Processing (DSP), 2015 IEEE International Conference on* (pp. 357-360). IEEE. 10.1109/ICDSP.2015.7251892

Mamatha, A. S., & Singh, V. (2014, September). Lossless hyperspectral image compression using intraband and interband predictors. In *Advances in Computing, Communications and Informatics (ICACCI, 2014 International Conference on* (pp. 332-337). IEEE.

Pathak, K. C., & Sarvaiya, J. N. (2017, March). Lossless medical image compression using transform domain adaptive prediction for telemedicine. In *Wireless Communications, Signal Processing and Networking (WiSPNET), 2017 International Conference on* (pp. 1026-1031). IEEE. 10.1109/WiSPNET.2017.8299918

Rad, R. M., Attar, A., & Shahbahrami, A. (2013). A predictive algorithm for multimedia data compression. *Multimedia Systems*, *19*(2), 103–115. doi:10.100700530-012-0282-0

Shirsat, T. G., & Bairagi, V. K. (2013, April). Lossless medical image compression by IWT and predictive coding. In *Energy Efficient Technologies for Sustainability (ICEETS), 2013 International Conference on* (pp. 1279-1283). IEEE. 10.1109/ICEETS.2013.6533571

Sophia, P. E., & Anitha, J. (2015). A systematic review on advances and perspectives of image compression in telemedicine. *International Journal of Advanced Intelligence Paradigms*, *7*(2), 136–155. doi:10.1504/IJAIP.2015.070768

Tiwari, A. K., & Kumar, R. R. (2009). A minimum entropy based switched adaptive predictor for lossless compression of images. *Signal, Image and Video Processing*, *3*(4), 307–318. doi:10.100711760-008-0068-1

Veeraswamy, K., Srinivaskumar, S., & Chatterji, B. N. (2007). Lossless Image Compression using Topological Pixel Re-ordering and Switched Predictor. *Journal of the Institution of Electronics and Telecommunication Engineers*, *53*(6), 505–512. doi:10.1080/03772063.2007.10876167

Weinberger, M. J., Seroussi, G., & Sapiro, G. (2000). The LOCO-I lossless image compression algorithm: Principles and standardization into JPEG-LS. *IEEE Transactions on Image Processing*, *9*(8), 1309–1324. doi:10.1109/83.855427 PMID:18262969

Wu, X., & Memon, N. (1997). Context-based, adaptive, lossless image coding. *IEEE Transactions on Communications*, *45*(4), 437–444. doi:10.1109/26.585919

ADDITIONAL READING

Antony, A., & Sreelekha, G. (2017). HEVC-based lossless intra coding for efficient still image compression. *Multimedia Tools and Applications, 76*(2), 1639–1658. doi:10.100711042-015-3138-8

Attar, A., Rad, R. M., & Shahbahrami, A. (2010, November). An accurate gradient-based predictive algorithm for image compression. In *Proceedings of the 8th International Conference on Advances in Mobile Computing and Multimedia* (pp. 374-377). ACM. 10.1145/1971519.1971582

Boulgouris, N. V., Tzovaras, D., & Strintzis, M. G. (2001). Lossless image compression based on optimal prediction, adaptive lifting, and conditional arithmetic coding. *IEEE Transactions on Image Processing, 10*(1), 1–14. doi:10.1109/83.892438 PMID:18249592

Chang, C. C., & Chen, G. I. (2003). Enhancement algorithm for nonlinear context-based predictors. *IEE Proceedings. Vision Image and Signal Processing, 150*(1), 15–19. doi:10.1049/ip-vis:20030163

Chen, Y. T., & Tseng, D. C. (2007). Wavelet-based medical image compression with adaptive prediction. *Computerized Medical Imaging and Graphics, 31*(1), 1–8. doi:10.1016/j.compmedimag.2006.08.003 PMID:17046200

Danesh, A. S., Rad, R. M., & Attar, A. (2010, March). A novel predictor function for lossless image compression. In *Advanced Computer Control (ICACC), 2010 2nd International Conference on* (Vol. 2, pp. 527-531). IEEE.

Memon, N., & Wu, X. (1997). Recent developments in context-based predictive techniques for lossless image compression. *The Computer Journal, 40*(2-3), 127-136

Przelaskowski, A. (2001). Lossloss encoding of medical images: Hybrid modification of statistical modelling-based conception. *Journal of Electronic Imaging, 10*(4), 966–977. doi:10.1117/1.1407261

Shahbahrami, A., Rad, R. M., & Attar, A. (2010, April). A study of predictive method and presentation of an improvement. In *Local Workshop in Department of Computer Engineering*. Rasht, Iran: Faculty of Engineering, University of Guilan.

Shukla, J., Alwani, M., & Tiwari, A. K. (2010, April). A survey on lossless image compression methods. In *Computer Engineering and Technology (ICCET), 2010 2nd International Conference on* (Vol. 6, pp. V6-136). IEEE. 10.1109/ICCET.2010.5486344

Son, J. D., & Song, B. C. (2016). Enhanced Prediction Algorithm for Near-lossless Image Compression with Low Complexity and Low Latency. *IEIE Transactions on Smart Processing & Computing*, *5*(2), 143–151. doi:10.5573/IEIESPC.2016.5.2.143

Song, X., Huang, Q., Chang, S., He, J., & Wang, H. (2017). Lossless medical image compression using geometry-adaptive partitioning and least square-based prediction. *Medical & Biological Engineering & Computing*, 1–10. PMID:29105018

Tang, H., & Kamata, S. I. (2006). A gradient based predictive coding for lossless image compression. *IEICE Transactions on Information and Systems*, *89*(7), 2250–2256. doi:10.1093/ietisy/e89-d.7.2250

Tiwari, A. K., & Kumar, R. R. (2007, September). Least-squares based switched adaptive predictors for lossless video coding. In *Image Processing, 2007. ICIP 2007. IEEE International Conference on* (Vol. 6, pp. VI-69). IEEE. 10.1109/ICIP.2007.4379523

Chapter 12
HE Stain Image Segmentation Using an Innovative Type-2 Fuzzy Set-Based Approach

Dibya Jyoti Bora
Kaziranga University, India

ABSTRACT

HE stain images are widely used in medical diagnosis and often considered a gold standard for histology and pathology laboratories. A proper analysis is needed to have a critical decision about the status of the diagnosis of the concerned patient. Segmentation is always considered as an advanced stage of image analysis where objects of similar properties are put in one segment. But segmentation of HE stain images is not an easy task as these images involve a high level of fuzziness with them mainly along the boundary edges. So, traditional techniques like hard clustering techniques are not suitable for segmenting these images. So, a new approach is proposed in this chapter to deal with this problem. The proposed approach is based on type-2 fuzzy set and is new. The experimental results prove the superiority of the proposed technique.

INTRODUCTION

Image Segmentation is the basic and critical tasks during any medical image analysis task (Ho, 2012). Segmentation means the formation of different homogeneous regions based on some homogeneity criteria. These homogeneity criteria may be texture, color etc. So, with the help of segmentation, it is possible to outline different ROIs(Region of Interests). This will help to focus on particular ROI which

DOI: 10.4018/978-1-5225-6316-7.ch012

is specific to one particular application. With the help of mathematical equations, we can define segmentation as follows:

$$\text{(i) } \bigcup_{i=1}^{n} R_i = R \tag{1}$$

$$\text{(ii) } R_i \cap R_j = \phi \tag{2}$$

$$\text{(iii) } H\left(R_i\right) = TRUE \forall i \tag{3}$$

$$\text{(iv) } H(R_i \cup R_j) = FALSE \forall R_i \ \& \ R_j adjacent \tag{4}$$

According to the property (i), the summation of all the divided regions will produce image back. Property (ii) stands on the fact that two separate regions should be disjoint. The Property (iii) implies that within a region the homogeneity criteria should be satisfied. And the property(iv), says that two adjacent regions should not be homogeneous.

HE Stain images are regarded as of gold standard in histology and pathology laboratories (Paxton et al, 2003). In general, most cells are colorless and transparent. There arise difficulties to analyze them. So, staining is done in the histological sections to make the cells distinct and visible (Paxton et al, 2003). One such popular and commonly adopted technique is HE stain which involves the usage of hematoxylin and eosin which color nuclei and cytoplasm differently (Paxton, et al, 2003). Hematoxylin is generally a dark blue or violet stain which is basic/ positive. Eosin is a red or pink stain and is Acidic / Negative. When hematoxylin and eosin are combined, then it produces blues, violets, and reds. Now, through segmentation, HE Stain image is divided into different segments. And from those segments, it will be easy to analyze the particular ROI for which diagnosis is conducted.

There exist many different techniques from different domains of segmentation (Jain et al, 1989). But, clustering is the most commonly adopted one. Clustering may be hard or soft (Bora, 2017). The main difference between the two is that in case of hard clustering an element should belong to only one particular cluster it has been assigned. While in case of soft clustering, one data element may contribute to more than one cluster depending on the membership grade it possesses. K-Means is a frequently adopted hard clustering technique for image segmentation (Bhanachandra et al, 2015; Bora et al, 2016). But, in case of medical images like HE Stain images, due to a large amount of fuzziness exist in the boundaries of ROI, it is not recommended to go for hard clustering based image segmentation techniques. Then, we have FCM (Bezdek et al, 1981) as a soft-computing counterpart of K-Means algorithm. As a soft computing based technique, FCM has the ability to deal with the vagueness of the boundaries to an extent since here grouping is performed the only basis of the membership grade. But what happens, if fuzziness exists even in the membership function of FCM itself. So, it is better to opt for an advanced fuzzy logic based technique while dealing with medical image segmentation. For that, we have adopted Type-2 fuzzy set (Zadeh, 1975) based technique to design an approach for HE Stain image segmentation. The remaining section of the paper is organized as follows: In Section 2, a review of the related work and motivation towards proposed work are presented. In section 3, the steps involved in the proposed work are discussed. In section 4 and its subsections, different methods and materials involved in the proposed work are elaborated. Section 5 is the experiment and result in the discussion section. Finally, the conclusion is drawn in section 6.

REVIEW OF RELATED WORKS AND MOTIVATION TOWARDS PROPOSED WORK

In this section, some noteworthy contributions in the field of HE Stain image segmentation are presented. This section is subdivided into two subsections: Literature Review and Motivation towards Proposed Work.

Literature Review

Dimitropoulos et al. (Dimitropoulos et al, 2017) proposed a framework for the detection and classification of centroblasts (CB) in follicular lymphoma (FL) tissue samples stained with PAX5 and H&E stains. The tissues are sliced at 1 Âµm thickness level. PAX5 immunohistochemistry is employed to facilitate the segmentation of nuclei. H&E staining is done to extract textual information related to histological characteristics used by pathologists in the diagnosis of FL grading. For the segmentation, the authors initially applied an energy minimization technique based on graph cuts. Also, an algorithm is proposed for the separation of overlapped nuclei inspired by the clustering of large-scale visual vocabularies. The morphological characteristics of nuclei extracted from PAX5-stained images are combined with a number of textural characteristics identified in H&E images through a Bayesian network classifier, which aims to model pathologist 's knowledge used in FL grading.

Experimental results have proved that the proposed approach has a great potential carrying an average F-score of 94.56%.

In (De Oliveria, 2013), the authors proposed a novel segmentation method for cuboidal cell nuclei in HE Stained images of prostate tissue. The proposed method consists of three steps: pre-processing, segmentation of cuboidal cell nuclei and post-processing. Here, in the pre-processing step, contrast stretching is applied to the red (R) channel and thereby highlight the contrast of cuboidal cell nuclei.In the second step, minimum cross-entropy based global thresholding is applied to generate a binary image with candidate regions for cuboidal cell nuclei. Then, in the last step, i.e., in the post-processing step, false positives are removed using the connected component method. The proposed method has been applied to an image bank with 105 samples and measures of sensitivity, specificity and accuracy were compared with those provided by another state of the art segmentation approaches. The experimental results are found promising and also verifies that proposed method allows the segmentation of cuboidal cell nuclei with a mean accuracy of 97%.

Nguyen et al. (2017) discussed segmenting histological structures in hematoxylin and eosin (H&E) stained images of breast tissues, e.g. invasive carcinoma, carcinoma in situ, atypical and normal ducts, adipose tissue, lymphocytes.Two graph-theoretic segmentation methods based on local spatial color and nuclei neighborhood statistics are introduced in this paper. A dataset of 232 high power field breast tissue images together with expertly annotated ground truth are considered for the experiments. To accurately model the preference for histological structures (ducts, vessels, tumor nets, adipose etc.) over the remaining connective tissue and non-tissue areas in ground truth annotations, a new region-based score for evaluating segmentation algorithms is proposed.The proposed approach has been found superior to another state of the art algorithms with respect to both region and boundary based performance measures.

Shi et al. (2016) proposed an automated quantitative image analysis pipeline based on hierarchical clustering of local correlations, which segmented the image into nuclei, cytoplasm and extracellular spaces by classifying image pixels on the basis of local correlation features.Then, the segmentation for precise nucleus boundaries was performed, and finally, a set of indicators characterizing tissue structures were extracted to complete quantification of HE images. The authors claim the superiority of the proposed approach through proper experiments and result in analysis.

In (2012), the author's Model-based approaches use a priori information on cell shape features to obtain the segmentation, which may introduce a bias favoring the detection of cell nuclei only with certain properties. In this study, we present a novel contour-based minimum-model cell detection and segmentation approach that uses minimal a priori information and detects contours independent of their shape. This approach avoids a segmentation bias with respect to shape features and allows for an accurate segmentation (precision50.908; recall50.859; validation based on,

8000 manually-labeled cells) of a broad spectrum of normal and disease-related morphological features without the requirement of prior training.

Liu et al. proposed a novel approach for automated segmentation of HE-stained skeletal muscle cross sections (2013). The proposed technique consists of two major steps: In the first step, they applied a learning-based seed detection method to find the geometric centers of the muscle fibers, and in the second step, a color gradient repulsive balloon snake deformable model is introduced which utilizes color gradient in Luv color space. The results of the proposed approach are experimentally proved accurate and efficient.

Veta et al. (2013) proposed an automated nuclei segmentation method for hematoxylin and eosin (H&E) stained breast cancer histopathology images. Their proposed technique mainly consists of four steps: In the first step,pre-processing with color unmixing and morphological operators is carried out, In the second step, segmentation with marker-controlled watershed algorithm at multiple scales and with different markers are processed, in the third step, which is exactly a post-processing step is carried out for rejection of false regions and in the final step, merging of the results from multiple scales is done to obtain the final results. The technique is found efficient for segmenting HE stained breast cancer histopathology images.

Motivation Towards Proposed Work

So, from the literature review, we have found that various researchers put efforts towards developing a technique for segmenting HE Stained images. But, the main problem they face is that it is very hard to distinctly segment the cells, i.e. cell boundaries are very hard to be detected. This is due to the fuzzy behavior of the boundary regions in almost every HE stained images. So, it is better to develop a segmentation technique which will be able to deal this vagueness efficiently and output a better-segmented version. Only, the advanced fuzzy set-based technique can provide the same. This is the reason why we have been motivated for developing the proposed technique. The type-2 fuzzy set-based logic is adapted for developing the segmentation technique. Also, only a very few such types of techniques are found in the literature.So, it is believed that the proposed technique will act as a novel framework for HE Stain image segmentation.

STEPS INVOLVED IN THE PROPOSED TECHNIQUE

The algorithm for the proposed approach consists of the following steps:

Step 1: Input the Color HE Stain Image

Step 2: The input RGB HE Stain image is converted into HSV image, and the V channel has been extracted from this converted image.

Step 3: Define the primary membership function as follows:

$$J_x = \frac{I - I_{min}}{I_{max} - I_{min}} \tag{5}$$

where I is the V-channel of the converted HSV version of the input HE Stain color image (say A) of the range 0 to L-1, I_{min} is the minimum value of intensities and I_{max} is the maximum value.

Step 4: Then find out upper and lower bounds of the above membership function (equation number 5) so that an interval based type-2 fuzzy set can be constructed. This task is completed with the following equations:

$$\mu_{upper}=[J_x]^{\alpha}, \mu_{lower}=[J_x]^{1/\alpha} \tag{6}$$

where

$$0<\alpha\leq 1 \tag{7}$$

A proper value of the α should be determined through trial and error strategy.

Step 5: The new membership function i.e. the type-2 fuzzy set based membership function is calculated using the following equation:

$$\widehat{\mu}_A = \frac{\mu_{low} \bullet \lambda + \mu_{high} \bullet (1-\lambda)}{1-(1-\lambda) \bullet \mu_{low} \bullet \mu_{high}} \tag{8}$$

Here λ can be found out using the following equation:

$$\lambda= I_{mean}/L \tag{9}$$

The above equation (8) is developed Bora (2014) by considering the fact that darker region should not be made further darker. Also, through this equation, it is found that fuzziness in the boundaries is removed to a maximum extent.

Step 6: Finally, the cluster centers are updated using the conventional FCM algorithm by considering the membership grade values produced by equation (8) . The equation for updating cluster centers is:

$$c_j = \frac{\sum_{i=1}^{N} \widehat{\mu}_A^{\,m} \bullet x_i}{\sum_{i=1}^{N} \widehat{\mu}_A^{\,m}} \tag{10}$$

So, cluster centers are updated using equation (10). The objective function (Bezdek, 1981) in this case is:

$$OBJ_m = \sum_{i=1}^{N} \sum_{j=1}^{C} \widehat{\mu}_A^{\,m} \, \| x_i - c_j \|^2 \quad {}_{1 \le m < \infty} \tag{11}$$

where m is the value of the exponent which is any real number greater than 1, and in our experiment, we have fixed m=2.1 (Bora et al, 2014).

Here, $\widehat{\mu}_A$ represents the degree of membership of x_i with respect to a particular cluster j, x_i is the ith of d-dimensional measured data, c_j is the d-dimension center of the cluster, and $\|*\|$ is representing any norm conveying the similarity between any considered data and the center (Bora, 2017).

So, a particular pattern p_i with a high membership value towards a certain cluster c_k will be assigned to this particular cluster.

As usual, the fuzzy clustering process will be carried on until the stopping criteria are reached up. In this case, the stopping criteria defined is:

$$|OBJ_m - OBJ_{m+1}| < \in \tag{12}$$

where OBJ_m and OBJ_{m+1} are the values of the objective functions at two consecutive events and $\in < 1$ is an arbitrarily small positive number.

Step 7: Replace the old V-channel obtained at Step 2 with the segmented version of the same obtained at Step 6. This way the segmented image is obtained in HSV color space.

Step 8: HSV to RGB color space conversion is carried out to obtain the segmented color HE Stain image in RGB color space. Output this version of the segmented image.

So, the proposed technique consists of the above steps. Now, in the next section, all the technical terminologies are illustrated in details.

METHODS AND MATERIALS INVOLVED IN THE PROPOSED TECHNIQUE

In this section, we are going to discuss the main techniques involved in the proposed technique. Here, the main focus is given on Type-2 interval based fuzzy set and the main material regarding this paper i.e. HE Stained image.

Type-2 Fuzzy Set

In 1965, Zadeh established the idea of fuzzy set in (Zadeh, 1965). But the membership function of the type-1 fuzzy set itself contains some uncertainty. So, fuzziness is not completely removed through the type-1 fuzzy set. Hence, to solve this problem, Zadeh introduced the idea of type-2 fuzzy set in 1975 (Zadeh, 1975). The type-2 fuzzy set can be thought as an expansion of the type-1 fuzzy set. It is found very useful in such cases when there arises obscurity to agree on the accuracy of the type-1 membership function due to uncertainty in its shape, location or other such parameters (Bora et al, 2018). Proper upper and lower bounds are used to bound the membership function. In other words, the type-1 membership function is blurred to obtain the type-2 membership function[Mendel] (Bora et al, 2018). The following figure [Mendel] more clearly depicts this fact of blurriness.

Mathematically, we can define type-2 fuzzy set as follows (Mendel et al, 2002):

$$A_{TYPEII} = \left\{x, \widehat{\mu}_A(\mathrm{x}, \mu) \mid \forall\, \mathrm{x} \in \mathrm{X}, \forall u \in \mathrm{J}_x \subseteq [0,1]\right\}$$

where $\widehat{\mu}_A(\mathrm{x}, \mu)$ is the Type II membership function, J_x is the prime one.

The relation of upper and lower bound in a type-2 fuzzy set with respect to type-1 fuzzy set can be shown with the help of the following figure:

One more terminology related to type-2 fuzzy set is the FOOTPRINT OF UNCERTAINTY (FOU) (Bora et al, 2018). This is used to illustrate the uncertainty in the primary membership of a type-2 fuzzy set. The following equation articulates the FOU in terms of the primary membership function J_x:

$$FOU(\mathrm{A}_{TYPEII}) = \bigcup_{x \in X} J_x \tag{13}$$

Figure 1. (a) Type-1 Membership Function, and (b) Fuzziness raises the type-2 membership function

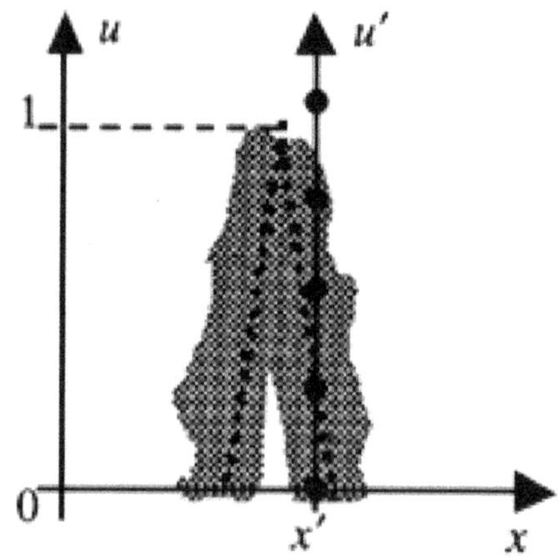

Figure 2. Upper and Lower Limit defining Membership area With Respect to Type-1 and Type-2 Fuzzy Set

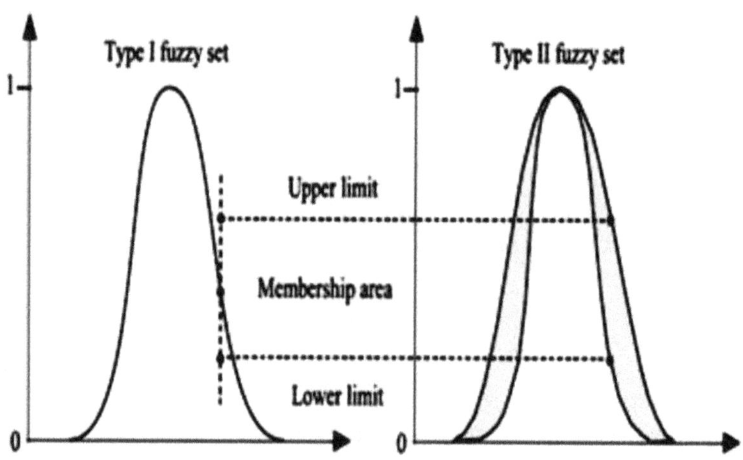

The type-2 fuzzy set has the ability to cope with uncertainty in a much better way than its counterparts like the type-1 fuzzy set, intuitionistic fuzzy set etc (Bora et al, 2018; Mendeal eta l, 2002; Chaira, 2014) so it has been adopted almost all the key areas of medical image processing like contrast improvement, edge detection, segmentation etc.

HE Stain Images

HE stain image is regarded as of gold standard in histology and pathology laboratories ("H&E Stain", 2018; "Wikipedia H0026E Stain", n.d.). These images are widely used in medical diagnosis as they lead to accurate diagnosis process. Normally, most cells are found colorless and transparent. So, it is a very difficult process to analyze them. In staining, the histological sections are stained in such a way these cells should be visible. HE stain is one of such popularly adopted staining technique. In this technique, hematoxylin and eosin are used to color nuclei and cytoplasm differently (Paxton et al, 2003). Hematoxylin is a dark blue or violet stain. This is basic/positive by nature. While, Eosin is a red or pink stain and is Acidic / Negative by nature. When, hematoxylin and eosin are combined, it produces blues, violets, and reds. It is a strong belief among many pathologists that as there exists a long history of H&E, well-established methods, and a good amount of data and publications, H&E will continue to be the universal practice over the next 50 years (Paxton et al, 2018). But, like other medical images, HE Stain images also suffer from fuzziness near or on the boundaries. Due to the high amount of vagueness, it is very hard to distinguish the boundaries separating different cells or ROIs. Because of this, segmentation of such images to analyze the ROIs become more complicated in the case if we employ some traditional hard clustering based techniques. So, there arises the need of a soft computing based technique cluster or segment different regions. Also, it is recommended to remove the fuzziness as much as possible or to a maximum possible before the final segmentation process. So, in this chapter we focus on such advanced fuzzy set-based technique which can result an efficient segmentation of HE stain images.

HSV Color Space

Color space is an abstract mathematical model used for representing colors in terms of intensity values with respect to a specific coordinate system which generally is a three dimensional system. There exists a number of different types of color spaces, each with a different feature or characteristic. RGB is the default color space. But, the main problem with RGB color space is that here intensity values are associated with each of the three channels: Red, Green and Blue. There is not any devoted channel for intensity level measurement. So, if changes occur to any channel, then color misclassification may take place. HSV color space is a good alternative in this case. Here, three channels are associated: Hue (H), Saturation(S) and Value (V) ("Wikipedia HSL and HSV", n.d.). Hue can be characterized as an angle in the range $[0,2\pi]$ and is straightly related to color (Bora eta l, 2016). With respect to different hue angles, different colors can be obtained. Saturation is used to describe how pure

Figure 3. A Sample HE stain image ("[Medisp.bme.teiath.g", 2018)

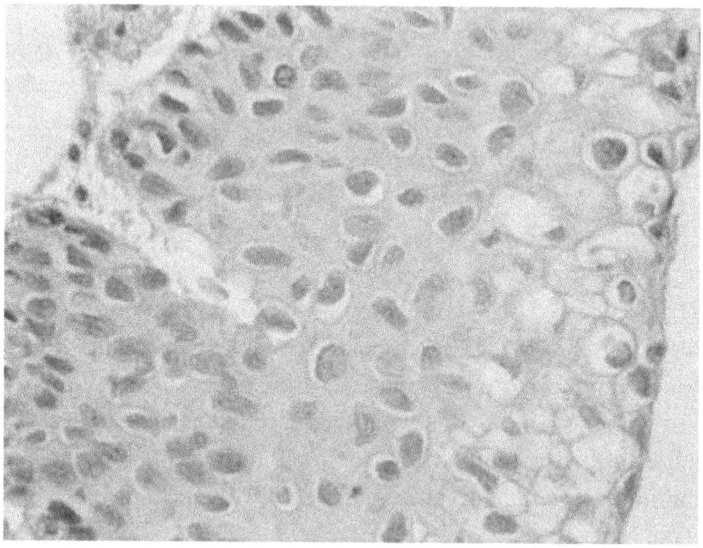

the hue is with respect to a white reference. This is calculated as a radial distance from the central axis with values between 0 at the center to 1 at the outer surface (Bora eta l, 2016). The V channel or value channel symbolizes a percentage value in the range from 0 to 100 which expresses the amount of light illuminating a color. The V channel in HSV color space operates as a devoted channel for intensity level measurements. This is the reason, why we have selected HSV color space for our proposed approach. The segmentation task is employed on the V-channel and hence there is not a chance for color miss-classification. A details and in-depth study on color space and HSV color space is presented in (Bora, 2017).

EXPERIMENT AND RESULT DISCUSSION SECTION

The proposed algorithm has been tested on over 30 different HE stain images. In this paper, results are shown for three HE stain images among them which are collected from the public data set (Shamir et al, 2008). To compare the efficiency of the proposed technique, we have adopted three frequently adopted algorithms K-Means, FCM and watershed algorithm. Watershed-based algorithm selected for segmentation is a recent one proposed in (Bora et al, 2015). The results are analyzed both subjectively and objectively.

Figure 4. Coordinate System for HSV Color Space

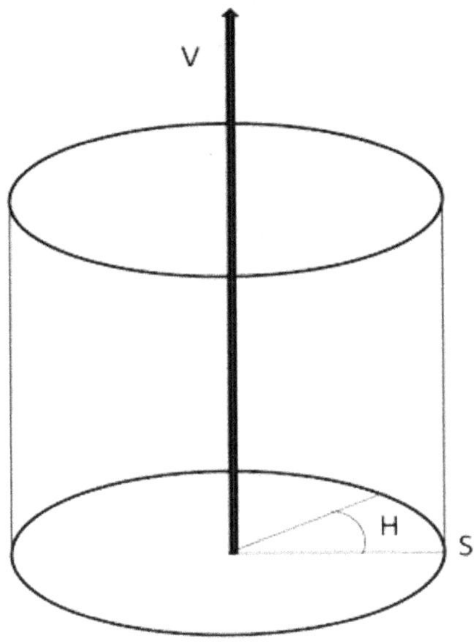

Subjective Evaluation

The subjective evaluation is carried out through the feedbacks obtained on the segmentation results by five different experts from the subject domain. They have given a Minimum Evaluation Score (MES) which is a value from the range 0 to 10 where o indicating worst segmentation and 10 as the best. While an MES value >=5 is desired to consider a segmentation technique as a good one. While an MES value <5 is considered as not a recommendable technique for the segmentation task.

So, on average, we have seen that MES values for K-Means algorithm is *5.4*, Watershed Algorithm is *2.6*, FCM is *6.2* and Proposed Algorithm is ***7.2***. So, from their opinion, K-Means,FCM, and Proposed algorithm are suitable for HE Stain Color image segmentation. As the proposed algorithm is possessing a highest MES value, so, it is the most recommended one for HE Stain image segmentation.

If the results are observed closely, then it is obvious that watershed algorithm is suffering from over segmentation as redundant regions are produced here making it difficult to analyze them. K-Means algorithm succeeds to isolate the different ROIs but still some noise sensitivity issues are there in between different ROIs. This is less in case of FCM, but here also, we can not say that fuzziness around the boundaries are removed fully as from the results it is clear that ambiguity lies on boundaries, darker regions are produced and hence, making it difficult to accurately analyze consecutive ROIs. But, in case of the proposed type-2 fuzzy set based segmentation

Figure 5. (a) Original HE Stain image (b) Segmentation by K-Means Algorithm; (c) Segmentation by Watershed Based Technique; (d) Segmentation by FCM Algorithm; (e) Segmentation by Our Proposed Technique

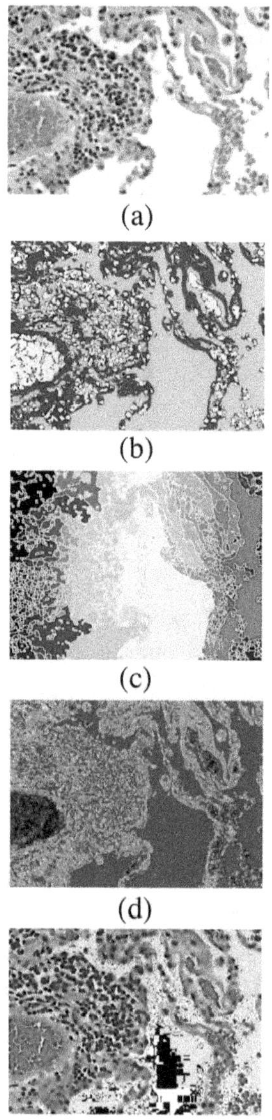

(a) (b) (c) (d) (e)

Figure 6. (a) Original HE Stain image (b) Segmentation by K-Means Algorithm; (c) Segmentation by Watershed Based Technique; (d) Segmentation by FCM Algorithm; (e) Segmentation by Our Proposed Technique

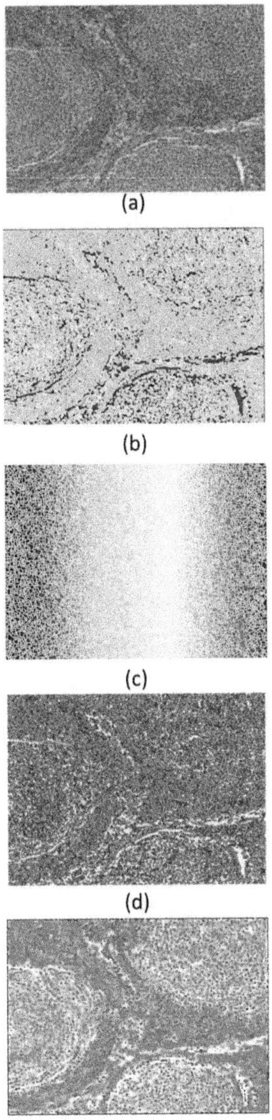

Figure 7. (a) Original HE Stain image (b) Segmentation by K-Means Algorithm; (c) Segmentation by Watershed Based Technique; (d) Segmentation by FCM Algorithm; (e) Segmentation by Our Proposed Technique

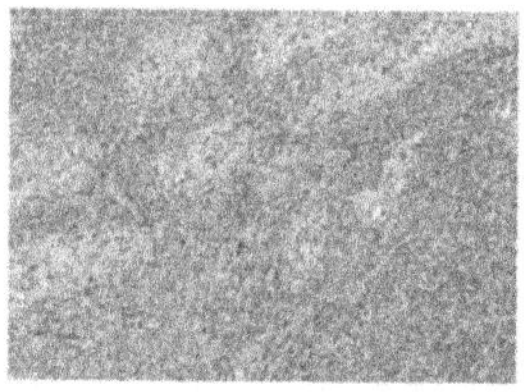

(a)

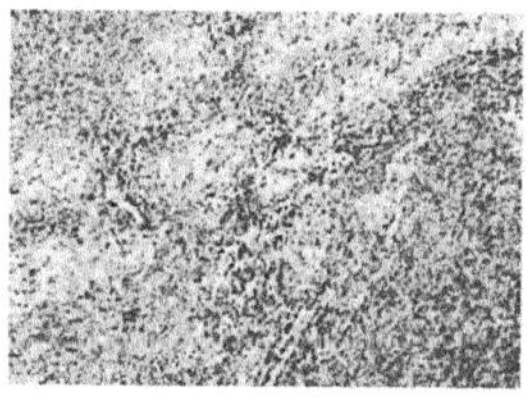

(b)

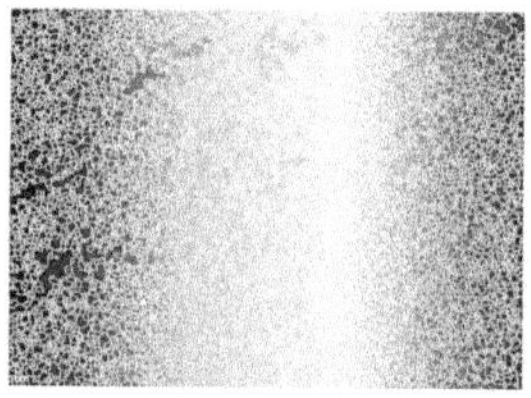

(c)

(d)

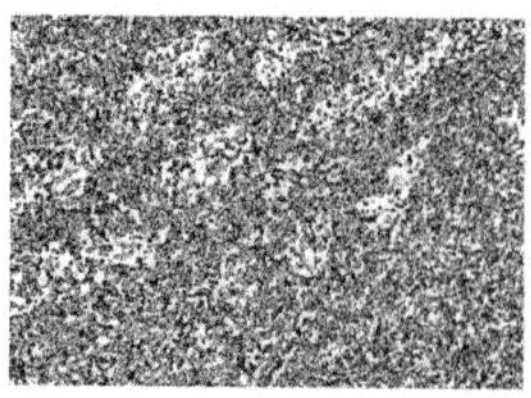

(e)

Table 1. Subjective Evaluation

	K-Means Algorithm	Watershed Algorithm	FCM Algorithm	Proposed Algorithm
Expert 1	6	3	6	7
Expert 2	5	2	5	7
Expert 3	5	3	6	6
Expert 4	6	3	7	8
Expert 5	5	2	7	8

technique, ambiguity is removed to a satisfactory level. Different ROIs are clearly distinguishable with more distinct edges.

Objective Analysis

When it comes to analysis of the segmentation results, subjective evaluation matters a lot as ultimately the results are going to be analyzed by some person of relevant expertise. But, the subjective evaluation may vary from person to person. So, it is suggested to claim the efficiency of a technique through some objective measures. Here, we have selected two metrics for objective evaluation: PSNR and MSSIM.

The PSNR value of an image is calculated using the following equation.

$$PSNR = 10\log_{10}(\frac{MAX_i^2}{MSE}) \quad (14)$$

where MAX_i the maximum possible pixel value of the image and MSE is the Mean Squared Error which is given by the following equation no.(15):

$$MSE = \sum_{y=1}^{M}\sum_{x=1}^{N}[\mathrm{I}(\mathrm{x},\mathrm{y}) - \mathrm{I}'(\mathrm{x},\mathrm{y})]^2 \quad (15)$$

where, M, N are the dimensions of the image and I(x,y) is the original image, I'(x,y) is the segmented version of it.

The Comparison can be observed more clearly from Figure 8.

So, the results from the proposed algorithm succeed to produce higher PSNR values than the other algorithms under consideration. So, this signifies that the segmentation results from the proposed algorithm are less suffering from noises and hence producing a better segmentation result.

Table 2. PSNR Values Comparison

	K-Means Algorithm	Watershed Algorithm	FCM Algorithm	Proposed Algorithm
Image: 1	15.31	11.13	17.05	19.81
Image: 2	15.63	14.41	20.66	21.24
Image: 3	17.3	15.54	17.9	19.98

Figure 8. Comparison of PSNR Values With Respect to The Concerned Algorithms

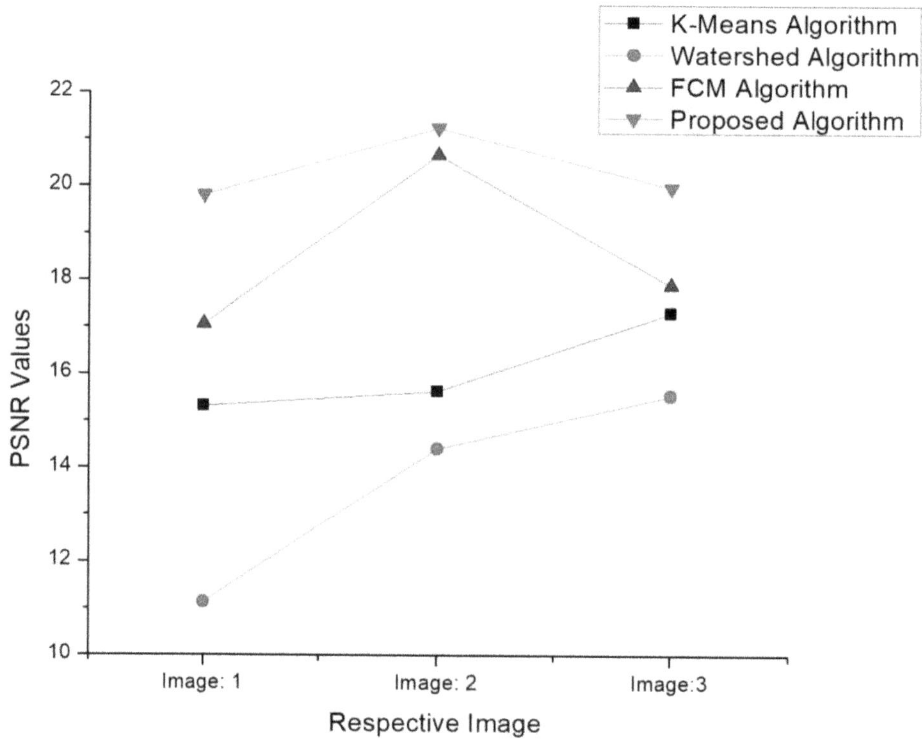

MSSIM

SSIM index was proposed by Zhou Wang et al (2004). SSIM has the ability to automatically predict perceived image quality(in our case, quality of the segmented version with respect to original HE stain image). We have used mean SSIM (MSSIM) index to estimate the overall image quality (Dey et al, 2017).

$$mssim(IMG1, IMG2) = \frac{1}{N}\sum_{i=1}^{N} ssim(img1_i, img2_i) \quad (16)$$

where IMG1 is the original image and IMG2 is its segmented version.; img1i and img2 i are the image contents in the ith local window and N is the total number of the local windows of the image. A higher value of mssim implies a better quality of segmentation. The MSSIM values for all the images with respect to the algorithms under consideration are shown in Table 3.

The Comparison can be observed more clearly from the Figure 9.

So, we have seen that the proposed algorithm is showing a comparatively higher MSSIM value than the other algorithms under consideration. This signifies a better quality of the segmentation result from the proposed algorithm. A better quality segmentation fuels a better analysis of inner structures of a medical image and thereby leads to an accurate diagnosis result (Rajinikanth et al, 2018).

Time

Now, to measure and compare the time complexities of the proposed algorithm with the other algorithms under consideration, we have calculated the time consumed by the algorithms during whole segmentation process and mentioned in the following table. It may be noted that this time calculations may slightly vary from system to system with respect to the processing power of the same. Hence, it should be considered as an approximate evaluation, not as a constant or fixed value.

The Comparison can be observed more clearly from Figure 10.

So, from Figure 10, it is clear that K-Means algorithm is taking least amount of time and FCM is taking a higher amount of time than K-Means algorithm. While watershed algorithm and our proposed algorithm is taking more time for the segmentation than K-Means and FCM.

Table 3. MSSIM Values Comparison

	K-Means Algorithm	Watershed Algorithm	FCM-Algorithm	The Proposed Algorithm
Image: 1	0.5315	0.4011	0.5813	0.6519
Image: 2	0.4243	0.4096	0.5671	0.7661
Image: 3	0.5985	0.4441	0.7509	0.7872

Figure 9. Comparison of MSSIM Values With Respect to The Concerned Algorithms

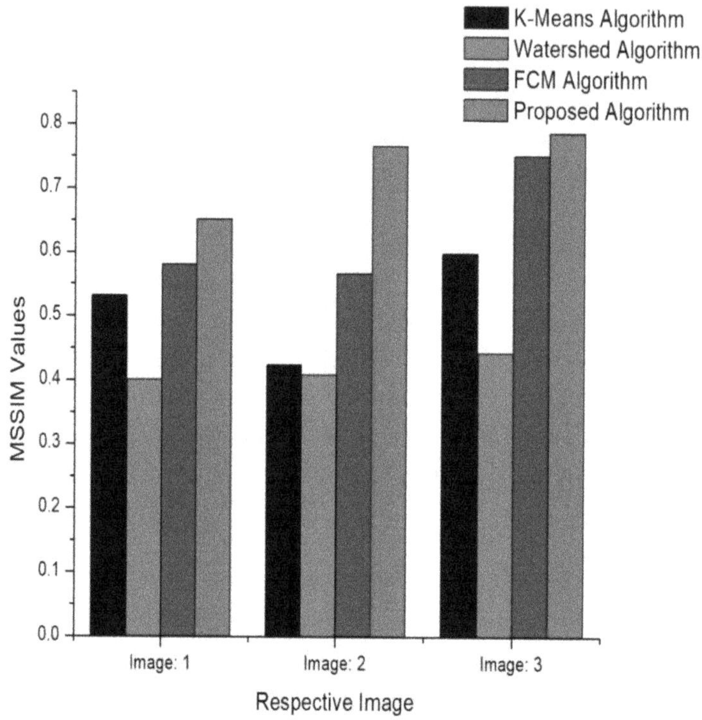

Table 4. Time Taken by The Respective Algorithms (in Seconds)

	K-Means Algorithm	Watershed Algorithm	FCM Algorithm	Proposed Algorithm
Image: 1	4.817440	17.218066	12.04142	17.825420
Image: 2	7.593150	17.018576	15.011287	15.332220
Image: 3	9.946874	11.983450	11.76424	11.828165

CONCLUSION AND SUGGESTIONS

HE Stain image helps to achieve an accurate diagnosis of different diseases. Segmentation is an advanced image processing technique which fuels the analysis process by isolating different regions of interests in an image. A proper segmentation of HE stain image is very crucial as these images involve a very high level of fuzziness with them. So, traditional hard clustering based algorithm may not be able to deal with such high level of ambiguity and as a result, over-segmentation may arise. This is the common case in the boundary areas surrounding the tissues

Figure 10. Comparison of time consumption by the concerned algorithms

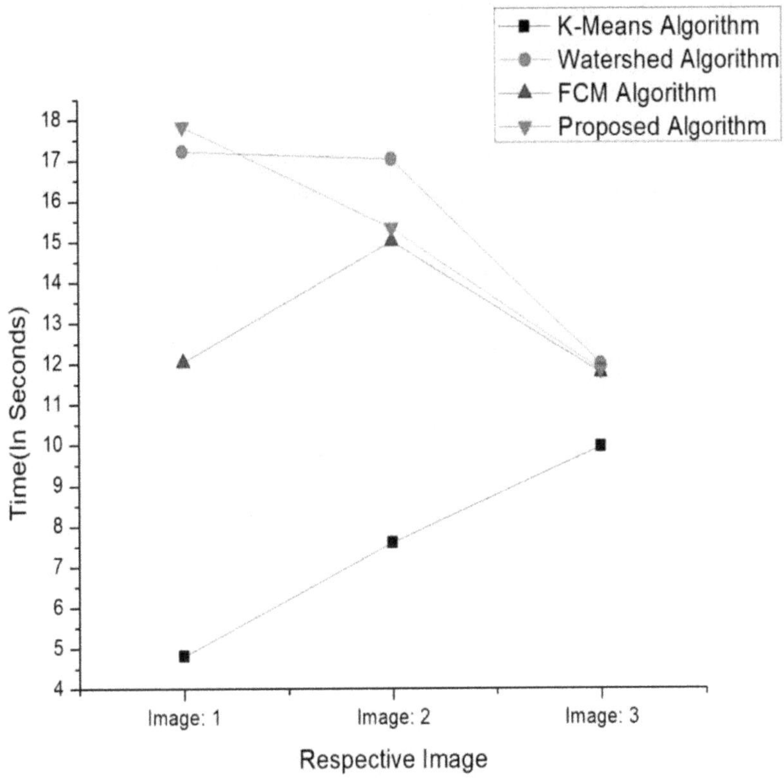

and nuclei in the image. So, a type-2 fuzzy set-based technique for HE Stain image segmentation is introduced in this chapter. Color computations are taken very seriously in this technique and HSV color space is chosen for the same. Such that no color miss-classification arise, the segmentation is done on V channel only. Results are compared with some popular and most frequently adapted algorithms for color image segmentation: K-Means, Watershed and FCM algorithm. After both the subjective and objective evaluations, it is found that the proposed technique succeeds to produce better segmentation results than the others algorithms under comparison. So, following suggestions are made with respect to HE Stain image segmentation:

1. It is suggested that while going for developing a technique for HE Stain image segmentation, an advanced fuzzy set-based technique like type-2 fuzzy set should be given more preference than the other clustering algorithms like K-Means algorithm, FCM algorithm. Even FCM is not suitable in this case as the membership function itself may contain a certain level of fuzziness.

2. Watershed algorithm alone can not deal with the high-level ambiguity presents in such images and hence usually results in over-segmentation. So, some measures should be taken in order to take care of this over segmentation problem.
3. Color space selection and a proper channel selection from the selected color space is a very important task and also an unavoidable issue in this case. As otherwise, color miss-classification may arise. So, a channel which is a devoted one especially for intensity level measurements should be selected for the segmentation task. V channel of HSV color space is a good choice in this case. Similarly, L channel in LAB color space also an alternative to this.

The only drawback of the proposed algorithm is that it involves a high level of time complexity, higher than FCM and K-Means algorithm. So, future study lies in minimizing the time complexity of the proposed approach. But, in case of an accurate image analysis and hence for a proper diagnosis process, this can be sacrificed since here getting an error-free result is more important than a few seconds of delay.

REFERENCES

Bezdek, J. C. (1981). Objective Function Clustering. In *Pattern recognition with fuzzy objective function algorithms* (pp. 43–93). Boston, MA: Springer. doi:10.1007/978-1-4757-0450-1_3

Bora, D. (2017). Performance Comparison of K-Means Algorithm and FCM Algorithm with Respect to Color Image Segmentation. *International Journal of Emerging Technology and Advanced Engineering, 7*, 460–470. doi:10.6084/m9.figshare.5394313

Bora, D. J. (2017). *Importance of image enhancement techniques in color image segmentation: A comprehensive and comparative study*. arXiv preprint arXiv:1708.05081

Bora, D. J. (2018). An Ideal Approach for Medical Color Image Enhancement. In *Advanced Computational and Communication Paradigms* (pp. 351–361). Singapore: Springer. doi:10.1007/978-981-10-8237-5_34

Bora, D. J., & Gupta, A. K. (2014). *Impact of exponent parameter value for the partition matrix on the performance of fuzzy C means Algorithm*. arXiv preprint arXiv:1406.4007

Bora, D. J., & Gupta, A. K. (2016, December). AERASCIS: An efficient and robust approach for satellite color image segmentation. In *Electrical Power and Energy Systems (ICEPES), International Conference on* (pp. 549-556). IEEE.

Bora, D. J., Gupta, A. K., & Khan, F. A. (2015). Color Image Segmentation Using An Efficient Fuzzy Based Watershed Approach. *Signal & Image Processing International Journal (Toronto, Ont.)*, *6*(5), 15–34.

Bora, D. J., & Thakur, R. S. (2018). An Efficient Technique for Medical Image Enhancement Based on Interval Type-2 Fuzzy Set Logic. In Progress in Computing, Analytics and Networking (pp. 667-678). Springer. doi:10.1007/978-981-10-7871-2_64

Chaira, T. (2014). An improved medical image enhancement scheme using Type II fuzzy set. *Applied Soft Computing*, *25*, 293–308. doi:10.1016/j.asoc.2014.09.004

De Oliveira, D. L. L., Do Nascimento, M. Z., Neves, L. A., De Godoy, M. F., De Arruda, P. F. F., & de Santi Neto, D. (2013). Unsupervised segmentation method for cuboidal cell nuclei in histological prostate images based on minimum cross entropy. *Expert Systems with Applications*, *40*(18), 7331–7340. doi:10.1016/j.eswa.2013.06.079

Dey, N., & Ashour, A. S. (2017). *Meta-Heuristic Algorithms in Medical Image Segmentation: A Review*. Advancements in Applied Metaheuristic Computing.

Dhanachandra, N., Manglem, K., & Chanu, Y. J. (2015). Image segmentation using K-means clustering algorithm and subtractive clustering algorithm. *Procedia Computer Science*, *54*, 764–771. doi:10.1016/j.procs.2015.06.090

Dimitropoulos, K., Barmpoutis, P., Koletsa, T., Kostopoulos, I., & Grammalidis, N. (2017). Automated detection and classification of nuclei in PAX5 and H&E-stained tissue sections of follicular lymphoma. *SIViP*, *11*(1), 145–153. doi:10.100711760-016-0913-6

en.wikipedia.org. (2018). *H0026E stain*. Available at: https://en.wikipedia.org/wiki/H

Gurcan, M. N., Boucheron, L. E., Can, A., Madabhushi, A., Rajpoot, N. M., & Yener, B. (2009). Histopathological image analysis: A review. *IEEE Reviews in Biomedical Engineering*, *2*, 147–171. doi:10.1109/RBME.2009.2034865 PMID:20671804

H&E Stain. (2018). Available at: https://cytoinformatics.com/Cyto/he-stain

HE Stain. (n.d.). Retrieved from https://en.wikipedia.org/wiki/H\%26E_stain

Jain, A. K. (1989). *Fundamentals of digital image processing*. Prentice-Hall, Inc.

Liu, F., Mackey, A. L., Srikuea, R., Esser, K. A., & Yang, L. (2013). Automated image segmentation of haematoxylin and eosin stained skeletal muscle crossâ€ sections. *Journal of Microscopy*, *252*(3), 275–285. doi:10.1111/jmi.12090 PMID:24118017

Mendel, J. M., & John, R. B. (2002). Type-2 fuzzy sets made simple. *IEEE Transactions on Fuzzy Systems*, *10*(2), 117–127. doi:10.1109/91.995115

Nguyen, L., Tosun, A.B., Fine, J.L., Lee, A.V., Taylor, D.L., & Chennubhotla, S.C. (2017). Spatial statistics for segmenting histological structures in H&E stained tissue images. *IEEE Transactions on Medical Imaging*, 1522-1532.

Paxton, S. A., & Peckham, M. (2003). *The Leeds Histology Guide.* Available at: http://www.histology.leeds.ac.uk/tissue_types/epithelia/epi_stratified.php

Pei-Gee, Ho. (2012). *Image Segmentation.* InTech. Retrieved from: http://www. intechopen. com/books/image-segmentation

Rajinikanth, V. (2018). DWT-PCA Image Fusion Technique to Improve Segmentation Accuracy in Brain Tumor Analysis. In *Microelectronics, Electromagnetics and Telecommunications* (pp. 453–462). Singapore: Springer. doi:10.1007/978-981-10-7329-8_46

Shamir, L., Orlov, N., Eckley, D. M., Macura, T. J., & Goldberg, I. G. (2008). IICBU 2008: A proposed benchmark suite for biological image analysis. *Medical & Biological Engineering & Computing*, *46*(9), 943–947. doi:10.100711517-008-0380-5 PMID:18668273

Shi, P., Zhong, J., Huang, R., & Lin, J. (2016, December). Automated Quantitative Image Analysis of Hematoxylin-Eosin Staining Slides in Lymphoma Based on Hierarchical Kmeans Clustering. In *Information Technology in Medicine and Education (ITME), 2016 8th International Conference on* (pp. 99-104). IEEE. 10.1109/ITME.2016.0031

Veta, M., van Diest, P. J., Kornegoor, R., Huisman, A., Viergever, M. A., & Pluim, J. P. (2013). Automatic nuclei segmentation in H&E stained breast cancer histopathology images. *PLoS One*, *8*(7), e70221. doi:10.1371/journal.pone.0070221 PMID:23922958

Wang, Z., Bovik, A. C., Sheikh, H. R., & Simoncelli, E. P. (2004). Image quality assessment: From error visibility to structural similarity. *IEEE Transactions on Image Processing*, *13*(4), 600–612. doi:10.1109/TIP.2003.819861 PMID:15376593

Wienert, S., Heim, D., Saeger, K., Stenzinger, A., Beil, M., Hufnagl, P., ... Klauschen, F. (2012). Detection and segmentation of cell nuclei in virtual microscopy images: A minimum-model approach. *Scientific Reports*, *2*(1), 503. doi:10.1038rep00503 PMID:22787560

Zadeh, L. (1965). Fuzzy sets. *Information and Control*, *8*(3), 338–353. doi:10.1016/S0019-9958(65)90241-X

Zadeh, L. A. (1975). The concept of a linguistic variable and its application to approximate reasoningâ€"I. *Information Sciences*, *8*(3), 199–249. doi:10.1016/0020-0255(75)90036-5

Compilation of References

Abadi, M., Agarwal, A., Barham, P., Brevdo, E., Chen, Z., Citro, C., … Zheng, X. (2015). *TensorFlow: Large-scale machine learning on heterogeneous systems*. Available from tensorflow.org

Abdaheer, S. M., & Khan, E. (2009). Shaped based classification of breast tumors using fractal analysis. In *Proceeding of IEEE conference of Multimedia, Signal Processing and Communication Technologies* (pp. 272-275). Aligarh, India: IEEE.

Abhinaya, B., & Raja, N. S. M. (2015). Solving multi-level image thresholding problem—an analysis with cuckoo search algorithm. *Advances In Intelligent Systems And Computing*, *339*, 177–186. doi:10.1007/978-81-322-2250-7_18

Abo-Zahhad, M., Gharieb, R. R., Ahmed, S. M., & Abd-Ellah, M. K. (2015). Huffman image compression incorporating DPCM and DWT. *Journal of Signal and Information Processing*, *6*(02), 123–135. doi:10.4236/jsip.2015.62012

Ada & Kaur, R. (2013). Feature extraction and principal component analysis for lung cancer detection in CT images. *International Journal of Advanced Research in Computer Science and Software Engineering*, *3*(3), 187–190.

Agrawal, M., & Choudhary, R. R. (2016, August). Median Edge Detector for Lossless Video Coding: An efficient prediction scheme for lossless video coding. In *Proceedings of the International Conference on Advances in Information Communication Technology & Computing* (p. 40). ACM. 10.1145/2979779.2979819

Aharon, M., Elad, M., & Bruckstein, A. (2006). K-SVD: An Algorithm for Designing Overcomplete Dictionaries for Sparse Representation. *IEEE Transactions on Signal Processing*, *54*(11), 4311–4322. doi:10.1109/TSP.2006.881199

Ahmad, M., & Alam, M. S. (2009). A New Algorithm of Encryption and Decryption of Images using Chaotic Mapping. *International Journal on Computer Science and Engineering*, *02*(01), 46–50.

Akramifard, H., Firouzmand, M., & Moghadam, R. A. (2012). Extracting, recognizing, and counting white blood cells from microscopic images by using complex-valued neural networks. *Journal of Medical Signals and Sensors*, *2*(3), 169–175. PMID:23717809

Al-amri, S. S., Kalyankar, N. V., & Khamitkar, S. D. (2010). Image Segmentation by using Thresholding Technique. *Journal of Computers*, *2*(5), 83–86.

Ali, U., Shaukat, A., Hussain, M., Ali, J., Khan, K., Khan, M. B., & Shah, M. A. (2016). Automatic Cancerous Tissue Classification using Discrete Wavelet Transformation and Support Vector Machine. *Journal of Basic and Applied Scientific Research*, *6*(7), 15–23.

Al-Kofahi, Y., Lassoued, W., Lee, W., & Roysam, B. (2010). Improved Automatic Detection and Segmentation of Cell Nuclei in Histopathology Images. *IEEE Transactions on Biomedical Engineering*, *57*(4), 841–852. doi:10.1109/TBME.2009.2035102 PMID:19884070

Alvarez-Ramos, C. M., Niño, E., & Santos, M. (2013). Automatic Classification of Nosema Pathogenic Agents through Machine Vision techniques and Kernel-based Vector Machines. *IEEE, 8th Computing Colombian Conference.*

Andrion, A., Magnani, C., Betta, P. G., Donna, A., Mollo, F., Scelsi, M., ... Terracini, B. (1995). Malignant mesothelioma of the pleura: Inter-observer variability. *Journal of Clinical Pathology*, *48*(9), 856–860. doi:10.1136/jcp.48.9.856 PMID:7490321

Anitha, P., Bindhiya, S., Abinaya, A., Satapathy, S. C., Dey, N., & Rajinikanth, V. (2017). RGB image multi-thresholding based on Kapur's entropy—A study with heuristic algorithms. *Second International Conference on Electrical, Computer and Communication Technologies (ICECCT).* 10.1109/ICECCT.2017.8117823

Anonymous. (2008). Bee mortality and bee surveillance in Europe. *EFSA Journal*, *154*, 1–28.

Anonymous. (2009). *Colony Collapse Disorder Progress Report.* CCD Steering Committee.

Anzalone, A., Fusco, G., Isgro, F., Orlandi, E., Prevete, R., Sciortino, G., ... Valenti, C. (2013). A System for the Automatic Measurement of the Nuchal Translucency Thickness from Ultrasound Video Stream of the Foetus. *Proceedings of the 26th IEEE International Symposium on Computer-Based Medical Systems*, 239-44. 10.1109/CBMS.2013.6627795

Araújo, T., Aresta, G., Castro, E., Rouco, J., Aguiar, P., Eloy, C., ... Campilho, A. (2017). Classification of breast cancer histology images using Convolutional. *Neural Networks*, *12*(6), e0177544. doi:10.1371/journal.pone.0177544 PMID:28570557

Arrowsmith, D. K., Cartwright, J. H. E., Lansbury, A. N., & Place, C. M. (1993). The Bogdanov Map: Bifurcations, Mode Locking, and Chaos in a Dissipative System. *International Journal of Bifurcation and Chaos in Applied Sciences and Engineering*, *3*(04), 803–842. doi:10.1142/S021812749300074X

Ashour, A. S., Samanta, S., Dey, N., Kausar, N., Abdessalemkaraa, W. B., & Hassanien, A. E. (2015). Computed tomography image enhancement using cuckoo search: A log transform based approach. *Journal of Signal and Information Processing*, *6*(3), 244–257. doi:10.4236/jsip.2015.63023

Asvestas, P., Matsopoulos, G. K., & Nikita, K. S. (1998). A power differentiation method of fractal dimension estimation for 2-D signals. *Journal of Visual Communication and Image Representation*, *9*(4), 392–400. doi:10.1006/jvci.1998.0394

Aswathy, M. A., & Jagannath, M. (2017). Detection of breast cancer on digital histopathology images: Present status and future possibilities. *Informatics in Medicine Unlocked*, *8*, 74–79. doi:10.1016/j.imu.2016.11.001

Avramović, A., & Savić, S. (2011). Lossless predictive compression of medical images. *Serbian Journal of Electrical Engineering*, *8*(1), 27–36. doi:10.2298/SJEE1101027A

Ayoobkhan, M. U. A., Chikkannan, E., & Ramakrishnan, K. (2017). Feed-Forward Neural Network-Based Predictive Image Coding for Medical Image Compression. *Arabian Journal for Science and Engineering*, 1–9.

Babu, P. S., & Sathappan, S. (2015). Efficient lossless image compression using modified hierarchical prediction and context adaptive coding. *Indian Journal of Science and Technology*, *8*(34), 1–6.

Bairagi, V. K., & Sapkal, A. M. (2013). ROI-based DICOM image compression for telemedicine. *Sadhana*, *38*(1), 123–131. doi:10.100712046-013-0126-4

Balan, N. S., Kumar, A. S., Raja, N. S. M., & Rajinikanth, V. (2016). Optimal multilevel image thresholding to improve the visibility of plasmodium sp. in blood smear images. *Advances in Intelligent Systems and Computing*, *397*, 563–571. doi:10.1007/978-81-322-2671-0_54

Balle, J., Laparra, V., & Simoncelli, E. P. (2016). End-to-end optimization of nonlinear transform codes for perceptual quality. In *Proceedings of Picture Coding Symposium (PCS)*, (*vol. 16*, pp. 1-5). Academic Press. 10.1109/PCS.2016.7906310

Banu, N. M., & Sujatha, S. (2015). 3D medical image compression: A review. *Indian Journal of Science and Technology*, *8*(12).

Barik, R. K., Dubey, H., Misra, C., Borthakur, D., Constant, N., Sasane, S. A., & Mankodiya, K. (2018). Fog Assisted Cloud Computing in Era of Big Data and Internet-of-Things: Systems, Architectures, and Applications. In *Cloud Computing for Optimization: Foundations, Applications, and Challenges* (pp. 367–394). Cham: Springer. doi:10.1007/978-3-319-73676-1_14

Basavanhallya, A., Yu, E., Xu, J., Ganesan, S., Feldman, M., Tomaszewski, J., Madabhushi, A. (2011). Incorporating Domain Knowledge for tubule detection in breast histopathology using O'Callaghan neighborhoods, *SPIE Medical Imaging, 7963: 796310.*

Base, A. M., Jancke, K., Wismuller, A., Foo, S., & Martinetz, T. (2005). Medical image compression using topology-preserving neural networks. *International Journal of Engineering Applications of Artificial Intelligence*, *18*(4), 383–392. doi:10.1016/j.engappai.2004.10.004

Belsare, A. (2012). Histopathological Image Analysis Using Image Processing Techniques: An Overview. *Signal and Image Processing: an International Journal*, *3*(4), 23–36. doi:10.5121ipij.2012.3403

Bezdek, J. C. (1981). Objective Function Clustering. In *Pattern recognition with fuzzy objective function algorithms* (pp. 43–93). Boston, MA: Springer. doi:10.1007/978-1-4757-0450-1_3

Bigdeli, N., Farid, Y., & Afshar, K. (2012). A novel image encryption/decryption scheme based on chaotic neural networks. *Engineering Applications of Artificial Intelligence, Elsevier, 25*(4), 753–765. doi:10.1016/j.engappai.2012.01.007

Biswas, M. K., Ghose, T., Guha, S., & Biswas, P. K. (1998). Fractal dimension estimation for texture images: A parallel approach. *Pattern Recognition Letters, 19*(3-4), 309–313. doi:10.1016/S0167-8655(98)00002-6

Blanton, R., Levitt, J., Thompson, P., Narr, K., Capetillo, C. L., Nobel, A., & Singerman, J. (2001). Mapping cortical asymmetry and complexity patterns in normal children. *Psychiatry Research, 107*(1), 29–43. doi:10.1016/S0925-4927(01)00091-9 PMID:11472862

Blessa Binolin Pepsi, M., & Bargavi, G. (2017). Analysis of Accuracy and Performance of Big Data using Data Mining Techniques in Hadoop Mapreduce. In *Advances and Applied Sciences* (Vol. 11). AENSI Publisher.

Bora, D. J. (2017). *Importance of image enhancement techniques in color image segmentation: A comprehensive and comparative study*. arXiv preprint arXiv:1708.05081

Bora, D. J., & Gupta, A. K. (2014). *Impact of exponent parameter value for the partition matrix on the performance of fuzzy C means Algorithm.* arXiv preprint arXiv:1406.4007

Bora, D. J., & Gupta, A. K. (2016, December). AERASCIS: An efficient and robust approach for satellite color image segmentation. In *Electrical Power and Energy Systems (ICEPES), International Conference on* (pp. 549-556). IEEE.

Bora, D. J., & Thakur, R. S. (2018). An Efficient Technique for Medical Image Enhancement Based on Interval Type-2 Fuzzy Set Logic. In Progress in Computing, Analytics and Networking (pp. 667-678). Springer. doi:10.1007/978-981-10-7871-2_64

Bora, D. (2017). Performance Comparison of K-Means Algorithm and FCM Algorithm with Respect to Color Image Segmentation. *International Journal of Emerging Technology and Advanced Engineering, 7*, 460–470. doi:10.6084/m9.figshare.5394313

Bora, D. J. (2018). An Ideal Approach for Medical Color Image Enhancement. In *Advanced Computational and Communication Paradigms* (pp. 351–361). Singapore: Springer. doi:10.1007/978-981-10-8237-5_34

Bora, D. J., Gupta, A. K., & Khan, F. A. (2015). Color Image Segmentation Using An Efficient Fuzzy Based Watershed Approach. *Signal & Image Processing International Journal (Toronto, Ont.), 6*(5), 15–34.

Borujeni, S. E., & Eshghi, M. (2009). *Chaotic Image Encryption Design using Tompkins-Paige Algorithm. Mathematical Problems in Engineering.*

Bovik, A. C., Wang, Z., & Simoncelli, E. P. (2003). Multiscale structural similarity for image quality assessment. In *Proceedings of the Thirty-Seventh Asilomar Conference on Signals, Systems and Computers* (vol. 2, pp. 1398–1402). IEEE.

Brajevic, I., Tuba, M., & Bacanin, N. (2012). Multilevel image thresholding selection based on the Cuckoo search algorithm. *Proceedings of the 5th International Conference on Visualization, Imaging and Simulation (VIS'12)*, 217–222.

Bravo, J., Carbonell, V., Valdebenedito, J. T., Figueroa, C., Valdovinos, C. E., Martín-Hérnandez, R., ... Delporte, C. (2014). Identification of Nosemaceranaein the Valparaíso District, Chile. *Archivos de Medicina Veterinaria*, *46*(3), 487–491. doi:10.4067/S0301-732X2014000300021

Buades, A., Coll, B., & Morel, J.-M. (2005). A Non-Local Algorithm for Image Denoising. *2005 IEEE Computer Society Conference on Computer Vision and Pattern Recognition (CVPR'05)*, *2*, 60-65. 10.1109/CVPR.2005.38

Bullmore, E., Brammer, M., Harvey, I., Persaud, R., Murray, R., & Ron, M. (1994). Fractal analysis of the boundary between white matter and cerebral cortex in magnetic resonance images: A controlled study of schizophrenic and manic-depressive patients. *Psychological Medicine*, *24*(03), 771–781. doi:10.1017/S0033291700027926 PMID:7991759

Cai, X., & Lim, J. S. (2015, March). Adaptive residual DPCM for lossless intra coding. In *Visual Information Processing and Communication VI* (Vol. 9410). International Society for Optics and Photonics.

Calderón, R. A., & Pichardo, J. (2011). *Nosemiasis en abejas melíferas: diagnóstico, control y prevalencia*. Heredia.

Calderón, R. A., & Ramírez, F. (2010). *Enfermedades de las abejas melíferas, con énfasis en abejas africanizadas* (Vol. 125). Heredia, Costa Rica: Ed. CINAT-UNA.

Calderón, R. A., & Sánchez, L. (2001). Diagnóstico de enfermedades en colmenas de abejas africanizadas en Costa Rica: Prevalencia y distribución de setiembre a noviembre del 2007. *Agronomia Costarricense*, *35*, 49–60.

Carlsson, S., Chen, J., & Mattsson, C. (1996). Heaps with bits. *Theoretical Computer Science*, *164*(1-2), 1–12. doi:10.1016/0304-3975(95)00152-2

Caselles, V., Catte, F., Coll, T., & Dibos, F. (1993). A geometric model for active contours in image processing. *Numerische Mathematik*, *66*(1), 1–31. doi:10.1007/BF01385685

Caughey, A. B., Lyell, D. J., Filly, R. A., Washington, E. A., & Norton, M. E. (2001). The Impact of the Use of the Isolated Echogenic Intracardiac Focus as a Screen for Down Syndrome in Women under the Age of 35 Years. *American Journal of Obstetrics and Gynecology*, *185*(5), 1021–1027. doi:10.1067/mob.2001.117674 PMID:11717625

Chaddad, A., & Tanougast, C. (2016). Quantitative evaluation of robust skull stripping and tumor detection applied to axial MR images. *Brain Informatics*, *3*(1), 53–61. doi:10.100740708-016-0033-7 PMID:27747598

Chaira, T. (2014). An improved medical image enhancement scheme using Type II fuzzy set. *Applied Soft Computing*, *25*, 293–308. doi:10.1016/j.asoc.2014.09.004

Chakraborty, S., Chatterjee, S., Ashour, A. S., Mali, K., & Dey, N. (2017). *Intelligent Computing in Medical Imaging: A Study*. Advancements in Applied Metaheuristic Computing.

Chakraborty, S., Chatterjee, S., Dey, N., Ashour, A. S., Ashour, A. S., Shi, F., & Mali, K. (2017). Modified cuckoo search algorithm in microscopic image segmentation of hippocampus. *Microscopy Research and Technique*, *80*(10), 1051–1072. doi:10.1002/jemt.22900 PMID:28557041

Chakraborty, S., Dey, N., Samanta, S., Ashour, A. S., Barna, C., & Balas, M. M. (2017). Optimization of non-rigid demons registration using cuckoo search algorithm. *Cognitive Computation*, *9*(6), 817–826. doi:10.100712559-017-9508-y

Chan, A., & Tuszynski, J. A. (2016). Automatic prediction of tumour malignancy in breast cancer with fractal dimension. *Royal Society Open Science*, *3*(12), 1–10. doi:10.1098/rsos.160558 PMID:28083100

Chan, Y. K., Tsai, M. H., Zheng, Z. H., & Hung, K. D. (2010). Leukocyte nucleus segmentation and nucleus lobe counting. *BMC Bioinformatics*, *11*(1), 558. doi:10.1186/1471-2105-11-558 PMID:21073711

Chatap, N., & Shibu, S. (2014). Analysis of blood samples for counting leukemia cells using Support vector machine and nearest neighbour. *IOSR Journal of Computer Engineering*, *16*(5), 79–87. doi:10.9790/0661-16537987

Chatterjee, S., Dey, N., Ashour, A. S., & Drugarin, C. V. A. (2017). Electrical energy output prediction using cuckoo search based artificial neural network. *Lecture Notes in Networks and Systems*, *18*, 277–285. doi:10.1007/978-981-10-6916-1_26

Chatterjee, S., Dey, N., Shi, F., Ashour, A. S., Fong, S. J., & Sen, S. (2017). Clinical application of modified bag-of-features coupled with hybrid neural-based classifier in dengue fever classification using gene expression data. *Medical & Biological Engineering & Computing*, 1–12. PMID:28891000

Chaudhuri, B., & Sarkar, N. (1995). Texture segmentation using fractal dimension. *IEEE Transaction on Pattern Analysis*, *17*(1), 72–77. doi:10.1109/34.368149

Chen, W. S., Yuan, S. Y., & Hsieh, C. M. (2003). Two algorithms to estimate fractal dimension of gray-level images. *Optical Engineering (Redondo Beach, Calif.)*, *42*(8), 2452–2464. doi:10.1117/1.1585061

Chen, Y. T., & Tseng, D. C. (2007). Wavelet-based medical image compression with adaptive prediction. *Computerized Medical Imaging and Graphics*, *31*(1), 1–8. doi:10.1016/j.compmedimag.2006.08.003 PMID:17046200

Cook, M., Free, S., Manford, M., Fish, D., Shorvon, S., & Stevens, J. (1995). Fractal description of cerebral cortical patterns in frontal lobe epilepsy. *European Neurology*, *35*(6), 327–335. doi:10.1159/000117155 PMID:8591799

Cox, I. J., Miller, M. L., Bloom, J. A., Fridrich, J., & Kalker, T. (2007). *Digital watermarking and steganography*. Morgan Kaufmann publisher.

Crane, E. (1990). *Bees and beekeeping: science, practice and world resources*. London, UK: HeinemannNewnes.

Crisan, D. A., Coculescu, C., & Stanica, J. L. (2009). Using fractal techniques to reduce haziness in medical imaging. In Proceedings of Computer Science and Information Technology (pp. 92-95). Beijing, China: Academic Press.

Cristina, D. R. (2011). Prenatal Diagnosis of Down Syndrome. In *Advances in Research on Down Syndrome* (pp. 75-92). INTECH. doi:10.5772/intechopen.71064

Da Costa, L. (2015). Digital image analysis of blood cells. *Clinics in Laboratory Medicine*, *35*(1), 105–122. doi:10.1016/j.cll.2014.10.005 PMID:25676375

Dabov, K., Foi, A., Katkovnik, V., & Egiazarian, K. (2009). BM3D image denoising with shape-adaptive principal component analysis. SPARS'09 - Signal Processing with Adaptive Sparse Structured Representations.

Dabov, K., Foi, A., Katkovnik, V., & Egiazarian, K. (2007). Image Denoising by Sparse 3-D Transform-Domain Collaborative Filtering. *IEEE Transactions on Image Processing*, *16*(8), 2080–2095. doi:10.1109/TIP.2007.901238 PMID:17688213

Dahinden, C. (2009). *An improved random forests approach with application to the performance prediction challenge datasets*. Zurich, Switzerland: Seminar fur Statistik. pp. 1-6

Dai, T., Lu, W., Wang, W., Wang, J., & Xia, S.-T. (2017). Entropy-based bilateral filtering with a new range kernel. *Signal Processing*, *137*(C), 223–234. doi:10.1016/j.sigpro.2017.02.005

Das, H., Jena, A. K., Badajena, J. C., Pradhan, C., & Barik, R. K. (2018). Resource Allocation in Cooperative Cloud Environments. In Progress in Computing, Analytics and Networking (pp. 825-841). Springer. doi:10.1007/978-981-10-7871-2_79

Das, H., Mishra, S. K., & Roy, D. S. (2013). The topological structure of the Odisha power grid: a complex network analysis. *IJMCA*, *1*(1), 012-016.

Das, H., Naik, B., & Behera, H. S. (2018). Classification of Diabetes Mellitus Disease (DMD): A Data Mining (DM) Approach. In Progress in Computing, Analytics and Networking (pp. 539-549). Springer.

Das, S. K., Nayak, S. R., & Mishra, J. (2017). Fractal Geometry: The Beauty of Computer Graphics. *Journal of Advanced Research in Dynamical and Control Systems*, *9*, 76-82.

Das, H., Jena, A. K., Nayak, J., Naik, B., & Behera, H. S. (2014). *A Novel PSO Based Back Propagation Learning-MLP (PSO-BP-MLP) for Classification. In Computational Intelligence in Data Mining* (Vol. 2, pp. 461–471). Smart Innovation, Systems and Technologies.

Das, H., Jena, A. K., Nayak, J., Naik, B., & Behera, H. S. (2015). A novel PSO based back propagation learning-MLP (PSO-BP-MLP) for classification. In *Computational Intelligence in Data Mining-Volume 2* (pp. 461–471). New Delhi: Springer. doi:10.1007/978-81-322-2208-8_42

Das, H., Jena, A. K., Rath, P. K., Muduli, B., & Das, S. R. (2015). Grid computing-based performance analysis of power system: a graph theoretic approach. In *Intelligent Computing, Communication and Devices* (pp. 259–266). New Delhi: Springer. doi:10.1007/978-81-322-2009-1_30

Das, H., Naik, B., & Behera, H. S. (2018). Classification of Diabetes Mellitus Disease (DMD): A Data Mining (DM) Approach. In *Progress in Computing, Analytics and Networking* (pp. 539–549). Singapore: Springer. doi:10.1007/978-981-10-7871-2_52

Das, H., Naik, B., Pati, B., & Panigrahi, C. R. (2014). A survey on virtual sensor networks framework. *International Journal of Grid and Distributed Computing*, *7*(5), 121–130. doi:10.14257/ijgdc.2014.7.5.11

Das, H., Panda, G. S., Muduli, B., & Rath, P. K. (2014). The complex network analysis of power grid: a case study of the West Bengal power network. In *Intelligent Computing, Networking, and Informatics* (pp. 17–29). New Delhi: Springer. doi:10.1007/978-81-322-1665-0_3

Das, H., & Roy, D. S. (2013). A grid computing service for power system monitoring. *International Journal of Computers and Applications*, *62*(20).

Das, M., Das, B., Das, A., Chatterjee, I., & Majumder, D. (2015). Computational analysis of ultrastructural images of red blood cells. *Journal of Oncology Translational Research*, *1*, 104. doi:10.4172/jotr.1000104

Das, M., & Majumder, D. (2016). An analytical approach for leukemia diagnosis from light microscopic images of RBCs. *Proceedings of 2nd International Conference of Next Generation Computing Technology*, 21-24. doi: 10.1109/NGCT.2016.7877383

de Fontes Guillermo, F., Barroso, A., Coupé, P., & Hellier, P. (2011). Article. *Journal of Real-Time Image Processing*, *6*(15), 15–22. doi:10.100711554-010-0158-5

De Oliveira, D. L. L., Do Nascimento, M. Z., Neves, L. A., De Godoy, M. F., De Arruda, P. F. F., & de Santi Neto, D. (2013). Unsupervised segmentation method for cuboidal cell nuclei in histological prostate images based on minimum cross entropy. *Expert Systems with Applications*, *40*(18), 7331–7340. doi:10.1016/j.eswa.2013.06.079

Demir, C., & Yener, B. (2005). Automated cancer diagnosis based on histopathological images: A systematic survey. *Technical Report, Rensselaer Polytechnic Institute, Department of Computer Science, TR 05-09*, 1–16.

Demir, C., & Yener, B. (2016). Automated cancer diagnosis based on histopathological images A systematic survey. *Technical Report, TR 05-09*, 1–16.

Demirkaya, O., Aysali, M. H., & Sahoo, P. K. (2009). Image processing with MATLAB applications in medicine and biology (pp. 53). London: CRC Press.

Deng, Y., Wang, Y., & Chen, P. (2010). Automated Detection of Fetal Nuchal Translucency Based on Hierarchical Structural Model. *2010 IEEE 23rd International Symposium on Computer-Based Medical Systems (CBMS),* 78-84. 10.1109/CBMS.2010.6042618

Dey, N., & Ashour, A. S. (2018). Computing in Medical Image Analysis. *Soft Computing Based Medical Image Analysis,* 3-11.

Dey, N., & Ashour, A. S. (2017). *Meta-Heuristic Algorithms in Medical Image Segmentation: A Review.* Advancements in Applied Metaheuristic Computing.

Dey, N., & Ashour, A. S. (2018). Computing in Medical Image Analysis. *Soft Computing Based Medical Image Analysis*, 3–11.

Dey, N., Ashour, A. S., & Borra, S. (Eds.). (2017). *Classification in BioApps: Automation of Decision Making* (Vol. 26). Springer.

Dey, N., Rajinikanth, V., Amira, S., Ashour, A. S., & Tavares, J. M. R. S. (2018). Social Group Optimization Supported Segmentation and Evaluation of Skin Melanoma Images. *Symmetry, 10*(2), 51. doi:10.3390ym10020051

Dhanachandra, N., Manglem, K., & Chanu, Y. J. (2015). Image segmentation using K-means clustering algorithm and subtractive clustering algorithm. *Procedia Computer Science, 54,* 764–771. doi:10.1016/j.procs.2015.06.090

Di Ruberto, C., Dempster, A., Khan, S., & Jarra, B. (2000). Segmentation of blood images using morphological operators. *Proceedings of 15th International Conference on Pattern Recognition,* 3, 397 –400. 10.1109/ICPR.2000.903568

Di Ruberto, C., Dempster, A., Khan, S., & Jarra, B. (2002). Analysis of infected blood cell images using morphological operators. *Image and Vision Computing, 20*(2), 133–146. doi:10.1016/S0262-8856(01)00092-0

Dimililer, K. (2013). Back propagation neural network implementation for medical image compression. *International Journal of Applied Mathematics.*

Dimitropoulos, K., Barmpoutis, P., Koletsa, T., Kostopoulos, I., & Grammalidis, N. (2017). Automated detection and classification of nuclei in PAX5 and H&E-stained tissue sections of follicular lymphoma. *SIViP, 11*(1), 145–153. doi:10.100711760-016-0913-6

Dong, W., Shi, G., & Li, X. (2013). Nonlocal image restoration with bilateral variance estimation: A low-rank approach. *IEEE Transactions on Image Processing, 22*(2), 700–711. doi:10.1109/TIP.2012.2221729 PMID:23047875

Don, S., Revathy, D., Chung, K., Choi, E., & Min, D. (2009). A Neural Network Approach to Mammogram Image Classification Using Fractal Features. In *Proceedings of IEEE International Conference of Intelligent Computing and Intelligent Systems* (pp. 444-447). Shanghai, China: IEEE. 10.1109/ICICISYS.2009.5357653

Dragoi, I. C., Coltuc, D., & Caciula, I. (2014, June). Gradient based prediction for reversible watermarking by difference expansion. In *Proceedings of the 2nd ACM workshop on Information hiding and multimedia security* (pp. 35-40). ACM. 10.1145/2600918.2600924

Du, Y., Ren, Y., Yan, Y., & Cao, L. (2017). Absent Fetal Nasal Bone in the Second Trimester and Risk of Abnormal Karyotype in a Prescreened Population of Chinese Women. *Acta Obstetricia et Gynecologica Scandinavica, 97*(2), 180–186. doi:10.1111/aogs.13263 PMID:29164604

Echogenic Intracardiac Focus. (2017, January) *Kaiser Permanente*. Retrieved from https://mydoctor.kaiserpermanente.org/ncal/Images/GEN_US EIF handout_tcm63-9941.pdf

Eiri, D., Suwannapong, G., Endler, M., & Nieh, J. (2015). Nosemaceranae can infect honeybee larvae and reduces subsequentadult longevity. *PLoS One, 10*(5), 1–17. doi:10.1371/journal.pone.0126330 PMID:26018139

Elizabeth, C., Heathe, H., Cresswell, J., & Tyler, C. (2015). Interactive effects of pesticideexposure and pathogen infection on bee health - a critical analysis: Pesticide-pathogen interactions on bee health. *Biological Reviews of the Cambridge Philosophical Society*.

en.wikipedia.org. (2018). *H0026E stain*. Available at: https://en.wikipedia.org/wiki/H

Espina, D., & Ordetx, G. (1984). Apicultura tropical. *Tecnológica de Costa Rica*, 506.

Fernandes, S. L., Gurupur, V. P., Lin, H., & Martis, R. J. (2017). A novel fusion approach for early lung cancer detection using computer aided diagnosis techniques. *Journal of Medical Imaging and Health Informatics, 7*(8), 1841–1850. doi:10.1166/jmihi.2017.2280

Free, S., Sisodiya, S., Cook, M., Fish, D., & Shorvon, S. (1996). Three-dimensional fractal analysis of the white matter surface from magnetic resonance images of the human brain. *Cerebral Cortex, 6*(6), 830–836. doi:10.1093/cercor/6.6.830 PMID:8922340

Gangepain, J. J., & Carmes, C. R. (1986). Fractal approach to two dimensional and three dimensional surface roughness. *Wear, 109*(1-4), 119–126. doi:10.1016/0043-1648(86)90257-7

Gao, L., Wang, G., & Liu, J. (2015). Image denoising based on edge detection and prethresholding Wiener filtering of multi-wavelets fusion. International Journal of Wavelets, Multiresolution and Information Processing, 13(5).

Gelasca, E. D., Byun, J., Obara, B., & Manjunath, B. (2008). Evaluation and benchmark for biological image segmentation. *2008 15th IEEE International Conference on Image Processing*.

Gillibert, L., & Jeulin, D. (1994). Stochastic multiscale segmentation constrained by image content, In J. Serra & P. Soille (Eds.), Mathematical morphology and its applications to image processing (pp. 132-138). Kluwer Academic Publishers.

Gisder, S., Schüler, V., Horchler, L. L., Groth, D., & Genersch, E. (2017). Long-Term28 Temporal Trends of Nosema spp. Infection Prevalence in Northeast Germany: Continuous Spread of Nosemaceranae, an Emerging Pathogen of Honeybees (Apismellifera), but No General Replacement of Nosemaapis. *Frontiers in Cellular and Infection Microbiology*.

Giuffre, C., Lubkin, S. R., & Tarpy, D. R. (2017). Automated Assay and Differential Model Of Western Honey Bee (Apis Mellifera) Autogrooming Using Digital Image Processing. *Computers and Electronics in Agriculture*, *135*, 338–344. doi:10.1016/j.compag.2017.02.003

Goel, A., Sahu, O. P., Gupta, R., & Gupta, S. (2010). Improved digital watermarking techniques and data embedding in multimedia. *International Journal on Computer Science and Engineering*, *02*(02), 164–168.

Gonzalez, R. C., & Woods, R. E. (2008). *Digital Image Processing*. Pearson Prentice Hall.

Gonzalez, R. C., Woods, R. E., & Eddins, S. L. (2009). Introduction. In *Digital Image Processing Using MATLAB* (3rd ed.; pp. 2–3). Knoxville, TN: Pearson.

Gu, K., Tao, D., Qiao, J.-F., & Lin, W. (2018). Learning a no-reference quality assessment model of enhanced images with big data. *IEEE Transactions on Neural Networks and Learning Systems*, *29*(4), 1301–1313. doi:10.1109/TNNLS.2017.2649101 PMID:28287984

Guo, Q., Shao, J., & Ruiz, V. F. (2009). Characterization and classification of tumor lesions using computerized fractal-based texture analysis and support vector machines in digital mammograms. *International Journal of Computer Assisted Radiology and Surgery*, *4*(1), 11–25. doi:10.100711548-008-0276-8 PMID:20033598

Guo, Q., Zhang, C., Zhang, Y., & Liu, H. (2016). An efficient SVD-based method for image denoising. *IEEE Transactions on Circuits and Systems for Video Technology*, *26*(5), 868–880. doi:10.1109/TCSVT.2015.2416631

Gupta, P., Srivastava, P., Bhardwaj, S., & Bhateja, V. (2011). A modified PSNR metric based on HVS for quality assessment of color images. In *Proceedings of International Conference on Communication and Industrial Application* (pp. 1-4). IEEE Xplore. 10.1109/ICCIndA.2011.6146669

Gurcan, M. N., Boucheron, L., Can, A., Madabhushi, A., Rajpoot, N., & Yener, B. (2009). Histopatological Image Analysis: A Review. *IEEE Reviews in Biomedical Engineering*, *2*, 147–171. doi:10.1109/RBME.2009.2034865 PMID:20671804

Gurcan, M. N., Pan, T., Shimada, H., & Saltz, J. (2006). Image analysis for neuroblastoma classification: Segmentation of cell nuclei. *Proceedings of IEEE International Conference on Engineering in Medicine and Biology Society*, *1*, 4844-4847. 10.1109/IEMBS.2006.260837

H&E Stain. (2018). Available at: https://cytoinformatics.com/Cyto/he-stain

Han, Y., Xu, C., Baciu, G., & Li, M. (2015). Lightness biased cartoon-and-texture decomposition for textile image segmentation. *Neurocomputing*, *168*(C), 575–587. doi:10.1016/j.neucom.2015.05.069

Han, Z., Wei, B., Zheng, Y., Yin, Y., Li, K., & Li, S. (2017). Breast Cancer Multi-classification from Histopathological Images with Structured Deep Learning Model. *Scientific Reports*, *7*(1). PMID:28646155

Haralick, R. M., Shanmugam, K., & Dinstein, I. (1973). Textural Features for Image Classification. *IEEE Transactions on Systems, Man, and Cybernetics*, *SMC-3*(6), 610–621. doi:10.1109/TSMC.1973.4309314

Haseena, S. (2015). Segmentation of Optic Disc and Hard Exudates. In *International Journal of Applied Engineering Research* (Vol. 10). Research India Publications.

Hassani, E., & Eshghi, M. (2013). Image encryption based on chaotic tent map in time and frequency domains. *The ISC International Journal of Information Security*, *5*(1), 97–110.

HE Stain. (n.d.). Retrieved from https://en.wikipedia.org/wiki/H\%26E_stain

He, Y., Gan, T., Chen, W., & Wang, H. (2011). Adaptive denoising by singular value decomposition. *IEEE Signal Processing Letters*, *18*(4), 215–218. doi:10.1109/LSP.2011.2109039

Higes, M., Martin-Hernández, R., & Meana, A. (2010). Nosema ceranae in Europe: An emergent type C Nosemosis. *Apidologie*, *41*(3), 375–392. doi:10.1051/apido/2010019

Higes, M., Martin, R., & Meana, A. (2006). Nosemaceranae, a new microsporidian parasite in honeybees in Europe. *Journal of Invertebrate Pathology*, *92*(2), 93–95. doi:10.1016/j.jip.2006.02.005 PMID:16574143

Hochreiter, S., & Schmidhuber, J. (1997). Long short-term memory. *International Journal of Neural Computation*, *9*(8), 1735–1780. doi:10.1162/neco.1997.9.8.1735 PMID:9377276

Hore, S., Chakroborty, S., Ashour, A. S., Dey, N., Ashour, A. S., Sifaki-Pistolla, D., ... Chaudhuri, S. R. (2015). Finding contours of hippocampus brain cell using microscopic image analysis. *Journal of Advanced Microscopy Research*, *10*(2), 93–103. doi:10.1166/jamr.2015.1245

Horning, N. (2010). Random forests: an algorithm for image classification and generation of continuous fields data sets. *Proceedings of International Conference on Geo-informatics for Spatial Infrastructure Development in Earth and Allied Science*, 1-6.

Hsu, W. Y., Lin, C. C., Ju, M. S., & Sun, Y. N. (2007). Wavelet-based fractal features with active segment selection: Application to single-trial EEG data. *Journal of Neuroscience Methods*, *163*(1), 145–160. doi:10.1016/j.jneumeth.2007.02.004 PMID:17379316

Hung, K.-W., & Siu, W.-C. (2012). Robust soft-decision interpolation using weighted least squares. *IEEE Transactions on Image Processing*, *21*(3), 1061–1069. doi:10.1109/TIP.2011.2168416 PMID:21937348

Hwang, H., & Haddad, R. A. (1995). Adaptive median filters: New algorithms and results. *IEEE Transactions on Image Processing*, *4*(4), 499–502. doi:10.1109/83.370679 PMID:18289998

Iftekharuddin, K. (2005). Techniques in fractal analysis and their applications in brain MRI. *Journal of Medical Imaging Systems: Technology and Applications, 1*, 63-86.

Irshad, H., Veillard, A., Roux, L., & Racoceanu, D. (2014). Methods for Nuclei Detection, Segmentation, and Classification in Digital Histopathology: A Review—Current Status and Future Potential. *IEEE Reviews in Biomedical Engineering*, *7*, 97–114. doi:10.1109/RBME.2013.2295804 PMID:24802905

Ismail, S. M., Colclough, A. B., Dinnen, J. S., Eakins, D., Evans, D. M., Gradwell, E., ... Newcombe, R. G. (1989). Observer variation in histopathological diagnosis and grading of cervical intraepithelial neoplasia. *British Medical Journal*, *298*(6675), 707–710. doi:10.1136/bmj.298.6675.707 PMID:2496816

Jain, A. K. (1989). *Fundamentals of digital image processing*. Prentice-Hall, Inc.

Jain, A., Atey, S., Vinayak, S., & Srivastava, V. (2014). Cancerous cell detection using histopathological image analysis. *International Journal of Innovative Research in Computer and Communication Engineering*, *2*(12), 7419–7426. doi:10.15680/IJIRCCE.2014.0212026

Jain, A., & Rajpal, N. (2012). A two layer chaotic network based image encryption technique. *National Conference on Computing and Communication Systems*, 1-5. 10.1109/NCCCS.2012.6413005

Jia, Z., Huang, X., Chang, E. I., & Xu, Y. (2017). Constrained Deep Weak Supervision for Histopathology Image Segmentation. *IEEE Transactions on Medical Imaging*, *36*(11), 2376–2388. doi:10.1109/TMI.2017.2724070 PMID:28692971

Jin, X. C., Ong, S. H., & Jayasooriah. (1995). A practical method for estimating fractal dimension. *Pattern Recognition Letters*, *16*(5), 457–464. doi:10.1016/0167-8655(94)00119-N

Jun, Y., Yoon, Y., & Yoon, H. (1994). ECG data compression using fractal interpolation. In *Proceedings of IEEE Conference of Engineering in Medicine and Biology Society* (pp. 161-162). Baltimore, MD: IEEE.

Kabi, K. K., Pradhan, C., Saha, B. J., & Bisoi, A. K. (2014). Comparative Study of Image Encryption using 2D Chaotic Map. *International Conference on Information Systems and Computer Networks*, 105-108. 10.1109/ICISCON.2014.6965227

Kadachha, S. L., & Patel, P. J. (2013). Cancer detection using modified watershed. *International Journal of Engineering Research & Technology*, *2*(5), 2161–2164.

Kaewaramsri, Y., & Woraratpanya, K. (2015). Improved triangle box counting method for fractal dimension estimation. In H. Unger, P. Meesad, & S. Boonkrong (Eds.), *Recent Advances in Information and Communication Technology, In Proceedings of Advances in Intelligent Systems and Computing* (Vol. 361, pp. 53–63). Cham: Springer. doi:10.1007/978-3-319-19024-2_6

Kalmanti, E., & Maris, T.G. (2007). Fractal dimension as an index of brain cortical changes throughout life. *Journal of Fractal Analysis, 21*, 641-646.

Kalra, G. S., Talwar, R., & Sadawarti, H. (2011). Robust blind digital image watermarking using DWT and dual encryption technique. *International Conference on Computational Intelligence, Communication Systems and Networks*, 225-230. 10.1109/CICSyN.2011.56

Kamalanand, K., & Jawahar, P. M. (2012). Coupled jumping frogs/particle swarm optimization for estimating the parameters of three dimensional HIV model. *BMC Infectious Diseases*, *12*(1), 82. doi:10.1186/1471-2334-12-S1-P82 PMID:22471518

Kamalanand, K., & Jawahar, P. M. (2015). Prediction of Human Immunodeficiency Virus-1 Viral Load from CD4 Cell Count Using Artificial Neural Networks. *Journal of Medical Imaging and Health Informatics*, *5*(3), 641–646. doi:10.1166/jmihi.2015.1430

Kannappan, P. L. (1972). On Shannon's entropy, directed divergence and inaccuracy. *Probability Theory and Related Fields*, *22*, 95–100.

Karimi, N., Samavi, S., Soroushmehr, S. R., Shirani, S., & Najarian, K. (2016). Toward practical guideline for design of image compression algorithms for biomedical applications. *Expert Systems with Applications*, *56*, 360–367. doi:10.1016/j.eswa.2016.02.047

Kaur, S., & Jindal, G. (2011). Watershed segmentation of lung ct scan images for early diagnosis of cancer. *International Journal of Computer and Electrical Engineering*, *3*, 850–855. doi:10.7763/IJCEE.2011.V3.431

Kavitha, Chellamuthu, & Rupa. (2012). An Efficient Approach for Brain Tumour Detection Based on Modified Region Growing and Neural Network in MRI Images. *2012 International Conference on Computing, Electronics and Electrical Technologies (ICCEET*). doi:.10.1109/icceet.2012.6203809

Kedzia, A., Rybaczuk, M., & Andrzejak, R. (2002). Fractal dimensions of human brain cortex vessels during the fetal period. *Medical Science Monitor*, *8*, 46–51. PMID:11887041

Kennedy, J., & Eberhart, R. C. (1995). Particle swarm optimization. In *Proceedings of the IEEE International Conference on Neural Networks, IV* (pp. 1942–1948). Piscataway, NJ: IEEE Service Center. 10.1109/ICNN.1995.488968

Kennedy, J., & Eberhart, R. C. (1997), A discrete binary version of the particle swarm algorithm, *Proceedings 1997 Conference on Systems, Man, and Cybernetics* (pp. 4104–4109). Piscataway, NJ: IEEE Service Center. 10.1109/ICSMC.1997.637339

Khan, A. (2016). Content based image retrieval using genetic algorithm. *International Journal Engineering Science and Computing*, *6*(7), 8144–8148.

Khashman, A., & Dimililer, K. (2009). Medical radiographs compression using neural networks and Haar wavelet. In *Proceedings of International Conference on IEEE EUROCON* (pp. 1448-1453). IEEE.

Khemis, K., Lazzouni, S. A., Messadi, M., Loudjedi, S., & Bessaid, A. (2016). New Algorithm for Fractal Dimension Estimation based on Texture Measurements: Application on Breast Tissue Characterization. *International Journal of Image, Graphics and Signal Processing*, *4*(4), 9–15. doi:10.5815/ijigsp.2016.04.02

Knezović, J., Kovač, M., Žagar, M., Mlinarić, H., & Hofman, D. (2011). Novel prediction based technique for efficient compression of medical imaging data. In *Telemedicine Techniques and Applications*. InTech. doi:10.5772/18126

Komura, D., & Ishikawa, S. (2018). Machine Learning Methods for Histopathological Image Analysis. *Computational and Structural Biotechnology Journal*, *16*, 34–42. doi:10.1016/j.csbj.2018.01.001

Ko, S. J., & Lee, Y. H. (1991). Center weighted median filters and their applications to image enhancement. *IEEE Transactions on Circuits and Systems*, *38*(9), 984–993. doi:10.1109/31.83870

Kumar, R., Srivastava, R., & Srivastava, S. (2015). Detection and classification of cancer from microscopic biopsy images using clinically significant and biologically interpretable features. *Journal of Medical Engineering* 457906: 1-14. doi: 10.1155/2015/457906

Kumar, M. D., Babaie, M., Zhu, S., Kalra, S., & Tizhoosh, H. R. (2017). A comparative study of CNN, BoVW and LBP for classification of histopathological images. *2017 IEEE Symposium Series on Computational Intelligence (SSCI)*. 10.1109/SSCI.2017.8285162

Kumar, S., Sinha, B., & Pradhan, C. (2015). Comparative Analysis of Color Image Encryption using 2D Chaotic Maps. *Information Systems Design and Intelligent Applications, Springer*, *2*, 379–387. doi:10.1007/978-81-322-2247-7_39

Kviesisa, A., & Zacepinsa, A. (2015). System Architectures for Real-time Bee Colony Temperature Monitoring. *Procedia Computer Science*, *43*, 86–94. doi:10.1016/j.procs.2014.12.012

Lakshmi, V.S., Tebby, S.G., Shriranjani, D., & Rajinikanth, V. (2016). Chaotic cuckoo search and Kapur/Tsallis approach in segmentation of T.cruzi from blood smear images. *Int. J. Comp. Sci. Infor. Sec.*, *14*, 51-56.

Larkin, K. G. (2015). Structural Similarity Index SSIMplified: Is there really a simpler concept at the heart of image quality measurement? *Occasional Texts in the Pursuit of Clarity and Simplicity in Research*, *1*(1), 1–4.

Ledda, A., Quintelier, J., Samyn, P., Baets, P. D., & Philips, W. (2000). Quantitative image analysis with mathematical morphology. *Proceeding of ProRISC2003*, (pp. 399-406), Veldhoven, Netherlands.

Li, X., & Bi, G. (2015, July). Image reconstruction based on the improved compressive sensing algorithm. In *Digital Signal Processing (DSP), 2015 IEEE International Conference on* (pp. 357-360). IEEE. 10.1109/ICDSP.2015.7251892

Liang, H., & Weller, D. S. (2016). Comparison-Based Image Quality Assessment for Selecting Image Restoration Parameters. *IEEE Transactions on Image Processing*, *25*(11), 5118–5130. doi:10.1109/TIP.2016.2601783 PMID:27552759

Lian, S. (2009). A block cipher based on chaotic neural networks. *Neurocomputing, Elsevier*, *72*(4), 1296–1301. doi:10.1016/j.neucom.2008.11.005

Li, C., Xu, C., Gui, C., & Fox, M. D. (2010). Distance regularized level set evolution and its application to image segmentation. *IEEE Transactions on Image Processing*, *19*(12), 3243–3254. doi:10.1109/TIP.2010.2069690 PMID:20801742

Li, H., Giger, M. L., Olopade, O. I., & Lan, L. (2007). Fractal analysis of mammographic parenchymal patterns in breast cancer risk assessment. *Academic Radiology*, *14*(5), 513–521. doi:10.1016/j.acra.2007.02.003 PMID:17434064

Li, H., Liu, K., & Lo, S. (1996). Enhancement of micro-calcifications on mammograms using a fractal modelling approach. In *Proceedings of the IEEE Conference on Engineering in Medicine and Biology Society* (vol. 3, pp. 1111-1112). Amsterdam: IEEE. 10.1109/IEMBS.1996.652732

Li, J., Du, Q., & Sun, C. (2009). An improved box-counting method for image fractal dimension estimation. *Pattern Recognition*, *42*(11), 2460–2469. doi:10.1016/j.patcog.2009.03.001

Lin, H., & Li, Y. (2017). Using EEG data analytics to measure meditation. *Lecture Notes in Computer Science*, *10287*, 270–280. doi:10.1007/978-3-319-58466-9_25

LISC. (n.d.). Retrieved from http://users.cecs.anu.edu.au/~hrezatofighi/Data/Leukocyte%20 Data.htm

Liu, F., Mackey, A. L., Srikuea, R., Esser, K. A., & Yang, L. (2013). Automated image segmentation of haematoxylin and eosin stained skeletal muscle crossâ€ sections. *Journal of Microscopy*, *252*(3), 275–285. doi:10.1111/jmi.12090 PMID:24118017

Liu, H., & Kadir, A. (2015). Asymmetric Color Image Encryption Scheme using 2D Discrete-Time Map. *Signal Processing, Elsevier*, *113*, 104–112. doi:10.1016/j.sigpro.2015.01.016

Liu, Y., Chen, L., Wang, H., Jiang, L., Zhang, Y., Zhao, J., ... Song, Y. (2014). An improved differential box-counting method to estimate fractal dimensions of gray-level images. *Journal of Visual Communication and Image Representation*, *25*(5), 1102–1111. doi:10.1016/j.jvcir.2014.03.008

Li, Z., Dey, N., Ashour, A. S., & Tang, Q. (2017). Discrete cuckoo search algorithms for two-sided robotic assembly line balancing problem. *Neural Computing & Applications*, 1–12. doi:10.100700521-017-2855-5

Lopes, R., & Betrouni, N. (2009). Fractal and multifractal analysis: A review. *Medical Image Analysis*, *13*(4), 634–649. doi:10.1016/j.media.2009.05.003 PMID:19535282

Lu, H., Kot, A. C., & Shi, Y. Q. (2004). Distance-reciprocal distortion measure for binary document images. *IEEE Signal Processing Letters*, *11*(2), 228–231. doi:10.1109/LSP.2003.821748

Lynch, L., Berkowitz, G. S., Chitkara, U., & Wilkins, I. A. (1989). Ultrasound Detection of Down Syndrome: Is It Really Possible? *Journal of Diagnostic Medical Sonography: JDMS*, *5*(4), 217. doi:10.1177/875647938900500445 PMID:2521379

Madavan, R., Balaraman, S., & Saroja, S. (2017). Multi-Criteria Decision Making Methods for Grading High-Performance Transformer Oil with Antioxidants Under Accelerated Ageing Conditions. In IET Generation, Transmission and Distribution (Vol. 11). IET Publisher.

Magota, K., Kubo, N., Kuge, Y., Nishijima, K., Zhao, S., & Tamaki, N. (2011). Performance characterization of the Inveon preclinical small-animal PET/SPECT/CT system for multimodality imaging. *European Journal of Nuclear Medicine and Molecular Imaging*, *38*(4), 742–752. doi:10.100700259-010-1683-y PMID:21153410

Mahdi, A., Jawad, A. K., & Hreshree, S. S. (2016). Digital Chaotic Scrambling of Voice Based on Duffing Map. *Communications Engineering Journal*, *1*(2), 16–21.

Mairal, J., Elad, M., & Sapiro, G. (2008). Sparse representation for color image restoration. *IEEE Transactions on Image Processing*, *17*(1), 53–69. doi:10.1109/TIP.2007.911828 PMID:18229804

Mairal, J., Sapiro, G., & Elad, M. (2008). Learning multiscale sparse representations for image and video restoration. *Multiscale Modeling & Simulation*, *7*(1), 214–241. doi:10.1137/070697653

Majumder, D., Banerjee, D., Chandra, S., Banerjee, S., & Chakrabarti, A. (2006). Red cell morphology in leukemia, hypoplastic anemia and myelodysplastic syndrome. *Pathophysiology*, *13*(4), 217–225. doi:10.1016/j.pathophys.2006.06.002 PMID:16876391

Majumder, D., Ray, D. K., Chatterjee, I., & Dhar, P. K. (2017). Translation of middle out rational approach (MORA) in an understanding of therapeutic outcome of cancer: Experience from India. *Journal of Translational Research*, *1*(1), 4–7.

Malladi, R., Sethian, J. A., & Vemuri, B. C. (1995). Shape modeling with front propagation: A level set approach. *IEEE T. Pattern Anal. Mac. Int.*, *17*(2), 158–175. doi:10.1109/34.368173

Mamatha, A. S., & Singh, V. (2014, September). Lossless hyperspectral image compression using intraband and interband predictors. In *Advances in Computing, Communications and Informatics (ICACCI, 2014 International Conference on* (pp. 332-337). IEEE.

Mandelbrot, B. (1967). How long is the coast of Britain? Statistical self-similarity and fractional dimension. *Science*, *156*(3775), 636–638. doi:10.1126cience.156.3775.636 PMID:17837158

Mandelbrot, B. (1982). *The fractal geometry of nature*. W.H. Freeman and Company.

Mandelbrot, B. (1985). Self-affine fractals and the fractal dimension. *Physica Scripta*, *32*(4), 257–260. doi:10.1088/0031-8949/32/4/001

Mandelbrot, B., & Wheeler, J. A. (1983). The Fractal Geometry of Nature. *American Journal of Physics*, *51*(3), 286–196. doi:10.1119/1.13295

Manickavasagam, K., Sutha, S., & Kamalanand, K. (2014). Development of systems for classification of different plasmodium species in thin blood smear microscopic images. *Journal of Advanced Microscopy Research*, *9*(2), 86–92. doi:10.1166/jamr.2014.1194

Mankoff, D. (2007). A definition of molecular imaging. *Journal of Nuclear Medicine*, *48*(6), 18N–21N. PMID:17536102

Marr, D., & Hildreth, E. (1980). Theory of Edge Detection. *Proceedings of the Royal Society of London*, *207*(1167), 187–217. doi:10.1098/rspb.1980.0020 PMID:6102765

Mathur, A., Tripathi, A. S., & Kuse, M. (2013). Scalable system for classification of white blood cells from Leishman stained blood stain images. *Journal of Pathology Informatics*, *4*(2), S15. doi:10.4103/2153-3539.109883 PMID:23766937

Mavroforakis, M. E., Georgiou, H. V., Dimitropoulos, N., Cavouras, D., & Theodoridis, S. (2006). Mammographic masses characterization based on localized texture and dataset fractal analysis using linear, neural and support vector machine classifiers. *Artificial Intelligence in Medicine*, *37*(2), 145–162. doi:10.1016/j.artmed.2006.03.002 PMID:16716579

Medina, C., Guzmán, E., Espinosa, L., Uribe, L., Gutiérrez, R., & Gutiérrez, F. (2014). Frecuencia de Varrosis y Nosemosis en colonias de abejas melíferas (*Apis mellifera*) en el estado de Zacatecas, México. *Revista Chapingo Serie Ciencias Forestales y del Ambiente*, 30–36.

Meléndez, V., Parra, V., Delfín, H., Ayala, R., Reyes, E., & Manrique, P. (2008). Abejas silvestres: Diversidad, el papel como polinizadores y la importancia de su conservación. *Bioagrociencias*, *1*, 38–45.

Mendel, J. M., & John, R. B. (2002). Type-2 fuzzy sets made simple. *IEEE Transactions on Fuzzy Systems*, *10*(2), 117–127. doi:10.1109/91.995115

Mishra, B. S. P., Das, H., Dehuri, S., & Jagadev, A. K. (2018). *Cloud Computing for Optimization: Foundations, Applications, and Challenges* (Vol. 39). Springer. doi:10.1007/978-3-319-73676-1

Moghaddam, R. F., & Cheriet, M. (2010). A multi-scale framework for adaptive binarization of degraded document images. *Pattern Recognition*, *43*(6), 2186–2198. doi:10.1016/j.patcog.2009.12.024

Molina, A., Guzmán, E., Message, D., Jong, D., Pesante, D., Mantilla, C., . . . Alvarado, F. (1990). Enfermedades y plagas de la abeja melífera occidental. OIRSA-BID, 147.

Moorthi, M., & Amutha, R. (2012). Medical image compression using adaptive neural network. In *Proceedings of International Conference on Emerging Trends in Science, Engineering and Technology (INCOSET)* (pp. 222-227). Academic Press. 10.1109/INCOSET.2012.6513909

Nabian, S., Ahmadi, K., Nazem-Shirazi, M. H., & Gerami-Sadeghian, A. (2011). First detection of Nosemaceranae, a microsporidian protozoa of european honeybees (Apismellifera) in Iran. *Iranian Journal of Parasitology*, *6*, 89–95. PMID:22347302

Naqi, S. M., Sharif, M., Yasmin, M., & Fernandes, S. L. (2018). Lung nodule detection using polygon approximation and hybrid features from CT images. *Current Medical Imaging Reviews*, *14*(1), 108–117. doi:10.2174/1573405613666170306114320

Nateghi, R., Danyali, H., Helfroush, M. S., & Tashk, A. (2014). Mitosis detection from breast cancer histology slide images using particle swarm optimization and support vector machine. *International Journal of Sciences: Basic and Applied Research*, *16*(2), 164–177.

Nayak, S. R., & Mishra, J. (2017). On calculation of fractal dimension of color images. *International Journal of Image, Graphics and Signal Processing*, *9*, 33-40.

Nayak, S. R., Mishra, J., & Jena, P. M. (2018). Fractal analysis of image sets using differential box counting techniques. *International Journal of Information Technology, 10*, 39-47.

Nayak, S. R., Padhy, R., & Mishra, J. (2016). On estimation of fractal dimension of gray scale images using modified differential box counting method. *International Journal of Computer Science and Information Security, 14*, 764-772.

Nayak, S. R., Khandual, A., & Mishra, J. (in press). Ground truth study of fractal dimension of color images of similar textures. *Journal of the Textile Institute.*

Nayak, S. R., & Mishra, J. (2016). An improved method to estimate the fractal dimension of colour images. *Perspectives on Science*, *8*, 412–416. doi:10.1016/j.pisc.2016.04.092

Nayak, S. R., & Mishra, J. (2017). On estimation of fractal dimension of noise images. *Indian Journal of Science and Technology*, *10*, 1–6.

Nayak, S. R., & Mishra, J. (2018). A modified triangle box-counting with precision in error fit. *Journal of Information and Optimization Sciences*, *39*(1), 113–128. doi:10.1080/02522667.2017.1372155

Nayak, S. R., Mishra, J., Khandual, A., & Palai, G. (2018). Fractal Dimension of RGB Color Images. *International Journal for Light and Electron Optics*, *161*, 136–145. doi:10.1016/j.ijleo.2018.02.024

Nayak, S. R., Mishra, J., & Padhy, R. (2016). An improved algorithm to estimate the fractal dimension of gray scale image. In *Proceedings of IEEE International conference on signal processing, Communication, Power and Embedded System* (pp. 1109-1114). IEEE. 10.1109/SCOPES.2016.7955614

Nayak, S. R., Mishra, J., & Palai, G. (2018). A modified approach to estimate fractal dimension of gray scale Images. *International Journal for Light and Electron Optics*, *162*, 196–205. doi:10.1016/j.ijleo.2018.02.066

Nayak, S. R., Mishra, J., & Palai, G. (2018). An extended DBC approach by using maximum Euclidian distance for fractal dimension of color images. *International Journal for Light and Electron Optics*, *166*, 110–115. doi:10.1016/j.ijleo.2018.03.106

Nayak, S. R., Mishra, J., & Routray, S. (2017). Effect of noise determination on estimation of fractal dimension of digital images. *International Journal of Pure and Applied Mathematics*, *117*, 57–63.

Nayak, S. R., Mishra, J., Sethy, A., & Mohapatra, S. (2017). A comparative analysis on estimation of fractal dimension of gray scale images. *International Journal of Pure and Applied Mathematics*, *117*, 323–329.

Nayak, S. R., Padhy, R., & Mishra, J. (2018). A new extended differential box counting method by adopting unequal partitioning of grid for estimation of fractal dimension of digital images. In *Proceedings of Computational Signal Processing and Analysis* (Vol. 490, pp. 45–57). LNEE Book Series. doi:10.1007/978-981-10-8354-9_5

Nayak, S. R., Ranganath, A., & Mishra, J. (2015). Analysing Fractal Dimension of color Images. In *Proceedings of IEEE International Conference on Computational Intelligence and Networks* (pp. 156-159). IEEE.

Nguyen, L., Tosun, A.B., Fine, J.L., Lee, A.V., Taylor, D.L., & Chennubhotla, S.C. (2017). Spatial statistics for segmenting histological structures in H&E stained tissue images. *IEEE Transactions on Medical Imaging*, 1522-1532.

Nguyen, T., & Rangayyan, R. (2005). Shape Analysis of Breast Masses in Mammograms via the Fractal Dimension. In *Proceedings of the IEEE Engineering in Medicine and Biology* Society (vol. 3, pp. 3210-3213). Shanghai, China: IEEE.

Nirmala, S., & Palanisamy, V. (2009, June 4). Measurement of Nuchal Translucency Thickness in First Trimester Ultrasound Fetal Images for Detection of Chromosomal Abnormalities. *International Conference on Control, Automation, Communication and Energy Conservation.* Retrieved from https://ieeexplore.ieee.org/document/5204467/media

Noble, W. S. (2004). Support vector machine applications in computational biology. In *Kernel Methods in Computational Biology* (pp. 71–92). Cambridge, MA: MIT Press.

Noble, W. S. (2006). What is a support vector machine? *Nature Biotechnology*, *24*(12), 1565–1567. doi:10.1038/nbt1206-1565 PMID:17160063

Omran, M. (2005). *Particle swarm optimization methods for pattern recognition and image processing* (Ph.D. Thesis Computer Science). University of Pretoria.

Organización Mundial de Sanidad Animal (OIE). (2013). Manual de las Pruebas de Diagnóstico y de las Vacunas para los Animales Terrestres. *Capítulo 2.2.4 Nosemosis de las abejas melíferas.*

Otsu, N. (1979). A threshold selection method from gray-level histograms. *IEEE Transactions on Systems, Man, and Cybernetics*, *9*(1), 62–66. doi:10.1109/TSMC.1979.4310076

Palani, T. K., Parvathavarthini, B., & Chitra, K. (2016). Segmentation of brain regions by integrating meta heuristic multilevel threshold with Markov random field. *Current Medical Imaging Reviews*, *12*(1), 4–12. doi:10.2174/1573394711666150827203434

Panigrahi, C. R., Tiwary, M., Pati, B., & Das, H. (2016). Big Data and Cyber Foraging: Future Scope and Challenges. In *Techniques and Environments for Big Data Analysis* (pp. 75–100). Cham: Springer. doi:10.1007/978-3-319-27520-8_5

Pan, X., Li, L., Yang, H., Liu, Z., Yang, J., Zhao, L., & Fan, Y. (2017). Accurate segmentation of nuclei in pathological images via sparse reconstruction and deep convolutional networks. *Neurocomputing*, *229*, 88–99. doi:10.1016/j.neucom.2016.08.103

Paramasivam, A., Kamalanand, K., Sundravadivelu, K., & Mannar, J. P. (2017). Effect of electrode contact area on the information content of the recorded electrogastrograms: An analysis based on Rényi entropy and Teager-Kaiser Energy. *Polish Journal of Medical Physics and Engineering*, *23*(2), 37–42.

Pathak, K. C., & Sarvaiya, J. N. (2017, March). Lossless medical image compression using transform domain adaptive prediction for telemedicine. In *Wireless Communications, Signal Processing and Networking (WiSPNET), 2017 International Conference on* (pp. 1026-1031). IEEE. 10.1109/WiSPNET.2017.8299918

P. K. Pattnaik, S. S. Rautaray, H. Das, & J. Nayak (Eds.). (2018). Progress in Computing, Analytics and Networking*: Proceedings of ICCAN 2017* (Vol. 710). Springer.

Paul, S., & Bandyopadhyay, B. (2014). A novel approach for image compression based on multi-level image thresholding using Shannon entropy and differential evolution. *Students' Technology Symposium (TechSym), IEEE*, 56 – 61. 10.1109/TechSym.2014.6807914

Paxton, S. A., & Peckham, M. (2003). *The Leeds Histology Guide*. Available at: http://www.histology.leeds.ac.uk/tissue_types/epithelia/epi_stratified.php

Pei-Gee, Ho. (2012). *Image Segmentation*. InTech. Retrieved from: http://www. intechopen.com/books/image-segmentation

Phothisonothai, M., & Nakagawa, M. (2007). Fractal-based EEG data analysis of body parts movement imagery tasks. *The Journal of Physiological Sciences; JPS*, *57*(4), 217–226. doi:10.2170/physiolsci.RP006307 PMID:17637165

Pichler, B., Kolb, A., Nagele, T., & Schlemmer, H. (2010). PET/MRI: Paving the way for the next generation of clinical multimodality imaging applications. *Journal of Nuclear Medicine*, *51*(3), 333–336. doi:10.2967/jnumed.109.061853 PMID:20150252

Pirk, C., Miranda, J. C., Kramer, W., Murray, T. E., Nazzi, F., Shutler, D., ... Dooremalen, C. (2013). Statistical guidelines for Apismellifera research. *Journal of Apicultural Research*, *52*(4), 1–24. doi:10.3896/IBRA.1.52.4.13

Pradhan, C., Rath, S., & Bisoi, A. K. (2012). Non blind digital watermarking technique using DWT and cross chaos. *Procedia Technology, Elsevier*, *6*, 897–904. doi:10.1016/j.protcy.2012.10.109

Prinyakupt, J., & Pluempitiwiriyawej, C. (2015). Segmentation of white blood cells and comparison of cell morphology by linear and naïve Bayes classifiers. *Biomedical Engineering Online*, *14*(1), 63. doi:10.118612938-015-0037-1 PMID:26123131

Putzu, L., & Ruberto, C. D. (2013). White blood cells identification and counting from microscopic blood image. *International Journal of Medical and Health Sciences*, *7*(1), 20–27.

Rad, R. M., Attar, A., & Shahbahrami, A. (2013). A predictive algorithm for multimedia data compression. *Multimedia Systems*, *19*(2), 103–115. doi:10.100700530-012-0282-0

Raja, N. S. M., Rajinikanth, V., & Latha, K. (2014). Otsu based optimal multilevel image thresholding using firefly algorithm. Modelling and Simulation in Engineering, Article ID 794574.

Rajgire, B., Khobragade, P., Haygune, B. K., & Dhoke, G. (2017). Formation of clusters with K –Means algorithm using tumor classification. *Proceedings of the International Conference on Recent Trends in Engineering Science and Technology*, *5*(1), 199-201.

Rajinikanth, V., Dey, N., Satapathy, S. C., & Ashour, A. S. (2018). An approach to examine magnetic resonance angiography based on Tsallis entropy and deformable snake model. *Future Generation Computer Systems*, *85*, 160–172. doi:10.1016/j.future.2018.03.025

Rajinikanth, V., Fernandes, S. L., Bhushan, B., & Sunder, N. R. (2018). Segmentation and analysis of brain tumor using Tsallis entropy and regularised level set. *Lecture Notes in Electrical Engineering*, *434*, 313–321. doi:10.1007/978-981-10-4280-5_33

Rajinikanth, V., Raja, N. S. M., & Satapathy, S. C. (2016). Robust color image multi-thresholding using between-class variance and cuckoo search algorithm. *Advances in Intelligent Systems and Computing*, *433*, 379–386. doi:10.1007/978-81-322-2755-7_40

Rajinikanth, V., Raja, N. S. M., Satapathy, S. C., & Fernandes, S. L. (2017). Otsu's multi-thresholding and active contour snake model to segment dermoscopy images. *Journal of Medical Imaging and Health Informatics*, *7*(8), 1837–1840. doi:10.1166/jmihi.2017.2265

Rajinikanth, V., & Satapathy, S. C. (2018). Segmentation of ischemic stroke lesion in brain MRI based on social group optimization and fuzzy-Tsallis entropy. *Arabian Journal for Science and Engineering*, 1–14. doi:10.100713369-017-3053-6

Rajinikanth, V., Satapathy, S. C., Dey, N., & Vijayarajan, R. (2018). DWT-PCA image fusion technique to improve segmentation accuracy in brain tumor analysis. *Lecture Notes in Electrical Engineering*, *471*, 453–462. doi:10.1007/978-981-10-7329-8_46

Rajinikanth, V., Satapathy, S. C., Fernandes, S. L., & Nachiappan, S. (2017). Entropy based segmentation of tumor from brain MR images–A study with teaching learning based optimization. *Pattern Recognition Letters*, *94*, 87–94. doi:10.1016/j.patrec.2017.05.028

Ramesh, N., Dangott, B., Salama, M. E., & Tasdizen, T. (2012). Isolation and two-step classification of normal white blood cells in peripheral blood smears. *Journal of Pathology Informatics*, *3*(1), 13. doi:10.4103/2153-3539.93895 PMID:22530181

Ramya, R., Shridhar, R., Latha, K. C., & Balasubramanian, S. (2016). Endometrial cancer detection using fractal based texture analysis: A box counting Algorithm. *International Journal of Applied Research, 2*, 243-245.

Rani, J., Kumar, R., Talukdar, F. A., & Dey, N. (2017). The Brain tumor segmentation using Fuzzy C-Means technique: A study. In Recent Advances in Applied Thermal Imaging for Industrial Applications. IGI Global.

Ranjan, R., Arya, R., Fernandes, S. L., Sravya, E., & Jain, V. (2018). A fuzzy neural network approach for automatic k-complex detection in sleep EEG signal. *Pattern Recognition Letters*. doi:10.1016/j.patrec.2018.01.001

Reddy, K. H. K., Das, H., & Roy, D. S. (2017). *A Data Aware Scheme for Scheduling Big-Data Applications with SAVANNA Hadoop. Futures of Network*. CRC Press.

Renato, K. (2000). A morphological view on traditional signal processing. In *Mathematical morphology & its applications to image & signal processing, Computational imaging & vision series* (Vol. 18, pp. 3–12). Springer.

Rezatofighi, S. H., & Zadeh, H. S. (2011). Automatic recognition of five types of white blood cells in peripheral blood. *Computerized Medical Imaging and Graphics*, *35*(4), 333–343. doi:10.1016/j.compmedimag.2011.01.003 PMID:21300521

Ringnér, M. (2008). What is principal component analysis? *Nature Biotechnology*, *26*(3), 303–304. doi:10.1038/nbt0308-303 PMID:18327243

Ripon, S., Chowdhury, L., Ashour, A. S., & Dey, N. (2018). Machine-Learning Approach for Ribonucleic Acid Primary and Secondary Structure Prediction from Images. *Soft Computing Based Medical Image Analysis*, 203–221.

Ritter, W. (2001). Enfermedades de las abejas. Acribia, Zaragoza, 146.

Rozenberg, P., Bussières, L., Chevret, S., Bernard, J. P., Malagrida, L., Cuckle, H., ... Ville, Y. (2006). Screening for Down Syndrome Using First-trimester Combined Screening Followed by Second-trimester Ultrasound Examination in an Unselected Population. *American Journal of Obstetrics and Gynecology*, *195*(5), 1379–1387. doi:10.1016/j.ajog.2006.02.046 PMID:16723105

Russel, D., Hanson, J., & Ott, E. (1980). Dimension of strange attractors. *Physical Review Letters*, *45*(14), 1175–1178. doi:10.1103/PhysRevLett.45.1175

Saha, M., Chakraborty, C., & Racoceanu, D. (2018). Efficient deep learning model for mitosis detection using breast histopathology images. *Computerized Medical Imaging and Graphics*, *64*, 29–40. doi:10.1016/j.compmedimag.2017.12.001 PMID:29409716

Sahani, R., Rout, C., Badajena, J. C., Jena, A. K., & Das, H. (2018). Classification of Intrusion Detection Using Data Mining Techniques. In Progress in Computing, Analytics and Networking (pp. 753-764). Springer. doi:10.1007/978-981-10-7871-2_72

Sánchez, L., & Herrera, E. (2009). Importancia de la biodiversidad apícola para la seguridad alimentaria de Costa Rica. *Memorias del X Congreso Nacional de Apicultura: Apicultura y su impacto en la seguridad alimentaria*, 66.

Sankar, D., & Thomas, T. (2009). Analysis of Mammograms using Fractal Features. In Proceedings of Nature & Biologically Inspired Computing (pp. 936-941). Coimbatore, India: Academic Press.

Sarkar, N., & Chaudhuri, B. B. (1984). An efficient differential box-counting approach to compute fractal dimension of image. *IEEE Transactions on Systems, Man, and Cybernetics*, *24*(1), 115–120. doi:10.1109/21.259692

Sarkhel, P., Das, H., & Vashishtha, L. K. (2017). Task-Scheduling Algorithms in Cloud Environment. In *Computational Intelligence in Data Mining* (pp. 553–562). Singapore: Springer. doi:10.1007/978-981-10-3874-7_52

Scholl, I., Aach, T., Deserno, T. M., & Kuhlen, T. (2011). Challenges of medical image processing. *Computer Science Research & Development*, *26*(1-2), 5–13. doi:10.100700450-010-0146-9

Sebastian, B., Unnikrishnan, A., & Balakrishnan, K. (2012). Grey Leve Co-Occurrence Matrices: Generalization and Some New Features. *International Journal of Computer Science, Engineering and Information Technology*, *2*(2), 151–157.

Sertel, O., Catalyurek, U. V., Shimada, H., & Gurcan, M. N. (2009). Computer-aided prognosis of neuroblastoma: Detection of mitosis and karyorrhexis cells in digitized histological images. In *Proceedings of IEEE Engineering in Medicine and Biology Society* (pp. 1433-1436). IEEE. 10.1109/IEMBS.2009.5332910

Servicio Nacional de Salud Animal (SENASA). (2012). *Protocolo Vigilancia Epidemiológica de Nosemosis*. Programa Nacional de Sanidad Apícola.

Shahin, A. I., Guo, Y., Amin, K. M., & Sharawi, A. A. (2018). A novel white blood cells segmentation algorithm based on adaptive neutrosophic similarity score. *Health Inf. Sci. Syst.*, *6*(1), 1. doi:10.100713755-017-0038-5 PMID:29279774

Shakoor, S., Ismail, H., & Munim, S. (2012). Intracardiac Echogenic Focus and Fetal Outcome – Review of Cases from a Tertiary Care Centre in Karachi, Pakistan. *The Journal of Maternal-Fetal & Neonatal Medicine*, *26*(1), 2–4. doi:10.3109/14767058.2012.703724 PMID:22708618

Shamir, L., Orlov, N., Eckley, D. M., Macura, T. J., & Goldberg, I. G. (2008). IICBU 2008: A proposed benchmark suite for biological image analysis. *Medical & Biological Engineering & Computing*, *46*(9), 943–947. doi:10.100711517-008-0380-5 PMID:18668273

Shantanu, B., Rangayyan, R. M., & Desautels, J. E. L. (2009). Detection of Architectural Distortion in Prior Mammograms of Interval-cancer Cases with Neural Networks. In *Proceedings of the IEEE Conference on Engineering in Medicine and Biology Society* (pp. 6667-6670). Minneapolis, MN: IEEE.

Sharma, D., & Jindal, G. (2011). Identifying lung cancer using image processing technique. *Proceedings of International Conference Computation Technique Artificial Intelligence*, 115-120.

Shi, P., Zhong, J., Huang, R., & Lin, J. (2016, December). Automated Quantitative Image Analysis of Hematoxylin-Eosin Staining Slides in Lymphoma Based on Hierarchical Kmeans Clustering. In *Information Technology in Medicine and Education (ITME), 2016 8th International Conference on* (pp. 99-104). IEEE. 10.1109/ITME.2016.0031

Shi, Y., & Eberhart, R. C. (1998a). Parameter selection in particle swarm optimization, In *Evolutionary Programming VII: Proc. EP98* (pp. 591-600). New York: Springer-Verlag.

Shirsat, T. G., & Bairagi, V. K. (2013, April). Lossless medical image compression by IWT and predictive coding. In *Energy Efficient Technologies for Sustainability (ICEETS), 2013 International Conference on* (pp. 1279-1283). IEEE. 10.1109/ICEETS.2013.6533571

Shi, Y., & Eberhart, R. C. (1998b). A Modified Particle Swarm Optimizer. In *IEEE International Conference on Evolutionary Computation* (pp. 69-73). Anchorage, AK: IEEE.

Shree, V. T. D., Revanth, K., Raja, N. S. M., & Rajinikanth, V. (2018). A hybrid image processing approach to examine abnormality in retinal optic disc. *Procedia Computer Science*, *125*, 157–164. doi:10.1016/j.procs.2017.12.022

Sirinukunwattana, K., Raza, S. E., Tsang, Y., Snead, D. R., Cree, I. A., & Rajpoot, N. M. (2016). Locality Sensitive Deep Learning for Detection and Classification of Nuclei in Routine Colon Cancer Histology Images. *IEEE Transactions on Medical Imaging*, *35*(5), 1196–1206. doi:10.1109/TMI.2016.2525803 PMID:26863654

Skretting, K., & Engan, K. (2010). Recursive least squares dictionary learning algorithm. *IEEE Transactions on Signal Processing*, *58*(4), 2121–2130. doi:10.1109/TSP.2010.2040671

Slaa, J., Sánchez, L., Malagodi-Braga, K., & Hofstede, F. (2006). Stingless bees in applied pollination: Practice and perspectives. *Apidologie*, *37*(2), 293–315. doi:10.1051/apido:2006022

Smith-Bindman, R., Hosmer, W., Feldstein, V. A., Deeks, J. J., & Goldberg, J. D. (2001). Second-Trimester Ultrasound to Detect Fetuses With Down Syndrome. *Journal of the American Medical Association*, *285*(8), 1044–1055. doi:10.1001/jama.285.8.1044 PMID:11209176

Sonia, R., & Shanthi, V. (2016). Early Detection of Down Syndrome Marker by Measuring Fetal Nuchal Translucency Thickness from Ultrasound Images during First Trimester. *Indian Journal of Science and Technology*, *9*(21), 1–6. doi:10.17485/ijst/2016/v9i21/95174

Sophia, P. E., & Anitha, J. (2015). A systematic review on advances and perspectives of image compression in telemedicine. *International Journal of Advanced Intelligence Paradigms*, *7*(2), 136–155. doi:10.1504/IJAIP.2015.070768

Spanhol, F. A., Oliveira, L. S., Petitjean, C., & Heutte, L. (2016). Breast cancer histopathological image classification using convolutional neural networks. *Proceedings of the International Joint Conference of Neural Networks (IJCNN 2016)*, 2560-2567. 10.1109/IJCNN.2016.7727519

Stehlik, M., Hermann, P., & Nikolis, O. (2016). Fractal based cancer modelling. *Revstat Statistical Journal*, *14*, 139–155.

Stoyanov, B., & Kordov, K. (2014). *Novel Image Encryption Scheme Based on Chebyshev Polynomial and Duffing Map. The Scientific World Journal*, 1–11.

Subashini, V. J., & Poornachandra, S. (2017). Chaos Based Image Encryption Using Bogdanov Map. *Journal of Computational and Theoretical Nanoscience*, *14*(9), 4508–4514. doi:10.1166/jctn.2017.6768

Sudhan, G. H. H., Aravind, R. G., Gowri, K., & Rajinikanth, V. (2017). Optic disc segmentation based on Otsu's thresholding and level set. *International Conference on Computer Communication and Informatics (ICCCI)*. 10.1109/ICCCI.2017.8117688

Sudha, V., & Jayashree, P. (2012). Lung nodule detection in CT images using thresholding and morphological operations. *International Journal of Emerging Science & Engineering*, *1*, 17–21.

Takahashi, T., Kosaka, H., Murata, T., Omori, M., Narita, K., Mitsuya, H., ... Wada, Y. (2009). Application of a multifractal analysis to study brain white matter abnormalities of schizophrenia on T2-weighted magnetic resonance imaging. *Psychiatry Res. NeuroImage*, *172*(3), 177–188. doi:10.1016/j.pscychresns.2008.03.009

Thai, L. H., Hai, T. S., & Thuy, N. T. (2012). Image classification using support vector machine and artificial neural network. *International Journal of Information Technology and Computer Science*, *5*(5), 32–38. doi:10.5815/ijitcs.2012.05.05

Thanki, R., Borra, S., Dey, N., & Ashour, A. S. (2018). Medical Imaging and Its Objective Quality Assessment: An Introduction. In *Classification in BioApps* (pp. 3–32). Cham: Springer. doi:10.1007/978-3-319-65981-7_1

Tiwari, A. K., & Kumar, R. R. (2009). A minimum entropy based switched adaptive predictor for lossless compression of images. *Signal, Image and Video Processing*, *3*(4), 307–318. doi:10.100711760-008-0068-1

Toderici, G., O'Malley, S. M., Hwang, S. J., Vincent, D., Minnen, D., Baluja, S., ... Sukthankar, R. (2015). Variable rate image compression with recurrent neural networks. *Proceedings of International Conference on Learning Representations.*

Toderici, G., Vincent, D., Johnston, N., Hwang, S. J., Minnen, D., Shor, J., & Covell, M. (2016). *Full Resolution Image Compression with Recurrent Neural Networks.* CVF.

Tolxdorff, T., Deserno, T. M., Handels, H., & Meinzer, H. P. (2004). Advances in bio-medical image analysis past, present and future challenges. *Methods of Information in Medicine*, *43*(4), 308–314. doi:10.1055-0038-1633873 PMID:15472739

Tomasi, C., & Manduchi, R. (1998). Bilateral Filtering for Gray and Color Images. In *6th International Conference on Computer Vision (ICCV '98)*. IEEE Computer Society. 10.1109/ICCV.1998.710815

Tourassi, G. D., Delong, D. M., & Floyd, C. E. Jr. (2006). A study on the computerized fractal analysis of architectural distortion in screening mammograms. *Physics in Medicine and Biology*, *51*(5), 1299–1312. doi:10.1088/0031-9155/51/5/018 PMID:16481695

Townsend, D., Carney, J., Yap, J., & Hall, N. (2004). PET/CT today and tomorrow. *Journal of Nuclear Medicine*, *45*(1), 4S–14S. PMID:14736831

Traver, B., & Fell, R. D. (2011). Prevalence and infection intensity of Nosema in honeybee (ApismelliferaL) colonies in Virginia. *Journal of Invertebrate Pathology*, *107*(1), 43–49. doi:10.1016/j.jip.2011.02.003 PMID:21345338

Tuan, T. M. (2018). Dental diagnosis from X-Ray images: An expert system based on fuzzy computing. *Biomedical Signal Processing and Control*, *39*, 64–73. doi:10.1016/j.bspc.2017.07.005

Tu, G. J., Hansen, M. K., Kryger, P., & Ahrendt, P. (2016). Automatic behaviour analysis system for honeybees using computer vision. *Computers and Electronics in Agriculture*, *122*, 10–18. doi:10.1016/j.compag.2016.01.011

Urban, J. (2016). *Information Entropy, Applications from Engineering with MATLAB Concepts Jan Valdman*. IntechOpen. doi:10.5772/63401

Vaishnavi, G. K., Jeevananthan, K., Begum, S. R., & Kamalanand, K. (2014). Geometrical analysis of schistosome egg images using distance regularized level set method for automated species identification. *J. Bioinformatics Intell. Cont*, *3*(2), 147–152. doi:10.1166/jbic.2014.1080

Veeraswamy, K., Srinivaskumar, S., & Chatterji, B. N. (2007). Lossless Image Compression using Topological Pixel Re-ordering and Switched Predictor. *Journal of the Institution of Electronics and Telecommunication Engineers*, *53*(6), 505–512. doi:10.1080/03772063.2007.10876167

Veta, M., van Diest, P. J., Kornegoor, R., Huisman, A., Viergever, M. A., & Pluim, J. P. (2013). Automatic nuclei segmentation in H&E stained breast cancer histopathology images. *PLoS One*, *8*(7), e70221. doi:10.1371/journal.pone.0070221 PMID:23922958

Vieira, S., Pinaya, W. H., & Mechelli, A. (2017). Using deep learning to investigate the neuroimaging correlates of psychiatric and neurological disorders: Methods and applications. *Neuroscience and Biobehavioral Reviews*, *74*, 58–75. doi:10.1016/j.neubiorev.2017.01.002 PMID:28087243

Vincey, J. M. V., & Saravana, K. E. (2013). Computer aided diagnosis for liver cancer using statistical model. *International Journal of Research in Engineering & Technology*, *2*(12), 84–89. doi:10.15623/ijret.2013.0212014

Vishnupriya, R., Raja, N. S. M., & Rajinikanth, V. (2017). An efficient clustering technique and analysis of infrared thermograms. *Third International Conference on Biosignals, Images and Instrumentation (ICBSII)*, 1-5. 10.1109/ICBSII.2017.8082275

Waheed, S., Moffitt, R. A., Chaudry, Q., Young, A. N., & Wang, M. D. (2007). Computer aided histopathological classification of cancer subtypes. *Proceedings of the 7th IEEE International Conference on Bioinformatics and Bioengineering*, 503-508. 10.1109/BIBE.2007.4375608

Walther, B., Hossin, S., Townend, J., Abernethy, N., Parker, D., & Jeffries, D. (2011). Comparison of electronic data capture (EDC) with the standard data capture method for clinical trial data. *PLoS One*, *6*(9), 1–11. doi:10.1371/journal.pone.0025348 PMID:21966505

Wang, G., Wang, Z., & Liu, J. (2017). A New Image Denoising Method Based on Adaptive Multiscale Morphological Edge Detection. Journal of Mathematical Problems in Engineering.

Wang, P., Hu, X., Li, Y., Liu, Q., & Zhu, X. (2016). Automatic cell nuclei segmentation and classification of breast cancer histopathology images. *Signal Processing*, *122*, 1–13. doi:10.1016/j.sigpro.2015.11.011

Wang, Yu., Shi, F., & Cao, L. (2018). Morphological segmentation analysis and texture-based support vector machines classification on mice liver fibrosis microscopic images. *Current Bioinformatics*.

Wang, Z., Bovik, A. C., Sheikh, H. R., & Simoncelli, E. P. (2004). Image Quality Assessment: From Error Visibility to Structural Similarity. *IEEE Transactions on Image Processing*, *13*(4), 1–13. doi:10.1109/TIP.2003.819861 PMID:15376593

Wee, L. K., Min, T. Y., Arooj, A., & Supriyanto, E. (2010, August). Nuchal Translucency Marker Detection Based on Artificial Neural Network and Measurement via Bidirectional Iteration Forward Propagation. *WSEAS Transactions on Information Science and Application*, *7*(8), 1025–1036.

Weinberger, M. J., Seroussi, G., & Sapiro, G. (2000). The LOCO-I lossless image compression algorithm: Principles and standardization into JPEG-LS. *IEEE Transactions on Image Processing*, *9*(8), 1309–1324. doi:10.1109/83.855427 PMID:18262969

What Is Down Syndrome? (n.d.). *Right Diagnosis*. Retrieved from http://www.rightdiagnosis.com/d/down_syndrome/basics.htm

Wienert, S., Heim, D., Saeger, K., Stenzinger, A., Beil, M., Hufnagl, P., ... Klauschen, F. (2012). Detection and segmentation of cell nuclei in virtual microscopy images: A minimum-model approach. *Scientific Reports*, *2*(1), 503. doi:10.1038rep00503 PMID:22787560

Winter, T. C., Anderson, A. M., Cheng, E. Y., Komarniski, C. A., Souter, V. L., Uhrich, S. B., & Nyberg, D. A. (2000). Echogenic Intracardiac Focus in 2nd-Trimester Fetuses with Trisomy 21: Usefulness as a US Marker. *Radiology*, *216*(2), 450–456. doi:10.1148/radiology.216.2.r00au32450 PMID:10924569

Woraratpanya, K., Kakanopas, D., & Varakulsiripunth, R. (2012). Triangle-box Counting Method for Fractal Dimension Estimation, *ASEAN. Engineering Journal (New York)*, (Part D): 1, 5–16.

Wu, Y., Noonan, J. P. & Agaian, S. (2011). NPCR and UACI Randomness Tests for Image Encryption. *Cyber Journals: Multidisciplinary Journals in Science and Technology, Journal of Selected Areas in Telecommunications*, 31-38.

Wu, C.-H., Wang, T.-D., Hsieh, C.-H., Huang, S.-H., Lin, J.-W., Hsu, S.-C., ... Liu, T.-M. (2016). Imaging Cytometry of Human Leukocytes with Third Harmonic Generation Microscopy. *Scientific Reports*, *6*(1), 37210. doi:10.1038rep37210 PMID:27845443

Wu, H.-T., Huang, J., & Shi, Y.-Q. (2015). A reversible data hiding method with contrast enhancement for medical images. *Journal of Visual Communication and Image Representation*, *31*(C), 46–153.

Wu, X., & Memon, N. (1997). Context-based, adaptive, lossless image coding. *IEEE Transactions on Communications*, *45*(4), 437–444. doi:10.1109/26.585919

Xu, J., Janowczyk, A., Chandran, S., & Madabhushi, A. (2010). A weighted mean shift, normalized cuts initialized color gradient based geodesic active contour model: Applications to histopathology image segmentation. *Proceeding SPIE Digital Library*, *7623*(76230Y), 1-12. Retrieved from http://spiedl.org/terms

Xu, J., Luo, X., Wang, G., Gilmore, H., & Madabhushi, A. (2016). A Deep Convolutional Neural Network for segmenting and classifying epithelial and stromal regions in histopathological images. *Neurocomputing*, *191*, 214–223. doi:10.1016/j.neucom.2016.01.034 PMID:28154470

Xu, Y., Jiao, L., Wang, S., Wei, J., Fan, Y., Lai, M., & Chang, E. I. (2013). Multi-label classification for colon cancer using histopathological images. *Microscopy Research and Technique*, *76*(12), 1266–1277. doi:10.1002/jemt.22294 PMID:24123468

Yang, J., Bouzerdoum, A., & Phung, S. L. (2009). A New Approach to Sparse Image Representation Using MMV and K-SVD. In *International Conference on Advanced Concepts for Intelligent Vision Systems*. Springer-Verlag. 10.1007/978-3-642-04697-1_19

Yang, X. S. (2008). *Nature-Inspired Metaheuristic Algorithms*. Frome, UK: Luniver Press.

Yang, X. S., & Deb, S. (2009). Cuckoo search via Lévy flights. In *Proceedings of World Congress on Nature and Biologically Inspired Computing (NaBIC 2009)*. IEEE Publications. 10.1109/NABIC.2009.5393690

Yeo, W. K., & David, F. W., & Oh, T.H. (2011).Grayscale medical image compression using feed forward neural networks. *Proceedings of IEEE International Conference on Computer Applications and Industrial Electronics (ICCAIE)*, 633-638. 10.1109/ICCAIE.2011.6162211

Yonekura, A., Kawanaka, H., Prasath, V. B., Aronow, B. J., & Takase, H. (2017). Improving the generalization of disease stage classification with deep CNN for Glioma histopathological images. *2017 IEEE International Conference on Bioinformatics and Biomedicine (BIBM)*. 10.1109/BIBM.2017.8217831

Yu, K-H., Zhang, C., Berry, G.J., Altman, R.B., Re,´C., Rubin, D.L., & Snyder, M. (2016). Predicting non-small cell lung cancer prognosis by fully automated microscopic pathology image features. *Nature Communications*, *7*. doi: 10.1038/ncomms12474

Zadeh, L. (1965). Fuzzy sets. *Information and Control*, *8*(3), 338–353. doi:10.1016/S0019-9958(65)90241-X

Zadeh, L. A. (1975). The concept of a linguistic variable and its application to approximate reasoningâ€"I. *Information Sciences*, *8*(3), 199–249. doi:10.1016/0020-0255(75)90036-5

Zaremba, W., Sutskever, I., & Vinyals, O. (2014). *Recurrent Neural Network Regularization*. Computing Research Repository (CoRR) which is part of arXiv e-print service.

Zhang, L., Dong, W., Zhang, D., & Shi, G. (2010). Two-stage image denoising by principal component analysis with local pixel grouping. *Pattern Recognition*, *43*(4), 1531–1549. doi:10.1016/j.patcog.2009.09.023

Zheng, Y., Jiang, Z., Xie, F., Zhang, H., Ma, Y., Shi, H., & Zhao, Y. (2017). Feature extraction from histopathological images based on nucleus-guided convolutional neural network for breast lesion classification. *Pattern Recognition*, *71*, 14–25. doi:10.1016/j.patcog.2017.05.010

Zook, J., & Iftekharuddin, K. (2005). Statistical analysis of fractal-based brain tumor detection algorithms. *Magnetic Resonance Imaging*, *23*(5), 671–678. doi:10.1016/j.mri.2005.04.002 PMID:16051042

About the Contributors

Nilanjan Dey is an Assistant Professor in Department of Information Technology at Techno India College of Technology (under Techno India Group), Kolkata, India. He is also a Visiting Professor at Duy Tan University, Vietnam, He was an honorary Visiting Scientist at Global Biomedical Technologies Inc., CA, USA (2012-2015), Research Scientist of Laboratory of Applied Mathematical Modeling in Human Physiology, Territorial Organization of- Scientific and Engineering Unions, Bulgaria. Associate Researcher of Laboratoire RIADI, University of Manouba, Tunisia. He is an associated Member of University of Reading, London, UK and Scientific Member of - Politécnica of Porto. In addition, he was awarded as one among the top 10 most published academics in the field of Computer Science in India during the period of consideration 2015-17 during 'Faculty Research Awards' organized by Careers 360 at New Delhi, India on March 20, 2018. Before he joined Techno India, he was Assistant Professor of JIS College of Engineering and Bengal College of Engineering and Technology.He has authored/edited more than 30 books with Elsevier, Wiley, CRC Press and Springer, and published more than 270 papers. His h-index is 26 with more than 3000 citations. He is the Editor-in-Chief of Int. J. f Ambient Computing and Intelligence (IJACI, IGI Global,UK, Scopus), Int. J. of Rough Sets and Data Analysis (IGI Global,US, DBLP,ACM dl), Co- Editor-in-Chief of Int. J. of Synthetic Emotions (IGI Global,US, DBLP,ACM dl) and International Journal of Natural Computing Research (IGI Global,US, DBLP,ACM dl). He is the Series Co-Editor of Advances in Ubiquitous Sensing Applications for Healthcare (AUSAH), Elsevier, Series Editor of Computational Intelligence in Engineering Problem Solving and Intelligent Signal processing and data analysis, CRC Press (FOCUS/Brief Series) and Advances in Geospatial Technologies (AGT) Book Series, (IGI Global), US, serves as an editorial board member of several international journals, including International Journal of Image Mining (IJIM), Inderscience, Associated Editor of IEEE Access (SCI-Indexed), and International Journal of Information Technology, Springer.His main research interests include Medical Imaging, Machine learning, Computer Aided Diagnosis as well as Data Mining. He has been on program committees of over 50 international conferences, a workshop organizer of 5 workshops, and acted as a program co-chair and/or advisory chair of more than 10 international conferences. He has given more than 40 invited lectures in 10 countries, including many invited plenary/keynote talks at the international conferences such as ITITS2017 (China), TIMEC2017 (Egypt) and SOFA2018 (Romania), BioCom2018 (UK), etc.

Amira S. Ashour is currently an Assistant Professor and Head of Department-EEC, Faculty of Engineering, Tanta University, Egypt. She has been the Vice Chair of Computer Engineering Department, Computers and Information Technology College, Taif University, KSA for one year from 2015. She has been the vice chair of CS department, CIT college, Taif University, KSA for 5 years. Her research interests are Smart antenna, Direction of arrival estimation, Targets tracking, Image processing, Medical imaging, Machine learning, Signal/image/video processing, Image analysis, Computer vision, and Optimization. She has 6 books and about 70 published journal papers. She is an Editor-in-Chief for the International Journal of Synthetic Emotions (IJSE), IGI Global, US. She is an Associate Editor for the IJRSDA, IGI Global, US as well as the IJACI, IGI Global, US. She is an Editorial Board Member of the International Journal of Image Mining (IJIM), Inderscience.

Harihar Kalia is an Assistant Professor in the Department of Computer Science and Engineering, Seemanta Engineering College, Jharpokharia, Mayurbhanj, Odisha. He received his M.Sc. degree in Mathematics from Ravenshaw University, Odisha in 1995, and the M.Tech degree in Computer Science from Utkal University, Vani Vihar, Odisha in 2002. He completed his PhD work in the area of Multi-Objective Fuzzy Rule Mining in Department Information and Communication Technology, Fakir Mohan University, Vyasa Vihar, Balasore, Odisha, in 2015. His area of interest includes: Data Mining, Multi-Objective Optimization, Fuzzy Logic, Evolutionary Algorithms, and Hybrid Systems. He has about 18 years teaching experience, in teaching both graduate and postgraduate students. He is a member of Editorial and Reviewer Board in International Journal of Rough Computing and Intelligent Systems (IJRCIS), Reviewer in International Journal of Uncertainty, Fuzziness and Knowledge Based Systems (World Scientific) and Reviewer in International Journal of Applied Meta heuristic Computing (IJAMC), IGI Global.

R. T. Goswami received Phd in Technology from Birla Institute of Technology Mesra Ranchi India. He is having 23 years of experience in the field of academics and research. He was the professor in Computer Science and Engineering and also the Director of BIT Mesra Kolkata Campus since 1995. He joined Techno India College of Technology Kolkata as a Director in September 1 2016 on 2 year lien from BIT Mesra. His research interest in the field of Network Security and BigData.

He has conducted almost 30 MDP and FDP program. He has guided more than 100 students in UG and PG projects. He is the visiting faculty of 10 Institutions and member of ACM, IEEE, CSI and NIPM. Published almost 30 research papers. He chaired many National and International conferences.

Himansu Das is working as an as Assistant Professor in the School of Computer Engineering, Kalinga Institute of Industrial Technology (KIIT) Deemed to be University, Bhubaneswar, India. He has received his B. Tech degree from Institute of Technical Education and Research, India and M. Tech degree in Computer Science and Engineering from National Institute of Science and Technology, India. He has published several research papers in various international journals and conferences. He has also edited several books of international repute like IGI Global, Springer and Elsevier. He is also serving many journals and conferences as editorial or reviewer board member and as member, international advisory board of several national and international journals and conferences. He is proficient in the field of Computer Science Engineering and served as an organizing chair, publicity chair and act as member of technical program committees of many national and international conferences. He is also associated with various educational and research societies like IET, IACSIT, ISTE, UACEE, CSI, IAENG, and ISCA. His research interest includes in the field of Grid and Cloud Computing, Wireless Sensor Network, Data Mining, Soft Computing and Machine Learning. He has also more than 10 years of teaching and research experience in different engineering colleges.

* * *

S. Arunmozhi is currently working as Asso. Prof. in Department of ECE. He has 15 publications in Journals and more than 20 conferences. His areas of interest are Wireless Communication and Image processing.

Madhumita Das received her Master's degree in Computer Science from KIIT University. Her research interest includes digital image processing. She has published three research papers. Presently she is pursuing her Ph.D. in West Bengal State University under supervision of Dr. Durjoy Majumder.

Geovanni Figueroa-Mata holds a M.Sc. in computer science from the Costa Rica Institute of Technology and a master's degree in mathematic from Costa Rica University. He is a full professor and research at the Mathematical School from Costa Rica Institute of Technology. His research interests are in the areas of machine learning, computer vision, pattern recognition and optimization.

Madhu G. is associated as a faculty member in the department of Information Technology, VNR VJIET, Hyderabad, India. He has more than 15 years of teaching experience and has several papers published at national and international conferences and refereed journals. He is a member of IEEE, ISTE, CSI. He obtained his doctoral degree from JNTUH in 2015. He has been at and presented papers at International conferences within and abroad and has also received several best paper awards. His areas of research interest are data mining, machine learning, statistical analysis.

A. R. Kavitha is working as a Professor in the Department of Information Technology, Jerusalem College of Engineering, Chennai-600100. She has totally 17 years of teaching experience in Computer Science & Engineering/ Information Technology field. She has published her research works in several international Scopus indexed list of Journals and pioneered several new research directions and published book in Intech publisher which is indexed in Web of Science. She is a recognized supervisor of Anna University, Chennai and currently five research scholars are pursuing Ph.D. under her guidance. She has applied funded projects to the funding agencies such as AICTE, SERB and Institute of Engineers. She is a professional life member of ISTE, IE and British Council Library and applied patent on 2016. She is contributing as reviewer in Journal of Informatics in Medicine Unlocked (IMU), Elsevier publication and Alloy Journal of Computing and Applications. She is continuing her research work with full of effort in inter-disciplinary fields such as CSE, IT, and BME which is relevant to the society.

Hong Lin received his PhD in Computer Science and was a postdoctoral research associate at Purdue University, an assistant research officer at the National Research Council, Canada, and a software engineer at Nokia, Inc. Dr. Lin is currently a professor and assistant chair with UHD. His research interests include parallel/ distributed computing, data analytics, and human-centered computing. He is a senior member of the ACM.

Blessa Binolin Pepsi M. is currently working as Assistant Professor in the department of Information Technology, Mepco Schlenk Engineering College. Her research area includes big data analytics and machine learning.

Durjoy Majumder is presently working as Assistant Professor of Physilogy in West Bengal State University. Before joining to his present position he was with School of Information Technology, Faculty of Engineering, Bengal Engineering & Science University, Shibpur (presently IIEST). He has received his Ph.D. from Saha Institute of Nuclear Physics. He trained in clinical cancer research from Calcutta School of Tropical Medicine and SGPGIMS, Lucknow. He has more than two decades of research experience on cancer. His present research interest on Medical Analytics, Systems Biology/Medicine and Translational Research. More than 50 research articles are in his credit. He has delivered several invited talks in different international seminars. So far he acted as Project Supervisors in many research projects on Medical Analyis and Systems Biology/Medicine. His research contribution has been highlighted by Royal Society of Chemistry, Nature India and different national dailies.

R. Meena Prakash, Associate Professor/ECE, Sethu Institute of Technology has 15 years of teaching experience and her research interests include Image Processing and Embedded Systems. She has more than 10 research publications in reputed international journals.

Jibitesh Mishra was born in odisha in 1968. He received his MCA degree from the Utkal University, Odisha India, and the Ph.D. degrees from the Utkal University, Odisha India, in 2001. Currently, he is a Associate Professor and Head, Department of Computer Science and Application, College of Engineering and Technology, Bhubaneswar, a constituent college of Biju Patnaik University of Technology, Odisha. He has more than 16 years of teaching experience in various universities throughout the world. He has authored four books of repute. His research interests are fractal graphics.

Trisiladevi C. Nagavi is an assistant professor in the Department of Computer Science and Engineering. She graduated from Karnataka University, Dharwad. She obtained her Master's and Doctoral degree from Visvesvaraya Technological University, Belgaum. She has an expertise in the area of Audio, Music, Speech and Image Signal Processing, Information Retrieval and Machine Learning. Her research outcome resulted in an Android App to play favorite tunes. It is designed to retrieve songs by listening to user hum based on music melody representation models. She is an Active member of IEEE India Special Interest Group on Communications Disability and worked on Real Time Text to Speech Conversion and Translation System in Collaboration with All India Institute of Speech and Hearing (AIISH) Mysore and IEEE Standards Association. She has published over 8 peer-reviewed journals papers and 13 peer reviewed conference papers. She is currently mentoring doctoral student in the area of audio signal processing. The Certificate of Appreciation has been awarded for mentoring students for The Great Mind Challenge – 2011 Annual National Software Development Program by IBM.

Soumya Ranjan Nayak was born in odisha in 1984. He received his B.Tech and M.Tech degree in computer science and engineering from Biju Patnaik University of Technology, Odisha, India in 2009 and 2012, respectively. And recently completed his research work (Ph.D) from College of Engineering and Technology. Currently, he is working as Assistant Professor in K L University, AP. His research interest includes image analysis by means of fractal geometry, color and texture features.

Mahesha P. is working as Assistant Professor in the department of Computer Science & Engineering. His areas of interest include Speech Signal Processing, Machine Learning, Data analytics and Web Technologies. He is currently involved in clinical speech processing research. He has presented and published research papers across conferences and Journals of repute, serves as a program committee member for International Conferences and reviewer for various journals and is on the advisory board for a couple of organizations. He is recognized as official reviewer for two Elsevier Journals, International Journal of Computer Methods and Programs in Biomedicine, International Journal of Biomedical Signal Processing and Control. He holds a Bachelor of Engineering degree from University of Mysore and M.Tech and Ph.D. from Visvesvaraya Technological University, Belgaum.

Ketki C. Pathak is assistant professor at SCET, Surat. She is currently persuing PhD from SVNIT Surat. She has completed her MTech in communication system from SVNIT Surat in 2009, She has completed her BE from VNSGU in 2000. Her area of interest are Signal processing, medical image procession, HEVC video compression and Digital VLSI Design.

Nithin Prabhu G. is currently pursuing Bachelor of Computer Science and Engineering at S. J. College of Engineering, Mysuru, Karnataka, India. He has worked as an intern at L&T Technology Services Ltd., Mysuru for two terms. In his first internship, as a data scientist intern he has built a Chat Bot using Python. In his second internship, he has designed a web page for Thermostat Project of Aprilaire. Currently he is working on Fault Detection & Diagnostics on Electronic & Mechanical Devices as an Intern in Artificial Intelligence Domain at L&T.

Shantha Selva Kumari R. is Senior Professor & Head, Department of Electronics and Communication Engineering, Mepco Schlenk Engineering College, Sivakasi, India. She has received her Ph.D., in the year 2008 from MS University. She is having 31 Years of Teaching and Research experience in the field of ECE. Her publications include more than 85 research papers in international journals and more than 200 in conferences. Presently she is guiding research scholars in the area of Biosignal Processing, Image Processing and Digital Communication. She is a life member of FIETE, ISTE and CSI. She also serves as Editorial Board Member and as program Committee Member for several International Journals and Conferences.

T. Revathi has more than 31 years of rich academic and research experience. Currently she is working as Senior Professor and Head in Information Technology Department of Mepco Schlenk Engineeriing College, Sivakasi in Tamilnadu, India. Her research interest includes Big data analytics, cloud computing and sensor networks.

Sudipta Rudra is a specialist in computer vision and imaging techniques. Correspondence with specialization in neural engineering and neural computation domain. More than 3 years experience in machine learning (deep learning, reinforcement learning, vector space modelling, quantum computation, dynamic spatiotemporal data analysis and model generation).

Haseena S. is currently working as Assistant Professor(Sr.Grade) in Department of Information Technology, Mepco Schlenk Engineering College, Sivakasi. She is currently doing her research in the field of large scale image processing.

Saroja S. is currently working as Senior Assistant Professor in the department of information technology, Mepco Schlenk Engineering College. She is currently pursuing her research in the field of scheduling.

Michael Dinesh Simon obtained his Bachelor's degree in Information Technology and Master's degree in Computer Science Engineering from Anna University, Chennai, India. He is currently doing his PhD in Computer Science Engineering majoring in image processing in Jerusalem Engineering College (Affiliated to Anna University). His specializations include image processing, data mining network, medical image processing and neural network.

N. Sri Madhava Raja has received his Ph.D. degree at Anna University, Chennai. His research was focussed on analysis of retinal image processing based on optimization technique. He obtained his B.E. and M.E. degree in the years 2001 and 2002 respectively. He was born in the year 1979. Currently, he is working as an Associate Professor in the Department of Electronics and Instrumentation Engineering, St. Joseph's College of Engineering, Chennai, India. His current area of research includes optimization techniques, medical image processing, and biomechanics.

Rajinikanth V. is currently working as Professor, Department of EIE, St. Joseph's College of Engineering, Chennai, TN, India. He received his Ph.D titled Heuristic algorithm based system identification and controller design in 2013 from Anna University, TN, India. He has published over 50 papers in the field of heuristic algorithm applications. His research interest is heuristic algorithm assisted medical image and signal processing.

Index

F

G

H

I

K

L

M

N

P

Q

R

S

T

W

www.ingramcontent.com/pod-product-compliance
Lightning Source LLC
LaVergne TN
LVHW080559300926
849162LV00005B/997
* 9 7 8 1 5 2 2 5 6 3 1 6 7 *